M000208781

Pocket SURGERY

Second Edition

Editor:

DANIEL B. JONES, MD, MS, FACS

Wolters Kluwer

Philadelphia • Baltimore • New York • London
Buenos Aires • Hong Kong • Sydney • Tokyo

Acquisitions Editor: Brian Brown
Development Editor: Brendan Huffman
Editorial Coordinator: Annette Ferran
Senior Production Manager: Alicia Jackson
Manufacturing Manager: Beth Welsh
Marketing Manager: Dan Dressler
Design Coordinator: Steve Druding
Production Service: Aptara, Inc.

2nd edition

Copyright © 2018 Wolters Kluwer

© 2011 by LIPPINCOTT WILLIAMS & WILKINS, a WOLTERS KLUWER business. All rights reserved. This book is protected by copyright. No part of this book may be reproduced in any form by any means, including photocopying, or utilized by any information storage and retrieval system without written permission from the copyright owner, except for brief quotations embodied in critical articles and reviews. Materials appearing in this book prepared by individuals as part of their official duties as U.S. government employees are not covered by the above-mentioned copyright.

9 8 7 6 5 4

Printed in China

Library of Congress Cataloging-in-Publication Data

Names: Jones, Daniel B., 1964- editor.
Title: Pocket surgery / editor, Daniel B. Jones.
Other titles: Pocket surgery (Goldfarb) | Pocket notebook.
Description: 2nd edition. | Philadelphia : Wolters Kluwer, 2017. | Series:
   Pocket notebook | Preceded by Pocket surgery : the Beth Israel Deaconess
   Medical Center handbook of surgery / editors, Melanie Goldfarb . . . [et al.].
c2011. | Includes bibliographical references.
Identifiers: LCCN 2017026170 | ISBN 9781496355393
Subjects: | MESH: Surgical Procedures, Operative | Handbooks
Classification: LCC RD31 | NLM WO 39 | DDC 617–dc23 LC record available at https://lccn.loc.gov/2017026170

DISCLAIMER

This work is provided "as is," and the publisher disclaims any and all warranties, express or implied, including any warranties as to accuracy, comprehensiveness, or currency of the content of this work.

This work is no substitute for individual patient assessment based upon healthcare professionals' examination of each patient and consideration of, among other things, age, weight, gender, current or prior medical conditions, medication history, laboratory data and other factors unique to the patient. The publisher does not provide medical advice or guidance and this work is merely a reference tool. Healthcare professionals, and not the publisher, are solely responsible for the use of this work including all medical judgments and for any resulting diagnosis and treatments.

Given continuous, rapid advances in medical science and health information, independent professional verification of medical diagnoses, indications, appropriate pharmaceutical selections and dosages, and treatment options should be made and healthcare professionals should consult a variety of sources. When prescribing medication, healthcare professionals are advised to consult the product information sheet (the manufacturer's package insert) accompanying each drug to verify, among other things, conditions of use, warnings and side effects and identify any changes in dosage schedule or contraindications, particularly if the medication to be administered is new, infrequently used or has a narrow therapeutic range. To the maximum extent permitted under applicable law, no responsibility is assumed by the publisher for any injury and/or damage to persons or property, as a matter of products liability, negligence law or otherwise, or from any reference to or use by any person of this work.

CONTRIBUTING AUTHORS

Robert D. Acton, MD
Professor of Surgery and Pediatrics
Associate Surgery Program Director
Surgeon-in-Chief University of Minnesota Masonic Children's
Hospital
Minneapolis, Minnesota

Partha Bhurtel, MBBS
Surgery Resident, Department of General Surgery
St. Elizabeth Medical Center, Tufts University School of Medicine
Boston, Massachusetts

Christopher Boyd, MD
Assistant Professor of Surgery, Harvard Medical School,
Beth Israel Deaconess Medical Center
Boston, Massachusetts

Morgan A. Bresnick, MD
Instructor in Surgery, General and Bariatric Surgery,
Beth Israel Deaconess Medical Center
Boston, Massachusetts

Michael Cahalane, MD
Associate Professor of Surgery, Harvard Medical School
Acting Chief, Acute Care Surgery Division
Director, Undergraduate Education, Department of Surgery,
Beth Israel Deaconess Medical Center
Boston, Massachusetts

Mark P. Callery, MD
Professor of Surgery, Harvard Medical School
Chief, Division of General Surgery, Beth Israel Deaconess Medical Center
Boston, Massachusetts

David S. Caradonna, MD, DMD
Assistant Professor, Harvard Medical School,
Beth Israel Deaconess Medical Center
Boston, Massachusetts

Thomas Cataldo
Instructor in Surgery, Harvard Medical School and
Division of Colon and Rectal Surgery
Beth Israel Deaconess Medical Center
Boston, Massachusetts

Alexander V. Chalphin, MD
General Surgery Resident, Harvard Medical School, Beth Israel
Deaconess Medical Center
Boston, Massachusetts

Oliver S. Chow, MD
Cardiothoracic Surgery Fellow, Harvard Medical School,
Beth Israel Deaconess Medical Center
Boston, Massachusetts

Charles Cook, MD, FACS, FCCM
Division Chief, Acute Care Surgery, Trauma, Surgical Critical Care,
Beth Israel Deaconess Medical Center
Associate Professor of Surgery, Harvard Medical School
Boston, Massachusetts

Jonathan Critchlow, MD
Associate Professor of Surgery, Harvard Medical School
Associate Chief, General Surgery, Beth Israel Deaconess Medical Center
Boston, Massachusetts

Roger Eduardo, MD
General Surgery Resident,
Beth Israel Deaconess Medical Center
Boston, Massachusetts

Nassrene Y. Elmadhun, MD
Surgical Resident, Beth Israel Deaconess Medical Center
Boston, Massachusetts

Mariam F. Eskander, MD, MPH
General Surgery Resident, Beth Israel Deaconess Medical Center
Boston, Massachusetts

Amy Evenson, MD, MPH
Assistant Professor of Surgery, Harvard Medical School, Beth Israel
Deaconess Medical Center
Boston, Massachusetts

Sidhu P. Gangadharan, MD
Chief, Division of Thoracic Surgery and Interventional Pulmonology
Beth Israel Deaconess Medical Center
Associate Professor of Surgery, Harvard Medical School
Boston, Massachusetts

Mark A. Gromski, MD
Fellow, Gastroenterology and Hepatology
Indiana University School of Medicine
Indianapolis, Indiana

Alok Gupta, MD, FACS
Acute Surgeon, Harvard Medical School, Beth Israel Deaconess Medical
Center
Boston, Massachusetts

Huzifa Haj-Ibrahim, MD
General Surgery Resident, Harvard Medical School, Beth Israel
Deaconess Medical Center
Boston, Massachusetts

Allen Hamdan, MD
Vice Chair, Department of Surgery and Associate Professor of Surgery, Harvard Medical School
Chairman, Board of Advisors, Greater Boston Food Bank
Boston, Massachusetts

Thomas Hamilton, MD
Assistant Program Director, Pediatric Surgery Fellowship Program, Department of Surgery, Boston Children's Hospital
Assistant Professor of Surgery, Harvard Medical School
Boston, Massachusetts

Daniel A. Hashimoto, MD, MS
Edward D. Churchill Surgical Education and Simulation Research Fellow, Massachusetts General Hospital
General Surgery Resident, Harvard Medical School
Boston, Massachusetts

Per-Olof Hasselgren, MD
Professor of Surgery, Harvard Medical School
Vice Chairman, Research, Director, Endocrine Surgery, Beth Israel Deaconess Medical Center
Boston, Massachusetts

Mary Jane Houlihan, MD
Assistant Professor of Surgery, Harvard Medical School, Beth Israel Deaconess Medical Center
Boston, Massachusetts

Dre M. Irizarry, MD
General Surgery Resident
Beth Israel Deaconess Medical Center
Boston, Massachusetts

Sayuri P. Jinadasa, MD
Critical Care Research Fellow and General Surgery Resident, Beth Israel Deaconess Medical Center
Teaching Fellow in Surgery, Harvard Medical School
Boston, Massachusetts

Katherine M. Johnson, MD
OBGYN Resident, Beth Israel Deaconess Medical Center
Boston, Massachusetts

Daniel B. Jones, MD, MS, FACS
Professor of Surgery, Harvard Medical School
Vice Chair of Surgery, Beth Israel Deaconess Medical Center
Boston, Massachusetts

Stephanie B. Jones, MD
Vice Chair for Education and Faculty Development, Department of Anesthesia, Critical Care and Pain Medicine, Beth Israel Deaconess Medical Center
Associate Professor of Anaesthesia, Harvard Medical School
Boston, Massachusetts

Tovy Haber Kamine, MD
Surgical Critical Care Fellow, Brigham and Women's Hospital
Boston, Massachusetts

Mark A. Kashtan, MD
Surgery Resident, Beth Israel Deaconess Medical Center
Boston, Massachusetts

Michael Kearney, MD
Instructor in Surgery, Harvard Medical School, Beth Israel Deaconess Medical Center
Boston, Massachusetts

Tara S. Kent, MD, MS
Associate Professor of Surgery, Harvard Medical School
Vice Chair for Education, BIDMC Department of Surgery
Program Director, BIDMC Surgery Residency, Beth Israel Deaconess Medical Center
Boston, Massachusetts

Kamal Khabbaz, MD
Chief, Division of Cardiac Surgery, Beth Israel Deaconess Medical Center
Boston, Massachusetts

Khalid Khwaja, MD
Assistant Professor of Surgery, Harvard Medical School
Surgical Director of Solid Organ Transplantation, Transplant Institute, Beth Israel Deaconess Medical Center
Boston, Massachusetts

Omar Yusef Kudsi, MD, MBA
Assistant Professor of Surgery, Tufts University School of Medicine
Boston, Massachusetts

Janet Li, MD, CM
Instructor in Obstetrics, Gynecology and Reproductive Biology
Harvard Medical School
Section Head, Female Pelvic Medicine and Reconstructive Surgery
Beth Israel Deaconess Medical Center
Boston, Massachusetts

Fei Lian
Beth Israel Deaconess Medical Center
Boston, Massachusetts

Patric Liang, MD
Vascular Surgery Resident, Beth Israel Deaconess Medical Center
Boston, Massachusetts

Samuel Lin, MD, MBA
Plastic Surgeon, Harvard Medical School, Beth Israel Deaconess Medical Center
Boston, Massachusetts

Ali Linsk, MD
General Surgery Resident, Beth Israel Deaconess Medical Center
Boston, Massachusetts

Alan Lisbon, MD
Associate Professor in Anesthesia, Harvard Medical School
Executive Vice Chair, Department of Anesthesia, Beth Israel Deaconess
Medical Center
Boston, Massachusetts

Deborah Nagle, MD
Instructor in Surgery, Harvard Medical School
Chief, Division of Colon & Rectal Surgery, Beth Israel Deaconess
Medical Center
Boston, Massachusetts

Bharath Nath, MD, PhD
Clinical Fellow in Pediatric General Surgery, Boston Children's Hospital,
Harvard Medical School
Boston, Massachusetts

Russell J. Nauta, MD, FACS
Professor of Surgery, Harvard Medical School,
Chairman of Surgery, Mount Auburn Hospital
Vice-Chairman of Surgery, Beth Israel-Deaconess Medical Center
Cambridge, Massachusetts

Saila T. Pillai MD, MPH
Assistant Professor of Surgery, Indiana School of Medicine
Cardiovascular Surgeon, The Division of Cardiothoracic Surgery
IU Health Methodist Hospital
Indianapolis, Indiana

Steven R. Odom, MD
Instructor of Surgery, Department of Surgery, Harvard Medical School
Acute Care and Trauma Surgeon, Department of Surgery, Beth Israel
Deaconess Medical Center
Boston, Massachusetts

Georgios Orthopoulos, MD, PhD
Surgery Resident, Department of General Surgery
St. Elizabeth Medical Center, Tufts University School of Medicine
Boston, Massachusetts

Caroline Park
General Surgery Resident
Beth Israel Deaconess Medical Center
Boston, Massachusetts

Jordan Pyda, MD
General Surgery Resident, Harvard Medical School, Beth Israel
Deaconess Medical School
Boston, Massachusetts

Kristin Raven, MD
Surgery Resident, Harvard Medical School, Beth Israel Deaconess
Medical School
Boston, Massachusetts

Kortney Robinson, MD
General Surgery Resident, Harvard Medical School, Beth Israel
Deaconess Medical Center
Boston, Massachusetts

Patrick J. Ross, MD
General Surgeon
Surgery Inc.
Tulsa, OK

Ashraf A. Sabe, MD
General Surgery Resident, Beth Israel Deaconess Medical Center
Boston, Massachusetts

Benjamin E. Schneider, MD
Instructor in Surgery, Harvard Medical School, Beth Israel Deaconess
Medical Center
Boston, Massachusetts

George A. Scangas, MD
Fellow, Rhinology and Anterior Skull Base Surgery
Massachusetts Eye and Ear Infirmary/Harvard Medical School
Boston, Massachusetts

Steven D. Schwaitzberg, MD FACS
Professor and Chairman
Department of Surgery
Professor of Biomedical Informatics
Jacobs School of Medicine and Biomedical Sciences
University at Buffalo
The State University of New York
New York, New York

Ranjna Sharma, MD, FACS
Assistant Professor of Surgery, Harvard Medical School
Beth Israel Deaconess Medical Center
Boston, Massachusetts

Kathryn A. Stackhouse, MD
General Surgery Resident, Beth Israel Deaconess Medical Center
Boston, Massachusetts

Nicholas E. Tawa, Jr, MD, PhD
Assistant Professor of Surgery (Cell Biology), Harvard Medical School
Attending Surgeon, Department of Surgery, Division of Surgical
Oncology, Beth Israel Deaconess Medical Center
Boston, Massachusetts

Bijan J. Teja, MD, MBA
Anesthesia Resident, Harvard Medical School, Beth Israel Deaconess
Medical Center
Boston, Massachusetts

John Tillou, MD
General Surgery Resident, Beth Israel Deaconess Medical Center
Boston, Massachusetts

David Tomich, MD
Resident Physician, General Surgery, Beth Israel Deaconess Medical
Center
Boston, Massachusetts

Jennifer F. Tseng, MD, MPH
Chair of the Department of Surgery, Boston University
Surgeon-in-Chief, Boston Medical Center
Boston, Massachusetts

Heath Walden, MD
Surgical Critical Fare Fellow, Beth Israel Deaconess Medical Center,
Harvard Medical School
Boston, Massachusetts

Jennifer L. Wilson, MD
Instructor in Surgery, Harvard Medical School
Department of Thoracic Surgery
Beth Israel Deaconess Medical Center, Boston, Massachusetts
Cambridge Health Alliance, Cambridge, Massachusetts

FOREWORD

"One doesn't discover new lands without consenting to lose sight of the shore for a very long time."

Andre Gide

"As you set out for Ithaka
hope the voyage is a long one,
full of adventure, full of discovery...
And if you find her poor, Ithaka won't have fooled you.
Wise as you will have become, so full of experience,
you will have understood by then what these Ithakas mean."

C. P. Cavafy

To be a surgeon is to dedicate one's life in the service of others through the application of acquired clinical wisdom in the broad domains of repair, reconstruction, and replacement. It means learning to use one's mind and one's hands and of interacting with others in new ways so as to meet the challenges that face our patients each and every day to the best of our ability. It means that while at times a surgeon may be an anatomist, physiologist, pathologist, or internist, as the leader of a surgical team, whether in the operating room or on the floor, surgeons must always see with their mind, as well as their eyes.

For over a century, a foundation of excellence in the Department of Surgery at Beth Israel Deaconess Medical Center has been nurtured and sustained by a variety of outstanding leaders of Harvard Medical School. Written by the surgical faculty and house staff of our department, this handbook is principally directed toward those students commencing their clinical work in the operating room, outpatient clinics, and surgical wards. It is intended as a *vade mecum*, which translated from the Latin means "go with me," a handbook to be carried at all times.

The emphasis of this handbook is to provide students with a critical summary of broad anatomic, physiologic, and pathologic principles that form the framework for surgical decision-making. The intent of this handbook is not to provide facts to be memorized, but a guide to better understand a select number of common problems, diagnostic approaches, and those operative interventions that can be called upon to cure or to relieve suffering. Building upon this initial foundation, we believe that future leaders in American medicine will be best able to challenge currently accepted truths, through their creativity, original thought, and innovations.

ELLIOT L. CHAIKOF, MD, PhD
Chairman, Department of Surgery
Beth Israel Deaconess Medical Center
Harvard Medical School

PREFACE

Pocket Surgery is the "go to" resource for medical students and Surgery house staff. The bulleted format gets the information usually found in a two-volume surgery textbook into one loose leaf notebook small enough to fit into your white coat pocket. *Pocket Surgery*, Second Edition builds on the success of the first edition. With this release we have updated content and added more illustrations. Every chapter has been written by surgery residents and fellows and coauthored by experts in the field. The goal is to make sure medical students excel in their surgery clerkship rotation and surgery shelf exam. Interns and junior surgery residents will appreciate having outlines for relevant facts, medication doses, and management algorithms. Residents will also find *Pocket Surgery* a nice review for the ABSITE exam.

Pocket Surgery is the one comprehensive surgery resource which is easier to navigate than the internet. Everything you need to know to care for the surgery patient is at your fingertips.

DANIEL B. JONES, MD, MS, FACS
Professor of Surgery
Harvard Medical School

DEDICATION

In memory of George Blackburn, MD, PhD, the S. Daniel Abraham Professor at Harvard Medical School. Dr. Blackburn pioneered the development of intravenous hyperalimentation formulations and the safe delivery of total parenteral nutrition. He established the field of Bariatric Surgery. He will be remembered as a thoughtful investigator and selfless mentor. Dr. Blackburn served as the Director of the Study of Nutrition Medicine at Beth Israel Deaconess Medical Center.

CONTENTS

KORTNEY ROBINSON • RUSSELL NAUTA

1-1: NUTRITION

The most important part of your preoperative assessment is a good history and physical exam. This will direct your work-up for that individual patient.

Screening

Laboratory Tests and Equations

- **Prealbumin:** $t_{1/2}$ 2 days: influenced by nutritional and inflammatory states
- **Albumin:** $t_{1/2}$ 21 days (>3.5 = adequate nutrition; <3.0 = malnutrition)
  - Other causes of low albumin: hepatic insufficiency, protein-losing nephropathy
- Creatinine: marker of renal status; reflects state of hydration and muscle mass
- Can see delayed cutaneous hypersensitivity: anergy to antigens in malnutrition, cancer, infection, renal or hepatic failure, chemotherapy, radiation (rarely used in clinical practice)
- Nitrogen balance: determines anabolic vs. catabolic; total IN–total OUT. Dietary protein is divided by 6.25 because there are 6.25 grams of protein per gram of nitrogen.
  - (dietary protein/6.25) – (UUN + 4)
    - UUN = Urine Urea Nitrogen losses over 24 hours
    - ~4 g of nitrogen is lost daily as insensible losses (skin and GI)—may need to be adjusted for burns, high GI output, fistulae, etc.
- **Harris–Benedict equation:** basal energy expenditure (BEE): kcal/day; estimates caloric needs

  Male: $66.5 + (13.8 \times wt/kg) + (5 \times ht/cm) - (6.8 \times age)$
  Female: $66.5 + (9.6 \times wt/kg) + (1.9 \times ht/cm) - (4.7 \times age)$
- (BEE) × (activity factor) × (injury factor): for increased energy needs in illness/injury; minor surgery 1.2, skeletal trauma 1.35, sepsis 1.6, burn 2.1 (all reported estimates that vary with severity)
  - Intent of calculation is to avoid over or underfeeding the patient
- **Indirect calorimetry:** "Gold standard" for resting energy expenditure

  $RQ = VCO_2$ (CO_2 made)/VO_2 (O_2 used)

  ($RQ < 0.7$ = starvation/underfeeding (ketosis); $RQ > 1.0$ = **overfeeding** (lipogenesis); $RQ = 1$ carbohydrate; $RQ = 0.7$ lipid; $RQ = 0.8$ mixed substrate/protein)

Subjective Global Assessment (SGA)

- Three parts
  - History
    - Weight loss in last 6 months
    - Dietary intake in relation to normal pattern
    - Gastrointestinal symptoms on a daily basis for more than 2 weeks
    - Functional capacity/energy level
    - Metabolic demands of underlying disease state
  - Physical exam
    - Loss of subcutaneous fat in triceps and mid-axillary line
    - Muscle wasting in quads and deltoids
    - Edema in ankles or sacral region
    - Ascites
  - Classification of patients as well nourished, moderately or severely malnourished

Enteral Nutrition (*J Parenter Enteral Nutr.* 2016;40(2):159–211)

Benefits Over Parenteral Nutrition

- It is preferable to feed patients by enteral means
- Even small amounts, "trophic tube feeds," can help
- Believed to support integrity of gut by maintaining tight junctions and protect the intestinal barrier
- Stimulates GALT and MALT (gut and mucosal associated lymphoid tissue)
- Shorter length of stay
- Less expensive
- Fewer septic complications

Disadvantages/Complications

- Noninfectious complications: abdominal distension, stomach retention, vomiting and diarrhea due to disturbance of normal motility, digestion, and absorption
- In septic and critically ill patients, there is a potential of intestinal pneumatosis with necrosis and gangrene. This is thought to be due to the hyperosmolar intestinal load of tube feeds combined with diminished blood flow to the gut

- Risk of aspiration when given via the stomach; risk decreased for postpyloric feeds
- Contraindications: intestinal obstruction, peritonitis, vomiting, ileus, diarrhea, gastrointestinal ischemia, hemodynamic instability (on unstable levels or multiple pressors)

Formulas (Fischer's Mastery of Surgery, 6th ed.)

- Polymeric formulas
  - Polymeric isotonic formulas are appropriate for most patients.
    Polymeric balanced; nutrient profiles mimic a healthy diet. It is the most common formula type.
  - 12–20% protein
  - Can have increased concentrations with higher caloric density (e.g., 1.5 or 2 kcal/mL). These are helpful for patients on fluid restriction or with high caloric needs.
- Elemental; hydrolyzed; predigested; chemically defined; elemental or semi elemental formulas
  - Require minimal digestion, and therefore are designed for patients with malabsorption and maldigestion
  - Proteins are in short-chain peptides and free amino acids; carbohydrates are as glucose oligosaccharides and fats are in long- and medium-chain triglycerides.
- Immune modulating formulas
  - Supplemented with arginine eicosapentaenoic acid, docosahexaenoic acid, glutamine and nucleic acid.
- Renal formulas
  - Generally lower in total protein (and therefore lower nitrogen loads) and have increased amounts of histidine and essential amino acids. Usually, they also have reduced levels of K, Mg, and Phos. Useful in patients with poor renal clearance and those trying to avoid dialysis.
  - Patients with adequate renal replacement therapy can be on standard formulas.
- Hepatic formulas
  - Have increased branch-chain amino acids and reduced aromatic amino acids (AAA's contribute to hepatic encephalopathy because they can act as a false neurotransmitter)
  - Can be useful in patients with hepatic encephalopathy that are resistant to standard treatments and are malnourished
- Pulmonary formulas
  - Low in carbs, high in fats to decrease the respiratory quotient
  - May not have as great of an effect on the respiratory quotient as overfeeding

Monitoring

- Monitor electrolytes, albumin, prealbumin, weight, etc.

Administration

- **Generally, start with an iso-osmolar formulation**
- Ensure the tube is flushed frequently and before/after intermittent feeds to help prevent clogging of the tube
- Some patients may benefit from using metoclopramide or erythromycin to help with motility.

Enteral Nutrition Access

- Nasoenteric: indicated for short-term use (weeks)
  - NGT: better for decompression and drainage
  - **Placement pearls: chin to chest, lubricate, warm water, topical anesthetic**
  - Have patient drink water and swallow during insertion (if cooperative)
  - **Secure tube in place (tape or bridle)**
  - Verify placement with radiograph **before** feeding or using for medications
  - Dobhoff: well tolerated for enteral feedings; but unsuitable for patients requiring gastric decompression
    - Leave stylet in place until position is confirmed by radiography
- Gastrostomy tube: indicated for long-term (>4 weeks) enteral access
  - Percutaneous endoscopic gastrostomy (PEG)
  - Surgical gastrostomy: **indicated when PEG placement is contraindicated or not possible**
- Surgical jejunostomy tube
  - Use when there is a need for long-term enteral access and the stomach cannot be used, or the patient is at increased risk for aspiration.
- Gastrojejunostomy
  - Indications: simultaneous jejunal feeding and gastric decompression
  - Benefits: reduces risk of aspiration
  - Technique: place a large-bore gastric tube in the stomach as in a standard gastrostomy → Pass a small-bore jejunal tube through the G-tube and advance distally into the duodenum/jejunum

PEG Technique

Pass the gastroscope into the stomach

Examine the esophagus, stomach, and duodenum to rule out abnormalities

⇩

Insufflate the stomach with air and keep it distended

⇩

Transilluminate the anterior abdominal wall and indent the stomach from the exterior to visualize a placement site in the LUQ just under the costal margin

⇩

Insert a small bore needle (on a syringe half filled with saline or local anesthetic) and apply suction while inserting. One should identify air in the syringe simultaneously with the appearance of the tip of the needle in the stomach. If air appears before the tip of the needle is visualized, there is concern for a loop of bowel between the stomach and the abdominal wall.

⇩

Once air is confirmed simultaneously with visualization, in the same location as the small needle, insert a large bore needle with a stylet or sheath under direct endoscopic vision into the stomach. Remove the stylet and introduce a string/wire

⇩

Create a ½–1-cm skin incision

⇩

Using a biopsy snare, grasp the string and remove via the patient's mouth

⇩

Attach the feeding tube to the string tip, pull it out through the patient's abdominal wall while reinserting the endoscope

⇩

Confirm proper positioning, secure an external crosspiece. Peg tube is usually 3–5 cm (depending on abdominal wall thickness); make sure it is not too tight and that the crosspiece/bumper/bolster can rotate freely.

Figure 1-1 (A) The site for gastric lumenal access should be carefully selected, using transillumination of the abdominal wall and gastric indentation with finger pressure as a guide. **(B)** The "safe tract" method will help to protect against inadvertent puncture of an adjacent viscus. The syringe is slowly advanced into the stomach until the needle is seen to enter the gastric lumen and air is seen to bubble into the syringe barrel. Should air appear in the barrel prior to the appearance of the needle in the gastric lumen, one may assume that there is a loop of bowel interposed between the stomach and the abdominal wall and that track should not be used. **(C)** Place the snare from the gastroscope around the needle. Then place the soft looped wire/suture through the needle. Grasp the wire with the snare and remove with the gastroscope. **(D)** The suture is affixed to the end of the gastrostomy catheter, and the catheter is pulled down the esophagus, into the stomach, and out of the abdominal wall. The scope is reintroduced to follow the progress of the tube, and care is taken to avoid undue tension. **(E)** In the "push" method, both ends of the guidewire are held taut as the tube is pushed over the wire and out of the abdominal wall. **(F)** The second passage of the instrument can be facilitated by snaring half the head of the gastrostomy catheter and following down with the endoscope into the esophagus. *(continued)*

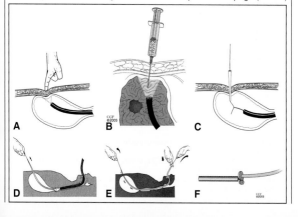

Figure 1-1 *(Continued)* (**G**) The head of the gastrostomy tube should be noted to lie in loose contact with the gastric mucosa. (**H**) An outer bolster is applied to prevent the tube from migrating inward. This should be placed several millimeters from the skin. (From Fischer JE, Bland KI. *Mastery of Surgery*, 5th ed. Philadelphia, PA: Lippincott Williams & Wilkins, 2007.)

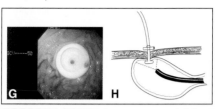

Parenteral (IV) Nutrition
Indications
- Nonfunctioning bowel: sepsis (with significant vasopressor support), inflammatory abdominal masses (i.e., diverticulitis, pancreatitis, appendicitis, IBD), incomplete obstruction
- Short-gut syndrome

Parenteral Nutrition Access
Peripherally Inserted Central Catheter (PICC)
- Can be used for months

Central Venous Line (CVL)
- Internal jugular vein: lower-risk of mechanical complications, increased rate of infection
- Subclavian vein: increased risk of pneumothorax, lower rate of infection
- Femoral Vein: Highest rate of infection

Seldinger Insertion Technique for Central Line Placement
- Prep and drape the patient. This is a sterile procedure and you need to maintain sterile technique.
- Place the patient in Trendelenburg Position.
- Use local anesthetic to infiltrate the area.
- Using a 16 or 18G needle attached to a syringe, with constant aspiration of the syringe guide the needle toward the vessel (with or without ultrasound guidance) (Figure 1-2A).
- When blood is aspirated, remove the syringe and introduce a flexible guide wire through the needle. Always maintain control of the wire (Figure 1-2B).
- Remove the needle, make a tiny incision in the skin at the point of wire entry.
- Introduce a dilator over the wire to create a track.
- Thread the central venous catheter over the wire and into the vessel.
- Check for blood return via ports.
- Flush ports of blood and cap.
- Secure line with suture and place a sterile dressing (Figure 1-2C&D).

Pearls:
- With subclavian lines, puncture the skin just inferior clavicle and direct the needle toward the sternal notch. Keep the angle of the needle at 10 degrees or less. Maintain negative pressure on the syringe and note any air filling the syringe (sign of inadvertent lung puncture).
- Best to use ultrasound guidance for internal jugular lines given close proximity to the carotid artery.
- Order and review the post procedure CXR to verify placement of the line and evaluate for possible pneumothorax.
  - For an IJ or Subclavian line, the tip of the catheter should be in the SVC just above the right atrium.

Figure 1-2 Seldinger technique for central venous cannulation by the subclavian approach. Using sterile technique, Trendelenburg positioning and local anesthesia, the sternal notch is identified. A small caliber needle is inserted through the infraclavicular skin at the junction of the clavicle's middle and lateral thirds. Once the vein is localized, a larger needle is used for subclavian cannulation (**A**). The syringe is detached, and a flexible guidewire is advanced through the needle under fluoroscopic guidance (**B**) and guided to a position in the superior vena cava, where it is secured with a suture (**C**), sterilely dressed and secured without kinking of the catheter (**D**). (From Fischer JE, Bland KI. *Mastery of Surgery*, 5th ed. Philadelphia, PA: Lippincott Williams & Wilkins, 2007.)

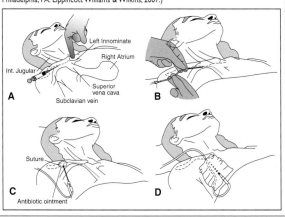

Tunneled Central Venous Catheter (TCVC)
- For long-term use
- Can be placed open via the cut down technique to the cephalic vein or percutaneously via the internal jugular or subclavian veins.
- Less likely to be dislodged and less infectious risk than traditional CVL
- TCVC (Hickman®, Broviac®, Groshong®): can have multiple lumens which are outside the body; need external site care
- "Ports" (PORT-A-CATH®, BardPort®, P.A.S. PORT®): often used for chemo. Are accessed by a noncoring needle.

Catheter-Related Complications
- Periprocedural: misplacement, pneumothorax, hemothorax, air embolism, and perforation of great vessels or heart
- Late: thrombosis, sepsis
- Incidence of thrombus is high, can be asymptomatic

CVL Infections
- Risk of infection highest with femoral lines, then internal jugular; lowest for subclavian line (*Crit Care.*, 2005;9(6):R631–R635)
- Suspected when clinical signs of infection without another source
- **Diagnosis: tip culture, peripheral and central blood cultures**
- If exit-site infection, i.e., erythema or purulence at skin, remove and resite line
- If signs of sepsis
  - Empiric antibiotics: cover *Staphylococcus* + gram negatives
  - Remove and resite catheter

Composition
- With both parenteral and enteral nutrition, feeds can be modified for the patient's comorbidities (i.e., renal, hepatic, pulmonary). See examples of modifications above under enteral formulas.
- Volume/energy: induce urinary output of 15 mL/kg/24 h and euvolemia in stable patient; in recovering patients, encourage negative fluid balance
- **Energy requirements: 25–30 kcal/kg IBW/24 h**
- Account for increased energy expenditure (ex: trauma, burn, critically ill patients)
- Fat = 9 kcal/g, protein = 4 kcal/g, glucose = 3.4 kcal/g

- **Fat: fat ~20% of calories**
- **Protein: 1.5 g/kg/24 h**
- Electrolytes: adjust daily/twice weekly depending on laboratory values and composition changes
- Trace elements/vitamins can be added to TPN: Zn, Cu, Mg, Se; Vit A, Vit C, B-vitamins

Monitoring
- Vital signs and finger sticks q6h for first 24–48 hours
- Mental state, muscle strength (hand grip or peak airway expiratory pressure), wound healing, regrowth of hair
- Daily (upon initiation of parenteral nutrition) to twice weekly (patients stabilized on a regimen) monitoring of: blood sugar, plasma electrolytes, renal function, hematology
- Weekly: liver enzymes, bilirubin, triglyceride, albumin, transferrin, CRP
- Every 2 weeks: trace elements and vitamins; longer intervals once stable

Complications
- **Infection** → improved with strict glucose control (80–110 μg/dL)
- Tendency to overfeed calories
- Liver steatosis, cholestasis, hypertriglyceridemia (treatment: decrease long chain fatty acids)
- **Refeeding syndrome: hypophosphatemia, hypokalemia, hypomagnesemia, low zinc**

An Example of How to Write TPN Orders

1. Determine the "feeding weight"
   - Calculate ideal body weight (IBW)
     - *Men:* **106 lbs for the first 5 feet and 6 lbs for each inch thereafter**
     - *Women:* **100 lbs for the first 5 feet and 5 lbs for each inch thereafter**
   - Compare with actual body weight or usual body weight if volume overloaded
   - If big discrepancy, calculate adjusted/feeding weight:
     - If patient is underweight, use ABW
     - **If patient is obese (120% IBW), then add 25% of the difference between the ABW and IBW to the IBW.**
     - Amputations: IBW less ~3% for BKA, less ~10% for AKA (Amputee-Coalition.org)

EXAMPLE: Using a 70-kg person ("feeding weight")
1. Calculate *GOAL* nutritional support.
   - Protein: 1.5 g/kg/day ($1.5 \times 70 = 105$ g)
   - Kilocalories: 25 kcal/kg/day ($25 \times 70 = 1,750$ kcal)
2. Determine the components of the GOAL TPN admixture
   - Start with total **kilocalories:** (1,750 kcal)
   - Calculate how much of total kilocalories will come from goal **protein** (1.5 g $\times 70$ kg $\times 4$ kcal/g $= 420$ kcal)
   - Subtract this amount of calories from the goal/total ($1,750 - 420 = 1,330$ kcal)
   - Make up the difference with **dextrose** ($1,330$ kcal ÷ 3.4 kcal/g $= 392$ g dextrose)

       OR

3. Determine the components of the GOAL TPN admixture **with lipids**
   - Start with total **kilocalories:** (1,750 kcal)
   - Calculate 20% of the total calories and provide this as **lipids** ($1,750 \times 0.2 = 350$ kcal → 350 kcal ÷ 9 kcal/g $= 38$ g. [round off to 35 g of lipids for easier calculation so lipids actually provide 315 cal])
   - Determine how much of total kilocalories will come from **protein** (105 g $\times 4$ kcal/g $= 420$ kcal)
   - Subtract the protein and fat calories from the total and administer the remaining calories as **dextrose** ($1750 - 315 - 420 = 1,015$ kcal → $1,015$ kcal ÷ 3.4 kcal/g $= 299$g [round to 300g for calculations] dextrose)
4. Final **volume** (*maximally* concentrated)
   - Amino acids (10% stock solution) 105 g = 1,050 cc
   - Dextrose (70% stock solution) 300 g = 430 cc
   - Lipids (20% stock solution) 35 g = 175 cc
   - Multivitamins/trace minerals/micronutrients 100 g = 100 cc

                                     1,650 cc total

How to Advance TPN
1. Day 1 starter formula: 1000 cc/70 g AA/150 g dextrose
2. If tolerated (BS < 150–180), advance to day 2 formula: 1,000 cc/70 g AA/210 g dextrose
3. If tolerated, advance protein to goal and then dextrose by 50–100 g/day until at goal:
   - If hyperglycemic, do not advance dextrose until blood sugars are controlled (around 150 mg/dL)
   - Try to cover dextrose in TPN with insulin

- Add up previous day's RISS; add two-thirds of total to what is in the current bag
- If advancing the dextrose amount, will need to increase the insulin
- Avoid aggressive additions of insulin to the TPN solution in order to avoid hypoglycemia, as well as the need to discard the TPN bag. If it is difficult to control blood sugars because of insulin resistance, be quick to switch to an insulin drip, especially in ICU patients.

Electrolytes
- Na, K, Cl, and acetate (depend on volume status, UOP, acid/base status and losses)
- Ca: RDA 10 mEq/day, Mg: RDA 10 mEq/day, Phos: RDA 30–40 mmol/day

Routine upon starting TPN (day 1)
- Start RISS and QID BS checks for goal around 150 mg/dL
- Check triglyceride level: lipids contraindicated if >400 mg/dL
- Can add famotidine to bag (150 mg/day if normal renal function)
- If on metoclopramide, can add to bag
- Remember to stop/adjust insulin when off TPN

Some things to remember
- Ca/Phos solubility curve
- TPN should only be cycled after blood sugar is well controlled, but before patient is discharged home
- Kilocalories *outside* of TPN:
  - You get 1 kcal/cc of propofol
  - D5W for meds and treatment of hypernatremia
  - Patients on CVVH(D) often have D5 solutions as return fluid
  - Protein/calories from concurrent enteral feeds

1-2: PREOPERATIVE ASSESSMENT

ASA Classification
ASA 1: healthy, no systemic disease, undergoing elective surgery, no extremes of age
ASA 2: one-system well-controlled disease not affecting daily activities
ASA 3: multisystem or well-controlled major system disease that limits daily activity
ASA 4: severe incapacitating disease that is a threat to life
ASA 5: imminent danger of death; operation last resort at preserving life
ASA 6: organ recovery

E, Emergency

Routine Preoperative Evaluation
- A good history and physical exam and knowledge of the planned procedure will determine what should be completed.
- Examples might include:
  - CBC: age >55–65, high expected blood loss, fatigue, h/o anemia, blood loss, or liver disease
  - Creatinine: age >40, h/o renal disease, DM, OSA, COPD, HTN, diuretics, chemo, known nephrotoxins
  - Coagulation studies: history, h/o VTE, anticoagulation use, liver disease
  - ECG: age >40 male, >50 female, HTN, CAD, CHF, DM, arrhythmias, family history
  - CXR: age >60, underlying cardiopulmonary disease, hospitalized
  - Urinalysis: signs of cystitis, GU, new hardware or implant procedure, hospitalized

Perioperative MI Risk
- Goldman criteria for cardiac risk in noncardiac surgery
  - Risk factors include: aortic stenosis, MI within 6 months, JVD, S3 gallop, ectopy, poor medical condition, emergency, thoracic or abdominal procedure, age >70, nonsinus rhythm
- Recent MI (<6 months) is a very important risk factor for elective surgery
  If possible, postpone elective surgeries to reduce risk of perioperative MI (J Am Coll Cardiol. 2014;64(22):e77).
- Perioperative β-blockade (J Am Coll Cardiol. 2014;64(22):e77)
  - Continue in patients chronically on β-blockade
  - Starting beta-blockers before surgery? Benefit may be limited to a small population of patients that have a significant risk of a cardiac event.
- National Surgical Quality Improvement Program (NSQIP) has an online risk calculator.
- POSSUM (Physiologic and Operative Scoring System for enUmeration of Mortality) (Br J Surg. 1991;78:356–360)

- Based on 12 physiologic factors and 6 operative factors. Originally published in 1991 and verified since.
- Risk of Mortality (R)
- Equation: Ln R/1–R = −7.04 + (0.13 × physiological score) + (0.16 × operative severity score)

Operative Severity Score			
	Score		
	1	2	4	8

	1	2	4	8
Operative severity	Minor	Moderate[a]	Major	Major[b]
Multiple procedures	1		2	>2
Total blood loss (mL)	≤100	101–500	501–999	≥1,000
Peritoneal soiling	None	Minor (serous fluid)	Local plus	Free bowel content, pus or blood
Malignancy	None	Primary only	Nodal metastases	Distant metastases
Mode of surgery	Elective		Emergency resuscitation of >2 h possible[c], Operation <24 h after admission	Emergency (immediate surgery <2 h needed)

Physiologic Score (to be scored at the time of surgery)			
	1	2	4	8

	1	2	4	8
Age (yrs)	≤60	61–70	≥71	
Cardiac signs	No failure	Diuretic, digoxin, antianginal or hypertensive therapy	Peripheral edema; warfarin therapy	Elevated jugular venous pressure
Chest x-ray			Borderline cardiomegaly	Cardiomegaly
Respiratory history	No dyspnea	Dyspnea on exertion	Limiting dyspnea (one flight). Moderate COAD	Dyspnea at rest (rate ≥30/min)
Chest x-ray		Mild COAD (Chronic Obstructive Airway Disease)	Moderate COAD	Fibrosis or consolidation
Blood pressure (systolic) (mm Hg)	110–130	131–170	≥171	—
		100–109	90–99	≤89
Pulse (beats/min)	50–80	81–100	101–120	≥121
		40–49		≤39
Glasgow Coma Score	15	12–14	9–11	≤8
Hemoglobin	13–16	11.5–12.9	10.0–11.4	≤9.9
		16.1–17.0	17.1–18.0	≥18.1
White cell count	4–10	10.1–20.0	≥20.1	
		3.1–4.0	≤3.0	
Urea (mmol/L)	≤7.5	7.6–10.0	10.1–15.0	≥15.1
Sodium (mmol/L)	≥136	131–135	126–130	≤125
Potassium (mmol/L)	3.5–5.0	3.2–3.4	2.9–3.1	≤2.8
		5.1–5.3	5.4–5.9	≥6.0
Electrocardiogram	Normal		Atrial fibrillation (rate 60–90)	Any abnormal rhythm or ≥5 ectopics/min, Q- or ST/T-wave changes

[a]Surgery of moderate severity includes appendectomy, ccy, mastectomy, TURP; major surgery includes any laparotomy, bowel resection, ccy with CBD exploration, peripheral vascular procedures, or major amputation.
[b]Major surgery includes any aortic procedure, APR, pancreas, or liver resection, esophagogastrectomy.
[c]Indicates that resuscitation is possible.
(See Copeland GP et al. POSSUM: a scoring system for surgical audit. Br J Surg. 1991;78:356–360.)

Bleeding Risk

History: Important Clues to Bleeding Risk

- ROS may include questions on epistaxis, easy bruising, bleeding, menorrhagia, bleeding with prior surgeries or dental extractions, prior blood transfusions
- Personal or family history of serious bleeding or clotting problems: uncontrolled nosebleeds, dental procedures, menses, minor cuts
- Current medications and last dose: aspirin/NSAIDs, Plavix, Coumadin
- Also vitamin E, supplements: ginseng (platelet inhibitor), St. John's wort, garlic
- Medical conditions: liver disease, biliary obstruction, renal disorder (uremia), blood dyscrasias, obstructive cancer, anemia, short gut, prosthetic valves

Lab Tests

- Platelet count
- PT/INR (extrinsic pathway); influenced by Coumadin
- aPTT (intrinsic pathway); influenced by heparin, lupus anticoagulant
- Vitamin K–dependent factors: II, VII, IX, X, Protein C and Protein S: influenced by warfarin
- Fibrinogen (low in liver failure, DIC, hereditary disorders)
- Bleeding time—generally not recommended preoperatively for evaluation
- Cross-matching: gets actual units ready to use
- Screening: analyzes patient's blood to prepare for future blood use

Bleeding Disorders			
	Etiology	Lab Abnormality	Treatment
Hemophilia A	• Factor VIII deficiency • X-linked recessive	• Prolonged PTT	• Factor VIII • DDAVP (releases Factor VIII) • Cryoprecipitate • FFP (small amount of factor VIII)
Hemophilia B (Christmas disease)	• Factor IX deficiency • X-linked recessive	• Prolonged PTT	• Factor IX concentrates
vWF (von Willebrand) disease	• Qualitative or Quantitative Deficiency of vWF	• Prolonged bleeding time (may be normal with mild to moderate severity) • Plasma vWF antigen • Plasma vWF activity (ristocetin cofactor) • Factor VIII activity	• DDAVP—small surgeries • Cryoprecipitate • vWF concentrate • Factor VIII concentrate
Vitamin K deficiency	Malnutrition Malabsorption Warfarin Biliary obstruction TPN, antibiotics	• Prolonged PT	• Vitamin K
Liver failure	Decreased clotting factors except factor VIII	• Prolonged PT • Prolonged PTT • Thrombocytopenia	• FFP • Vit K • Platelets • Cryoprecipitate
Renal failure	Uremic bleeding 2/2 platelet dysfunction		• Dialysis • DDAVP • Conjugated Estrogens • Cryoprecipitate
Hypothermia	e.g., trauma patient, cold exposure, etc.		• Fluid warmers and heating blankets

Blood Components	
RBC	Transfusion goals vary with patient condition, but per TRICC trial findings, most defer to the recommendation of keeping the hemoglobin above 7 (N Engl J Med. 1999;340:409–417)
FFP	Contains coagulation factors and protein
Cryoprecipitate	Concentrated preparation of vWF + VIII, fibrinogen
Platelets	Transfuse to >50 K if having major surgery. Can be a source of bacterial infection and sepsis (Ann Intern Med. 2015;162(3):205–213)

Transfusion Complications

	Etiology	Symptoms	Signs
Acute hemolytic transfusion reaction	• Most commonly from ABO incompatibility as a result of 2/2 clerical error	Fever, flank pain, red/brown urine	Shock, AKI, fever, rigors; intraoperative: hypotension and bleeding
Febrile nonhemolytic transfusion reaction	• Most common transfusion reaction • Caused by cytokines	Fever, chills, dyspnea, myalgias, malaise	Fever
Anaphylaxis	• One mechanism is anti-IgA in a patient that is IgA deficient	Bronchospasm, dyspnea	Pulmonary edema, wheezing
Transfusion-related acute lung injury (TRALI)	• Neutrophils likely effector cells • Increase in pulmonary capillary permeability with leakage of fluids	Dyspnea	Hypoxia, bilateral (pulmonary infiltrates, fever, hypotension)
Complications of massive transfusion	• Hypothermia • Alkalosis: citrate metabolized to HCO_3 but unable to be excreted in renal failure • Acidosis: if citrate is unable to be converted to HCO_3 by the liver due to acute or chronic liver disease • Hypocalcemia: citrate binding of ionized calcium • Hypo- or hyperkalemia: initial increase secondary to increased potassium in RBC supernatant, later it moves back to intracellular space or moves intracellularly in exchange for hydrogen ions to minimize alkalosis		

(Silvergleid, AJ. Immunologic blood transfusion reactions In: UpToDate, Post TW (Ed.) Waltham, MA. Accessed July 25, 2016.
Contin Educ Anaesth Crit Care Pain. 2006;6(6):225–229. doi: 10.1093/bjaceaccp/mkl053)

All blood transfusion reactions must be investigated. If there is concern for a transfusion reaction, stop the blood transfusion immediately. Treat the patient appropriately (based upon symptoms and likely reaction). Contact the blood bank for the appropriate transfusion reaction investigation to be initiated and give them the blood product that was infusing at the time of the reaction.

1-3: PROPHYLAXIS

Steroids

Cortisone 25 = hydrocortisone 20 = prednisone/prednisolone 5 = methylprednisolone 4 = dexamethasone 0.75

Perioperative "stress dose" steroids are a controversial topic
• Patients who have a suppressed HPA axis: those taking >20 mg prednisone/day for over 3 wks, patients with a cushingoid appearance.
• If unsure if the HPA axis is suppressed and patient needs an elective surgery; evaluate with an AM cortisol level. If >10, unlikely to have HPA axis suppression. If 5–10, proceed with ACTH stimulation test. If <5, likely to have a suppressed HPA axis.
• Minor surgery: outpatient (e.g., open inguinal hernia under local, colonoscopy)—most will not require stress dose steroids.
• Moderate surgery (e.g., total joint)
  50 mg hydrocortisone just prior to surgery and 25 q8h for 24 h.
• Major surgery (e.g., CABG, Whipple, liver resection)
  100 mg hydrocortisone just prior to surgery and 50 mg q8h for 24 h—may need to taper to home dose

(Hamrahian AH, Roman S, Milan S. The surgical patient taking glucocorticoids. In: UpToDate, Post TW (Ed.) Waltham, MA. Accessed July 25, 2016.)

Surgical Site Infections

(April 2013 CDC/NHSN Protocol Corrections, Clarification, and Additions. http://www.cdc.gov/nhsn/PDFs/pscManual/9pscSSIcurrent.pdf. Accessed June 10, 2016)

Factors contributing to surgical site infections
• Extremes of age, malnutrition, decreased blood flow to wound, steroids, cirrhosis, immunosuppression, foreign body (prosthetic implant), leukopenia, diabetes, cancer, radiation, etc.
• Duration of operation
• Break in sterile technique
• Dirty or infected wound classification

- Patient comorbidities
- Poor intraoperative glucose and temperature control

Surgical Wound Classification

- Class I/clean wounds: uninfected operative wound that does not enter the respiratory, alimentary or genital tract. Wound is closed primarily.
- Class II/clean-contaminated wounds: respiratory, alimentary, genital or urinary tracts are entered.
- Class III/contaminated wounds: fresh open wounds; operations with major breaks in sterile technique or gross spillage.
- Class IV/dirty-infected wounds: old traumatic wounds, retained devitalized tissue, existing clinical infection or perforated viscus.

Prevention

(Mangram AJ, Horan TC, Pearson ML, et al. Guideline for prevention of surgical site infection, 1999; Centers for Disease Control and Prevention (CDC) Hospital Infection Control Practices Advisory Committee. *Am J Infect Control* 1999;27:97.)

- Identify and treat infections remote to surgical site for elective operations.
- Hair removal: Only if at or around the incision. Clippers (not razor): best done immediately preoperatively (least risk of infection)
- Adequate control of blood glucose.
- Encourage tobacco cessation 30 days prior to elective operations.
- Have patients scrub preoperatively.
- Use skin preparation (chlorhexidine).
- Colonic surgery: The role of mechanical bowel preparation and enteral nonabsorbable antibiotics is controversial. However, perioperative IV antibiotics targeting gram-negative aerobes and anaerobes are standard.
- Antibiotic selection when indicated: based on procedure, individual hospital infection, and sensitivity rates
  - Timing: need to be administered close to the incision time

Antibiotic Classification

Penicillins: bactericidal; blocks bacterial cell wall synthesis; β-lactam ring
- Pen G,V: Strep pyogenes and clostridia
- Methicillin, oxacillin, nafcillin, dicloxacillin: *Staphylococcus aureus* and *Staphylococcus epidermidis*
- Ampicillin, amoxicillin: above + Enterococcus and some gram-negative rods (*E. coli, Proteus, Salmonella, Shigella, H. flu*)
- Piperacillin–tazobactam (Zosyn), ampicillin–sulbactam (Unasyn), amoxicillin–clavulanate (Augmentin): gram positive + bacteroides + gram-negative aerobes. Zosyn is effective against *Pseudomonas*

Cephalosporins: bactericidal; blocks cell wall synthesis; some allergic cross-rxn with penicillins
- First generation (i.e., cefazolin): Staph, Strep
- Second generation (cefuroxime, cefoxitin, cefotetan): increased gram negative coverage
- Third generation (cefotaxime, ceftriaxone, ceftazidime): broad GNR coverage. Ceftazidime has activity against *Pseudomonas*
- Fourth generation (cefepime)—cefepime also has activity against *Pseudomonas*
- Fifth generation (ceftaroline)—improved gram positive activity including MRSA

Monobactams: bactericidal; β-lactam
- Aztreonam: most gram-negative aerobes (incl. *Pseudomonas*)

Carbapenems: effective for those that produce ESBL (extended spectrum β-lactamases)
- Imipenem and meropenem: broad spectrum
- Ertapenem: narrower spectrum; less active against *Psuedomonas* and *Acinetobacter*. Long $T_{1/2}$, so able to do once daily dosing

Aminoglycosides: bactericidal; inhibit protein synthesis 30S subunit
- Gentamicin, tobramycin, amikacin: gram positives, gram negatives, and mycobacteria; poor activity against anaerobes

Trimethoprim and sulfonamides: bactericidal together; inhibit tetrahydrofolic acid synthesis
- Aerobic gram positive and negative coverage

Fluoroquinolones: bactericidal; inhibit DNA gyrase (replication)
- Ciprofloxacin, levofloxacin, moxifloxacin: broad spectrum (strong gram-negative coverage)
Other
- Vancomycin: inhibits cell wall synthesis; bactericidal. For MRSA. Treatment of *Clostridium difficile* with PO vancomycin. Resistance secondary to change in cell wall binding protein
- Linezolid: inhibits protein synthesis 50S subunit: gram positives
- Metronidazole: anaerobes, a few gram negatives; bactericidal

Macrolides: inhibit protein synthesis (act at 50S)
- Clarithromycin, azithromycin: used for community acquired respiratory tract infections. Have activity against *Streptococcus pneumonia, Haemophilis, Moraxella catarrhalis, Legionella pneumophlia, Chlamydia pneumoniae* and *Mycoplasma pneumoniae*.
- Erythromycin: common for bowel prep or motility agent

Lincosamides: Binds 50S ribosomal subunit
- Clindamycin: *Staphylococcus, Streptococci, Bacteroides fragilis, Clostridum perfringes*, etc.
- Associated with *Clostridum difficile* colitis

Antifungal
- Amphotericin B: Kills by binding cell wall sterols and causing cell death via lysis.
  - Effective but toxic!
- Azoles: imidazoles and triazoles: inhibit ergosterol synthesis; less toxic
- Echinocandins: inhibit cell wall synthesis

Bacterial Endocarditis Prophylaxis (*Circulation.* 2007;116(15):1736–54)
- Indications: prosthetic valve, history of endocarditis, unrepaired cyanotic heart disease (CHD) or repaired CHD within 6 months after repair, repaired CHD with residual defects, valvulopathy in a transplanted heart.
- Use in: dental, upper respiratory if it involves an incision or biopsy
- Not indicated for GU or GI procedures

DVT Prophylaxis
Virchow's Triad
- Venous stasis
- Endothelial injury
- Hypercoagulable state

Caprini Score (*Dis Mon.* 2005;51(2–3):70–78)
Risk factors worth one point
- Age 41–60
- Minor surgery planned
- History of prior major surgery within past month
- Varicose veins
- History of inflammatory bowel disease
- Current swollen legs
- BMI >25
- Acute MI
- CHF (<1 month)
- Sepsis (<1 month)
- Abnormal pulmonary function
- Patient currently at bed rest
- Oral contraceptives or hormone replacement therapy
- Pregnancy or postpartum (<1 month)
- History of >3 spontaneous abortions, unexplained stillborn infants, premature birth with toxemia or growth restricted infant

Risk factors worth two points
- Age 60–74
- Arthroscopic surgery
- Malignancy (prior or current)
- Major surgery (>45 minutes)
- Laparoscopic Surgery (>45 minutes)
- Patient confined to bed (>72 hours)
- Immobilizing plaster cast (<1 month)
- Central venous access

Risk factors worth three points
- Age >75
- History of DVT/PE
- Family history of thrombosis
- Positive factor V Leiden
- Positive prothrombin 20210A
- Elevated serum homocysteine
- Positive lupus anticoagulant
- Elevated anticardiolipin antibodies
- HIT (heparin-induced thrombocytopenia)
- Other congenital or acquired thrombophilia

Risk factors worth five points
- Elective major lower extremity arthroplasty

- Hip, pelvis, or leg fracture (<1 month)
- Stroke (<1 month)
- Multiple trauma (<1 month)
- Acute spinal cord injury (<1 month)

DVT Prophylaxis (Chest. 2012;141(2 Suppl):e227S–77S)
- **Very low risk:** Caprini score of 0.
  Early ambulation only
- **Low risk:** Caprini score of 1–2
  Pneumatic compression boots
- **Moderate risk:** Caprini score 3–4
  Pneumatic compression boots, subcutaneous heparin (HSC), or low–molecular-weight heparin (LMWH)
- **High risk:** Caprini score >5
  Mechanical (pneumatic compression boots or elastic stockings) combined with pharmacologic prophylaxis (HSC or LMWH)
- **High risk undergoing abdominal or pelvic surgery for cancer:** extended duration pharmacologic prophylaxis.

Anticoagulants
- Warfarin: Vitamin K antagonist
  - Monitor PT/INR (usual goal 2–3)
  - Therapeutic range is narrow and dosing is affected by many things, including genetics, other medications, and dietary intake.
    - Examples
      - Meds increasing metabolism: rifampin, antiepileptics,
      - Meds decreasing metabolism: Cipro, Flagyl, amiodarone
  - Complications: severe hemorrhage (more likely with supratherapeutic INR), warfarin-induced skin necrosis (because protein C and S decrease first)
- Unfractionated heparin: accentuates antithrombin to inactivate thrombin and factor Xa
  - "Low dose" = 5000 U SQ preoperatively and then every 8–12 hours postoperatively (depending on patient's size)
  - Rapidly reversible with protamine sulfate
  - If giving therapeutic dose (IVgtt), monitor with PTT's
  - Metabolized by reticuloendothelial system
  - Complications: HIT+ (heparin-induced thrombocytopenia): antibodies to PF4; usually develops 5–10 days into heparin therapy; see thrombocytopenia and may see thrombosis. 4 T scoring system for risk assessment. Can confirm with antibody testing. As with all anticoagulants, can have major hemorrhage
- LMWH
  - Equivalent inhibition of factor Xa (compared to unfractionated heparin), less inhibition of thrombin
  - Longer half-life; can do daily to BID dosing, may monitor by anti-factor Xa levels if needed
  - Excreted renally, so if used at all in renal insufficiency, must adjust dose
  - Decreased risk of HIT
  - Does not cross placenta and can be used in pregnancy
- Argatroban: thrombin inhibitor given as a gtt in patients with HIT
  - Follow PTTs; also raises INR (so care when bridging to INR)
- Fondaparinux: factor Xa inhibition through antithrombin III. Long half-life, allowing daily dosing.
- Dabigatran: oral direct thrombin inhibitor
- Rivaroxaban and Apixiban are oral direct Xa inhibitors

Caval filters
- Indications: thromboembolic disease with anticoagulation contraindication, DVT/ while on appropriate therapy, complications from anticoagulation
- Access: most common right or left femoral vein; right internal jugular can be used (for an IVC thrombus)
- Complications
  - Insertion: bleeding (hematoma or superficial infection), access-site thrombosis
  - Rare: filter migration, caval penetration, infection
  - Recurrent pulmonary emboli
- PREPIC trial (Circulation. 2005;112(3):416–422): long-term randomized study of caval filters for PE prevention
  - Showed that caval filters provided significant additional short- and long-term protection from PE when compared with anticoagulation alone but increased the incidence of DVT without a mortality benefit

DVTs
- Upper extremity DVT:
  - Spontaneous UE DVTs are rare; can be due to abnormalities of the thoracic outlet causing axillosubclavian compression and subsequent thrombosis (Pagent Schroetter syndrome)
  - Generally associated with axillary or subclavian vein thrombosis from indwelling catheters
  - Signs and symptoms: swelling and/or pain, SVC syndrome, loss of UE venous access
- Lower extremity DVT:
  - Signs and symptoms: swelling, tenderness, calf pain on ankle dorsiflexion, fever
  - Diagnosis: Doppler ultrasound

PE Clinical Presentation
- Pulmonary embolus: dyspnea, tachypnea, tachycardia, chest pain, fever, EKG changes (tachycardia, prominent S wave in lead 1, Q wave and inverted T in lead 3)
- Diagnosis: CTA or alternatively a V/Q scan
- May start treatment if high clinical suspicion prior to diagnostic imaging

DVT/PE Treatment
- Anticoagulation
  - IV heparin: Titrate drip to a PTT of 60–80; check PTT q6h until stable and therapeutic. If bridging to Coumadin, start after 1 or 2 days of heparin and continue heparin until warfarin dose is in the therapeutic range
  - Treat for 3+ months
  - Other anticoagulants discussed above.

Stress Ulcer Prophylaxis (Crit Care Med. 2016;44(7):1395–405)
Pathophysiology
- Hypoperfusion, mucosal ischemia, and loss of host defenses
- Decreased production of cytoprotectant factors (e.g., prostaglandins), increased permeability, loss of reparative capacity
- Gastric acidity and decrease in gastric mucosal barrier

Acute Risk Factors
- Mechanical ventilation >48 hours, renal replacement therapy
- Coagulopathy, renal failure, hypoperfusion, liver failure
- Brain/spinal cord injury, significant burn injury
- Multiple organ failure, major surgical procedures or trauma
- Other potential risks: concomitant NSAIDs, history of upper gastrointestinal hemorrhage, peptic ulcer disease, or gastritis

Treatment
- Controversial on which medication class to use (efficacy vs. possible side effects); pooled evidence is not clear
- H_2 blocker: famotidine, cimetidine, ranitidine.
- Proton pump inhibitor (PPI): omeprazole, pantoprazole.
- Sucralfate (Carafate): forms a protective barrier.

Complications of Medications for PPx
- Pneumonia—debated in literature. Most report greatest risk with PPI > H_2 blockers.
- *Clostridium difficile* infection rates appear to be higher in patients treated with PPIs

---

1-4: ELECTROLYTES AND ACID/BASE DISTURBANCES

Water Composition		
Total Body Water	Body Weight (%)	Total Body Water (%)
Total	60	100
Intracellular	40	67
Extracellular	20	33
Intravascular	5	8
Interstitial	15	25

Total Body Water (TBW)
- Men = $0.6 \times$ wt (kg)
- Women/older = $0.5 \times$ wt (kg)
- Infant = 0.7–$0.8 \times$ wt (kg)

Requirements
(NICE Clinical Guidelines on Intravenous Fluid Therapy, 2013)

Pediatric Volume Requirements
- First 0–10 kg: 100 mL/kg/day or 4 mL/kg/h
- Next 10–20 kg: an additional 50 mL/kg/day or 2 mL/kg/h
- For >20 kg: an additional 20 mL/kg/day or 1 mL/kg/h

Adult Volume Requirements
- ~25–30 mL/kg/day

Increased fluid requirement for:
- Fever
- Tachypnea
- Evaporation: ventilator, open abdominal wound, diaphoresis
- Gastrointestinal: diarrhea, fistula, tube drainage (NGT, chole tube, PTC)
- Third space losses, operative losses

Chloride/sodium/potassium requirements ~1 mmol/kg/day

Calcium: Total calcium is not reliable with a low albumin. If no ionized calcium on labs, follow below formula to identify patient's corrected calcium
- Corrected Ca = $(4 - albumin) \times 0.8 + Ca^{2+}$

Losses (NICE Clinical Guidelines on Intravenous Fluid Therapy, 2013)

Electrolytes Losses (mmol/L)					
Secretion	Na$^+$	K$^+$	Cl$^-$	HCO$_3$$^-$	H$^+$
Gastric	20–60	14	140	—	60–80
Bile	145	5	105	30	—
Pancreatic	125–138	8	56	85	—
Jejunal	140	5	135	8	—
Ileum	50–140	4–5	25–75	0–30	—
Colon	30–140	30–70		20–80	—

Volume Status
Total body water deficit = %BW × mass in kg [(Current Na − 140)/140)]
Osmolality = $2Na^+ + (glucose/18) + (BUN/2.8)$

Monitoring In's and Out's
- Primary goal is to maintain euvolemia and adequate urine output
  - I's and O's need to be closely monitored to ensure that one has their losses adequately repleted.
- As shown above, depending on the site of losses, the electrolyte losses may be great. Therefore, one must use replete both fluids and electrolytes.

Hypovolemia
- Etiologies: trauma, GI losses (vomiting, diarrhea, NGT), dehydration, third spacing (ascites, effusions, bowel obstruction, crush/burn injuries), insensible, diuretics
- Indications: systolic BP <100, HR >90, cap refill delayed, passive leg raise suggests fluid responsiveness, low UOP, elevated BUN/creatinine

Hypervolemia
- Increase interstitial > increase plasma volume
- Etiologies: iatrogenic, CHF, resuscitation, cirrhosis, CRF
- Diagnosis: decreased HCT and albumin, clinical exam (edema, crackles on auscultation), pulmonary edema on imaging

Acid–Base Disorders			
Disorder	pH	HCO$_3$$^-$	PCO$_2$
Metabolic acidosis	↓	↓	↓
Metabolic alkalosis	↑	↑	↑
Respiratory acidosis	↓	↑	↑
Respiratory alkalosis	↑	↓	↓

Metabolic Acidosis: Overproduction/Under Excretion of Acid, Depletion of Buffer Store
- **Anion gap (AG) = Na − (Cl + HCO$_3$)**
- High AG metabolic acidosis (>12): (MUDPILES) methanol, uremia, DKA, paraldehyde, INH, lactic acid (sepsis, MI, hemorrhage, infection), ethanol/ethylene glycol, salicylate

- No AG/hyperchloremic metabolic acidosis: usually due to loss of bicarbonate rich fluid or decreased excretion of acid renally. (CAGE) chloride excess, acetazolamide/ Addison's, GI losses/diarrhea, extras (RTA, ingestion of oral acidifying salts, etc.)

Metabolic Alkalosis: Loss of Acid or Gain in Base
- Chloride responsive (low U_{Cl}): contraction, diuretic, NGT, hyperemesis
- Chloride nonresponsive (high U_{Cl}): hypokalemia, hypomagnesemia, hyperaldosterone, steroids/Cushing's

Respiratory Acidosis: Hypoventilation/Hypercapnia
- Pulmonary (PTX, effusions, COPD, pneumonia)
- Pain, opioids, obesity, hypophosphatemia

Respiratory Alkalosis: Hyperventilation/Hypocapnia
- Early ASA OD, CHF, cirrhosis, pregnancy, PE, hyperparathyroidism, anxiety, pain

IV Fluid Composition					
Solution	Na^1	K^1	Ca^{21}	Cl^2	HCO_3^1
0.9% NS	154	—	—	154	—
0.45% NS	77	—	—	77	—
LR	130	4	2.7	109	28
3.0% NS	513	—	—	513	—

Electrolyte Imbalance
Hyperkalemia
- Etiologies: ARF/ESRD, ACE-I, spironolactone, cyclosporine, tacrolimus, tissue damage
- **EKG: peaked T-waves, shortened QT, increased PR and QRS intervals, P-wave flattens and can disappear**
- Treatments: calcium (gluconate or chloride) to stabilize heart, 10 U IV insulin w/50 mL D50W (transient decrease in potassium by moving K^+ intracellularly), Na bicarb, Kayexalate (GI excretion as a cation exchange resin; takes hours), β_2 agonists i.e., albuterol (also shifts K^+ intracellularly), loop diuretic (excretion of K), dialysis

Hypokalemia
- Etiologies: unreplenished GI or GU losses; hypomagnesemia
- Symptoms of muscle weakness
- **EKG: T-wave depression, U-wave, prolonged QT, PACs and PVCs**
- **Treatment: give potassium (and magnesium if low)**

Hypernatremia
- Etiologies: unreplenished loss of water (sweat, insensible losses, GI losses), diabetes insipidus, diuretic use, hypertonic saline administration.
- Symptoms: irritability, ataxia, seizures
- To avoid cerebral edema/herniation: correct at <0.5 mEq/L/h if patient has been hypernatremic for over 48 hours

Hyponatremia
- Etiologies: generally increased intake of water or retention of water; impaired renal excretion of water, adrenal insufficiency, SIADH, cirrhosis, heart failure, primary polydipsia.
- In hyperglycemia, can have psuedohyponatremia: for each 100 mg/dL glucose >100, Na is decreased by ~2.4 mEg/L (*Am J Med.* 1999;106(4):339–403)
- To avoid central pontine myelinolysis: correct at 6–8mmol/L increase over 24 hours (*Semin Nephrol.* 2009;29(3):282–99)
- Symptoms: CNS (weakness, fatigue, confusion, delirium, obtundation, seizures) > GI (nausea/vomiting)

Hypercalcemia
- Parathyroid mediated causes: primary hyperparathyroidism, familial hypocalciuric hypercalcemia, tertiary hyperparathyroidism (renal failure)
- Nonparathyroid causes: malignancy, PRHrP, osteolytic processes, Vitamin D intoxication, granulomatous disease, thiazide diuretics, adrenal insufficiency, milk alkali syndrome, and immobilization
- Symptoms: weakness, mental status changes, polyuria, nausea, vomiting, pancreatitis
- Treatment: saline hydration, hemodialysis, calcitonin, bisphosphonates, furosemide—controversial

Hypocalcemia
- Etiologies: pancreatitis, tumor lysis syndrome, hypoparathyroid, rhabdomyolysis, Vitamin D deficiency

- Signs/symptoms: paresthesias, muscle spasms, seizures, increased QT interval
  - Trousseau sign—carpedal spasm with inflation of a blood pressure cuff for 3 minutes
  - Chvostek's sign—contraction of ipsilateral facial muscle with tapping over the facial nerve
- Treatment: IV calcium chloride, IV calcium gluconate, PO calcium, calcitriol, Vitamin D, correction of concurrent hypomagnesemia

Hypermagnesemia
- Etiologies: renal failure, burns, crush injuries, rhabdomyolysis, tumor lysis syndrome, infusion, ingestion, or rectal magnesium administration
- Symptoms: loss of DTRs, nausea/vomiting, mental status changes
- Treatment: stop intake of magnesium, loop diuretics, dialysis

Zinc Deficiency
- Etiologies: malnutrition/malabsorption, trauma, Crohn's
- Symptoms: growth failure, dermatitis, impaired immunity

1-5: POSTOPERATIVE FEVER

(Weed H & Baddour L. Postoperative Fever. In: UpToDate, Post TW (Ed), UpToDate, Waltham, MA, Accessed September 9, 2016)

Most early postoperative fevers are not due to infection, but are caused by the inflammatory reaction caused by the surgery itself.
5 W's
- Wind (lung)
- Water (urine)
- Wound
- Walking (DVT/PE)
- Wonder/ What did we do? Infusions, blood transfusions, drug (reactions), sites of catheters, lines or indwelling drains, etc.

Workup: physical exam (look at wound), blood cultures, UA/U culture, CXR, CBC

Frequent Postoperative complications

Surgical Site Infection (April 2013 CDC/NHSN Protocol Corrections, Clarification, and Additions. http://www. cdc.gov/nhsn/PDFs/pscManual/9pscSSIcurrent.pdf. Accessed June 10, 2016)
- Symptoms: fever, erythema, purulent drainage, pain, leukocytosis
- Depth of infection:
  - Superficial infection: <30 days from surgery that involves the skin and subcutaneous tissue
    - Treatment: open wound if fluctuance; possible debridement, possible negative pressure wound therapy; antibiotics if only cellulitis
  - Deep infection: involves the fascia and muscle layers
    - Treatment: open wound, possible debridement, possible negative pressure wound therapy; may need antibiotics if contiguous cellulitis
  - Organ Space infection: ex intra-abdominal abscess; usually diagnosed via CT
    - Treatment: drainage and antibiotics

Postoperative Pneumonia
- RF: intubation/extubation, impaired consciousness, dysphagia, Trendelenburg position, nonfunctioning NGT, emergent intubation on full stomach
- Signs and symptoms: fever, purulent sputum, leukocytosis or leukopenia, worsening of oxygenation, new infiltrate on imaging
- Diagnosis: clinical exam, CXR, sputum gram stain and culture, bronchoalveolar lavage with quantitative culture
- Treatment (Am J Respir Crit Care Med. 2005:171:388–416)
  - Antibiotics—start empiric therapy if patient has a new or progressing infiltrate on CXR plus 2 of fever (above 38°C), leukocytosis or leukopenia, purulent sputum
  - Initial empiric therapy (while cultures pending) in patients with no known risk factors for multidrug resistant infections: ceftriaxone, levofloxacin, moxifloxacin, ampicillin/sulbactam, ertapenem
- Postoperative respiratory complications can be reduced by implementing multidisciplinary approach to respiratory care (JAMA Surg. 2013;148(8):740–745)
  - I COUGH: Incentive spirometry, Coughing and deep breathing, Oral care, Understanding (patient and family education), Getting out of bed three times daily and Head of bed elevation

Anastomotic Leak (J Am Coll Surg. 2009;208(2):269–278)

- Risk factors includes malnutrition, cardiovascular disease, steroids, bowel obstruction, tobacco use, ASA score, diverticulitis, low anastomoses or suboptimal anastomotic blood supply, operative time >2 hours, septic conditions
- Signs/symptoms: pain, peritonitis, feculent or purulent drainage, leukocytosis, fever
- Detected 3–45 days postoperatively
  - Two peaks: 7 days when diagnosis is usually made clinically and 16 days when diagnosis is usually made radiographically.
- Diagnosis: clinical picture, x-ray (sometimes free air), CT with fluid collections and air outside of the bowel.
- Treatment: resuscitation, antibiotics, and source control → return to OR
  - Of note: controversial, but for small/contained leaks, there is literature on treatment with a combination of bowel rest, percutaneous drainage, and/or colonic stenting

POD 3–5

Urinary Tract Infection (CID. 2010:50:625–663)

- No. 1 healthcare-associated infection
- Should not keep an indwelling catheter in longer than necessary
- Signs and symptoms: classic symptoms of frequent urination, urgent urination, suprapubic pain/tenderness may not be present in catheterized patients. Other signs and symptoms include hematuria, flank or costovertebral tenderness, lethargy, fevers, rigors, altered mental status
- Diagnosis:
  - UA: + nitrite (from bacteria), + leukocyte esterase, bacteria
  - Culture
    Organisms: most common: *Escherichia coli*; Others: *Klebsiella, Serratia, Citrobacter, Enterobacter, Staphylococci, Enterococci*
    Treatment: appropriate antibiotics; remove or exchange Foley

Peritoneal Abscess

- Signs: fever (spiking), abdominal pain, mass, ileus, anorexia, tachycardia
- Diagnosis: CT shows fluid collection with fibrinous ring, gas
- Treatment: drainage and antibiotics

Pseudomembranous colitis (Clostridium difficile in adults: Treatment. In: UpToDate, Post TW (Ed.), UpToDate, Waltham, MA. Accessed July 31, 2016)

- Colonization occurs by fecal–oral route which is facilitated by disruption of the normal intestinal flora (as a result of antimicrobial therapy). Overgrowth of *C. difficile* occurs, which produces a toxin that disrupts the epithelial integrity and causes an inflammatory infiltrate
- Risk factors: exposure to antibiotics (clindamycin, penicillins, cephalosporins, fluoroquinolones), older age, hospitalization, chemotherapy, PPIs
- Clinical presentation: abdominal pain, foul-smelling diarrhea, leukocytosis, fever, nausea/vomiting.
- Diagnosis: most commonly by stool assay for toxin
- Treatment: stop culprit antibiotic if possible; start metronidazole or PO vancomycin. For severe disease, vancomycin is generally recommended over metronidazole, but if concurrent ileus, add IV metronidazole. Fidaxomicin can be considered for recurrent infection. Fecal transplant is another option.
- Surgery (subtotal colectomy) is indicated with severe disease as evidenced by megacolon, perforation, necrotizing colitis, rapidly progressing disease, refractory disease.
  - As an alternative to the classic subtotal colectomy, there is literature on using a diverting loop ileostomy with colonic lavage (Ann Surg. 2011;254(3):423–427)

HEATH WALDEN • ALAN LISBON

2-1: CARDIOPULMONARY MONITORS

PA Catheters
- Invasive monitoring catheter floated intravascularly through the right ventricle to the pulmonary artery
- Allows for direct measurement of pulmonary artery pressure, central venous pressure, cardiac output, pulmonary artery saturation, mixed venous oxygen saturation, and core temperature
- Allows for calculation of systemic vascular resistance, stroke volume, oxygen delivery, oxygen consumption, pulmonary vascular resistance, left ventricular stroke work index, and right ventricular stroke work index
- Indications for use has decreased over time with the greater availability of noninvasive measurements
- Increased mortality in ICU patients in different studies
- **Complications of PA catheters**
  - Insertion: minor arrhythmias, sustained arrhythmias, arterial puncture, pneumothorax
  - Indwelling: infection at insertion site, catheter-related bloodstream infection mural thrombus, pulmonary artery rupture, pulmonary infarction
  - Misinterpretation and use of data

PiCCO
- Invasive cardiac output monitor that combines pulse contour analysis and transpulmonary thermodilution technique
- Catheter is an arterial line with a thermistor on the end, patient must also have a central line in place
- Contraindications: intracardiac shunts, aortic aneurysm, aortic stenosis, pneumonectomy, pulmonary embolism (PE), intra-aortic balloon pump, unstable arrhythmias
- Allows for measurement and calculation of cardiac output, cardiac index, global end-diastolic volume, global ejection fraction, intrathoracic blood volume, extravascular lung water, pule continuous cardiac output, systemic vascular resistance, stroke volume variation, dP_{max} (slope of pressure vs. time trace, closely approximating LV contractility), $ScvO_2$
- **Complications of PiCCO:** those associated with arterial line placement and an indwelling arterial line, complications associated with central lines, misinterpretation, and use of data

FloTrac
- Cardiac output monitor that uses pulse contour analysis
- Specialized sensor that attaches to a previously inserted radial arterial line
- Uses manufacturer's patented algorithm to calculate cardiac output, cardiac index, stroke volume, systemic vascular resistance, and stroke volume variation
- Accuracy remains controversial especially in the presence of extreme vasodilatation with hyperdynamic circulation, hepatic cirrhosis, aortic regurgitation, arrhythmias, and intra-aorta balloon pump (IABP) counterpulsation
- **Complications of FloTrac:** those associated with arterial line placement and with an indwelling arterial line, misinterpretation, and use of data

NICOM
- Enables continuous noninvasive hemodynamic monitoring based on phase shifts.
- Uses four sensors applied to the right and left sides of the chest. Each sensor has a double electrode configuration (one to receive, one to transmit).
- A low-amplitude AC current with a frequency of 75 kHz is applied and the return voltage is measured. The thorax resists the passage of current and causes a time delay between the current and voltage resulting in a phase shift. This phase shift correlates to aortic blood flow and allows calculation of the stroke volume.
- The system uses aortic blood flow as an indirect measurement of strength of contractility. Stroke volume variation over time is also measured.
- **Complications:** misinterpretation and use of data

Common Measurements: Normal Ranges
- Central venous pressure (CVP): 1–10 mm Hg
- Pulmonary capillary wedge pressure (PCWP): 6–12 mm Hg

- Cardiac output (CO): 4–6 L/min
  - CO = Stroke volume (SV) × heart rate (HR)
- Cardiac index (CI): 2.4–4 L/min/m^2
  - CI = CO/body surface area
- Pressure measurements
  - Right atrium: 3–6 mm Hg
  - Right ventricle: systolic: 20–30; diastolic: 2–8 mm Hg
  - Pulmonary artery: systolic: 20–30; diastolic: 5–15; mean: 10–20 mm Hg
- Systemic vascular resistance (SVR): 800–1200 dynes/s/cm^5
- Mixed venous saturation (SvO$_2$): 60–80%
  - a-vO$_2$ difference = oxygen delivered – oxygen consumed
- Stroke volume variability (SVV)
- Extrapolated equations
  - Oxygen delivery (DO$_2$) = CO × CaO$_2$
  - Oxygen content (CaO$_2$) = 1.34 × Hb × SaO$_2$ (oxygen saturation)

2-2: Shock

Definition
- An abnormality of the circulatory system that results in low blood perfusion to the tissues resulting in cellular injury and inadequate tissue function.

Stages of Shock
- **Initial:** hypoperfusion causes hypoxia
- **Compensatory:** body attempts to compensate for the resulting acidosis
- **Progressive:** natural compensatory mechanisms start to fail
- **Refractory:** irreversible organ failure

Hypovolemic Shock
Pathophysiology
- Severe intravascular volume loss that leads to a state of inadequate tissue perfusion leading to anaerobic metabolism
- Causes: **bleeding**, dehydration, or third-space losses
- Intravascular volume loss leads to decreased oxygen delivery (DO$_2$) from a decreased CO

Clinical Presentation
- Signs of decreased intravascular volume
- Tachycardia: body compensating to maintain cardiac output
- Hypotension: reflection of intravascular depletion
- Altered mental status due to inadequate DO$_2$ to the brain
- Decreased urine output

Classes of Hypovolemic Shock				
	Class I	Class II	Class III	Class IV
Blood loss (mL)	≤750	750–1,500	1,500–2,000	>2,000
Blood loss (%)	≤15%	15–30%	30–40%	>40%
Heart rate	<100	>100	>120	>140
Blood pressure	Normal	Normal	Decreased	Decreased
Respiratory rate	14–20	20–30	30–40	>35
Urine output (cc/h)	>30	20–30	5–15	Negligible
Mental status	Normal, slightly anxious	Anxious	Confused, anxious	Lethargic
Replacement fluid	Crystalloid	Crystalloid	Crystalloid and blood	Crystalloid and blood

Treatment
- Ensure there is adequate intravascular access
  - Two large bores (14–16 gauge): IVs—infusion rate 240 mL/min per IV
  - If unable to obtain IVs, central access with Cordis®/introducer (~8.5 Fr)—infusion rate 126 mL/min on gravity, 333 mL/min on pressure bag infusion
- Fluids (should be warmed)
- Rapid infuser pumps may be necessary
- If nonhemorrhagic, resuscitate with crystalloid and identify the source of loss (i.e., ongoing GI loss or dehydration)

- If hemorrhagic, balanced resuscitation between blood products, **identify and control** the source of bleeding

Distributive Shock

Etiologies
- Sepsis
- Anaphylaxis
- Neurogenic
- Adrenal crisis

Sepsis
- Sepsis: life-threatening organ dysfunction caused by a dysregulated host response to infection
- Septic shock: sepsis that has circulatory, cellular, and metabolic abnormalities that are associated with a greater risk of mortality than sepsis alone (*JAMA*. 2016;315(8):801–810)
  - Clinically: patients who fulfill criteria for sepsis that despite adequate fluid resuscitation, still require vasopressors to have MAP ≥65 mm Hg and have a lactate >2
- **Common sources in the ICU:** central line–associated bloodstream infection (CLABSI), pneumonia, UTI, *Clostridium difficile* infection, and intra-abdominal infection (abscess, perforated viscus)

Pathophysiology
- Bacterial endotoxins—i.e., lipopolysaccharides of gram-negative bacilli
  - Lipopolysaccharides contain an immunogenic lipid A core which binds to CD14 and activates monocytes, macrophages, and endothelial cells
  - High-dose release of secondary cytokines TNF and IL-1/6/8 leads to a decrease in vascular tone and general vasodilatation with hypotension
- Systemic endothelial injury leads to "leaky" capillary beds and loss of intravascular volume (i.e., pulmonary edema and acute respiratory distress syndrome [ARDS])
- Ultimately, activation of the coagulation cascade leads to disseminated intravascular coagulation and generalized hypoperfusion

Treatment
- Diagnostic sequence
  - Obtain cultures from all possible sources
  - Start broad-spectrum antibiotics targeted toward presumed source
  - Obtain imaging as indicated to help with identification/management
  - Source control: e.g., drain an abscess, remove infected line or resect perforated viscus
  - De-escalate antibiotics as appropriate based on culture data
- Volume resuscitation: initially replace intravascular volume with crystalloid
- Vasopressors: only use after adequate volume resuscitation
  - Norepinephrine (Levophed) is generally first choice for patients with septic shock
- General supportive care of all systems as indicated/needed (e.g., intubation, HD or CVVHD, glucose control, nutrition)

Anaphylaxis
- Type I hypersensitivity reaction
- Immune-mediated vasodilatory response leading to hypotension, edema, and bronchoconstriction
- Can be either immediate (occurs minutes after exposure, vasoactive amines, and lipid mediators) or late (2–4 hours, cytokines)

Pathophysiology
- Mediated by IgE
- Patient must have a previous exposure to the allergen, becoming "sensitized"
- Release of vasoactive amines from mast cells and basophils (histamines, leukotrienes, and prostaglandins)
  - Leads to vasodilation, increased permeability, smooth muscle spasm, and leukocyte extravasation
- Anaphylactoid reactions refer to the degranulation of mast cells without IgE

Clinical Presentation
- Hypotension
- Respiratory compromise (begins with wheezing and bronchoconstriction)
- Tracheal edema
- GI distress
- Angioedema
- Urticaria

Treatment
- Antihistamines for mild symptoms
- Bronchodilators for pulmonary bronchospasm (moderate symptoms)
- Epinephrine for threatened airway (severe symptoms)—mainstay of treatment
- Early intubation for stridor and laryngeal edema
- Volume resuscitation for hypotension
- Vasopressors +/– steroids if adequately resuscitated with persistent hypotension

Neurogenic Shock
Pathophysiology
- Loss of autonomic innervation of the vasculature
  - Spinal cord injury above T6, regional anesthesia, adrenergic nervous system blocking drugs in certain neurologic disorders
- Intrinsic blood volume becomes insufficient to fill the dilated intravascular space
- End result: relative hypovolemia

Clinical Presentation
- Decreased MAP from arteriolar dilation
- Warm extremities
- Venous pooling
- **Bradycardia**
- Decreased CO

Treatment
- Trendelenburg position: causes blood to be translocated from the denervated lower extremities back to the heart
  - Increases ventricular end-diastolic volume, stroke volume, cardiac output, and blood pressure
- Fluid resuscitation
- Can institute vasopressors earlier to avoid volume overload
  - Norepinephrine or fixed-dose dopamine (5 µg/kg/min)
  - Phenylephrine only in patients without reflex bradycardia

Adrenal Crisis
Pathophysiology
- Patients with undiagnosed primary adrenal insufficiency with a serious infection or acute, major stress
- Patient with known primary adrenal insufficiency who miss dosage of glucocorticoid
- Bilateral adrenal infarction or hemorrhage
- Patient with abrupt withdrawal of steroids
- Dysfunctional hypothalamic–pituitary–adrenal axis
- Primarily a mineralocorticoid deficiency causing shock

Clinical Presentation
- Shock
- Anorexia, nausea, vomiting, abdominal pain
- Weakness, fatigue, or lethargy
- Confusion or coma
- Hyponatremia, hyperkalemia, and hypoglycemia

Treatment
- Resuscitation with saline-containing solution
- Patient without known adrenal insufficiency is treated with dexamethasone (4 mg IV bolus)
  - Dexamethasone is undetectable on serum cortisol assays
- Patients with known adrenal insufficiency treat with hydrocortisone (100 mg IV bolus) or dexamethasone will need maintenance replacement

Cardiogenic Shock (Left Heart Failure)
Pathophysiology
- Failure of left ventricle to function effectively leading to inadequate circulation
- Common causes: myocardial infarction, cardiomyopathy, valvular disease, and arrhythmias
- Leads to decreased cardiac output and shock

Clinical Presentation
- Altered mentation, pale/mottled skin, hypotension, oliguria, and pulmonary edema
- Event sequence
  1. Increase in PCWP
  2. Decrease in SV + tachycardia
  3. Decrease in CO

Treatment
- Maintain CO
- Cardiac output monitoring
- Pharmacologic intervention with inotropes and vasopressors as needed
- Normalize filling pressures
- Keep HCT >30%
- May need mechanical assisting devices, i.e., IABP or extracorporeal membrane oxygenation (ECMO)
  - Balloon counterpulsation augments CO by inflating during diastole and deflating during systole; contraindicated if aortic regurgitation
- Ventilatory support as needed
- Surgical intervention: CABG, angioplasty, valve replacement

Obstructive Shock
Pathophysiology
- Anything that results in the prevention of blood outflow from the heart
- Can be external compressive forces:
- Pericardial tamponade, tension pneumothorax, excessive positive end-expiratory pressure (PEEP), ruptured or elevated diaphragm, or abdominal compartment syndrome
- Can be related to blood flow directly
- Pulmonary embolus, severe pulmonary artery hypertension (PAH), severe aortic stenosis, or aortic dissections

Clinical Presentation
- Hypotension
- Decreased cardiac output
- Symptoms related to primary etiology

Treatment
- If caused by external force need to relieve force
  - Drain pericardial effusion
  - Chest tube decompression of pneumothorax
  - Decrease PEEP
  - Relief of compartment syndrome
- If related to blood flow
  - Treat PE (anticoagulation, thrombolysis or mechanical thrombectomy)
  - Medical management of PAH—vasodilators, endothelin receptor antagonists, phosphodiesterase inhibitors, etc.
  - Surgical replacement of aortic valve or replacement of aortic arch

Hemodynamic Parameters in Shock			
Type of Shock	CO	SVR	CVP
Hypovolemic	↑	↑	↓↓↓
Distributive	↑↑	↓↓	↔ or ↓
Cardiogenic	↓↓	↑↑	↑↑
Obstructive	↓	↑	↑↑

2-3: VASOACTIVE DRUGS

Inotropic Agents and Vasopressors

Drug	Dose	Receptor	Action	Indication	Clinical Effect
Dopamine	Low dose: 1–5 mcg/kg/min Medium: 6–10 mcg/kg/min High: >10 mcg/kg/min	Dose: L M H α + ++ β_1 + ++ +++ $D_{1/2}$ +++ ++ ++	L: Renal/splanchnic vasodilatation M: Increases heart contractility H: vasoconstriction/increases BP	Second-line agent for patients with bradycardia and low risk for tachyarrhythmias	Low—↑ CO Medium—↑ CO and ↑ SVR High—↑↑ SVR
Dobutamine	5–20 mcg/kg/min	$\alpha_0/+$ β_1 +++ β_2 ++	Increases contractility Vasodilatation	Medically refractory heart failure and cardiogenic shock	↑ CO Decreased SVR
Epinephrine	Epinephrine 0.01–0.2 mcg/kg/min	α +++ β_1 +++ β_2 ++	At low doses increased CO from β_1 activity while α and β_2 offset Higher doses α effect overcomes β_2 and increases SVR	Anaphylaxis Second-line agent in septic shock Cardiogenic shock Post-CABG hypotension	↑↑ CO Low dose may ↓ SVR High dose ↑ SVR
Milrinone	Milrinone 0.125–0.75 µg/kg/min	N/A	Inhibits phosphodiesterase, increases calcium influx, increasing contractility	Used in cases of low cardiac output May be used as single agent	↑ CO ↓ SVR
Norepinephrine	0.01–0.5 mcg/kg/min	α +++ β_1 ++	Potent vasoconstriction and modest increase in CO	First line agent for septic, cardiogenic and hypovolemic shock	↑↑ SVR ↔/↑ CO
Phenylephrine	0.5–5 mcg/kg/min	α +++	Purely α vasoconstriction Increased SVR → increased afterload	First line in patients with tachyarrhythmias Additional agent in refractory shock Contraindicated if SVR >1,200	↑↑ SVR ↔/↑ CO
Vasopressin	0.02–0.06 unit/min	V_{1a} Receptor +	Pure vasoconstrictor, may decrease stroke volume and CO	Add-on agent to augment efficacy in refractory vasodilatory shock Can cause hyponatremia and pulmonary vasoconstriction	↑ SVR ↔/↓ CO

2-4: VENTILATOR MANAGEMENT

- Modern mechanical ventilators have evolved and become more complex with new modes, settings, and capabilities
- All of these modes control three variables: trigger, limit, and cycle

Ventilator Variables

Trigger

- Variable that serves as the signal to initiate the inspiratory phase
- Flow trigger: deliver a continuous flow of gas across the circuit and initiate inspiratory phase when patient effort leads to change in this flow
- Pressure trigger: the patient's spontaneous respiratory effort leads to a change in pressure in the circuit initiating the inspiratory phase
- Time trigger: starts inspiratory phase in mandatory or assisted modes

Limit

- Variable that is the maximal set inspiratory pressure or flow
- Pressure-controlled and pressure-support ventilation are based on set pressure limits
- Volume-controlled ventilation is flow-limited ventilation during the inspiratory phase since volume is the product of flow and time

Cycle

- The variable that determines what terminates the inspiratory cycle
- Time, flow, pressure, or volume

Volume-Limited Versus Pressure-Limited Ventilation

Volume-Limited

- Clinician sets the peak flow rate, flow pattern, tidal volume (V_T), respiratory rate (RR), PEEP, and FiO_2
- Airway pressures vary depending on ventilator settings and patient-related variables (i.e., compliance, airway resistance)

Pressure-Limited

- Clinician sets the inspiratory pressure level, inspiratory to expiratory ration (I:E), RR, PEEP, and FiO_2
- Peak airway pressure is constant and is the sum of inspiratory pressure and PEEP
- Delivered V_T is variable and is related to inspiratory pressure, compliance, airway resistance, and tubing resistance

Common Ventilator Modes

Volume Control

- Ventilator is set to deliver a preset volume of gas regardless of the amount of pressure needed to deliver the volume

Pressure Control

- Ventilator is set to deliver gas until a preset airway pressure is reached
- V_T varies based on patient factors

Pressure-Regulated Volume Control (PRVC)

- Adaptive mode that adjusts the inspiratory time and pressure to maintain a preset V_T based on changing lung compliance

Assist Control (AC)

- Ventilator supports every breath independent of trigger
- If patient initiates breath (either flow or pressure triggered) then the ventilator delivers the set V_T
- If ventilator does not sense a patient-based trigger over a set time period, then the ventilator delivers the set V_T
- If patient is anxious and frequently triggers ventilator above set RR, then can easily hyperventilate

Synchronized Intermittent Mandatory Ventilation (SIMV)

- Not all patient-triggered breaths are assisted
- If SIMV rate is set at 10 bpm, then the patient received ventilator-assisted breaths every 6 seconds
- In between these breaths, patient can take their own breaths

Indications for Intubation
• Hypoxia
• Hypercapnea
• Inability to clear and manage oropharyngeal secretions
• Depressed level of consciousness (GCS ≤8, intractable seizures, medication related)
• Periprocedural or to facilitate a necessary workup

General Ventilator Management

Monitoring

- Goal is to avoid lung damage, e.g., avoid volutrauma and barotrauma
- V_T: set at 5–10 cc/kg
- RR: 10–20 breaths/min
- PEEP: start at 5 cm H_2O
  - Increases functional residual capacity
  - Increase as needed to maintain PaO_2
- Pressure support: provides an amount of pressure during inspiration to help patient draw in a breath, can help overcome the resistance of the system (airway tubing, ET tube)
- Inspired fractionated O_2 (FiO_2): try to keep below 60%
- Plateau airway pressure <30 cm H_2O

Making Ventilator Adjustments

- Hypercapnea: increase the RR or the V_T
- Hypocapnea: decrease the RR or the V_T
- Hypoxia: increase the FiO_2 or the PEEP
- Hyperoxia: decrease FiO_2 and PEEP as tolerated to minimal settings

Discontinuation of Mechanical Ventilation

Evaluate Two Aspects

- Readiness: evaluation of objective clinical criteria in order to decide if you can start the process of discontinuation
- Weaning: process of decreasing ventilator support that has patient take over greater portion of ventilation

General Requirements to Perform a Spontaneous Breathing Trial

- Basic criteria: hemodynamic stability, awake, and responding to commands
- Physiologic criteria: PEEP <10, SaO_2 ≥90%, FiO_2 ≤0.60, pH >7.30
- Decrease FiO_2 and PEEP to physiologic levels, transition to pressure support ventilation, initiate SBT (protocols vary by institution)
- Check the Rapid Shallow Breathing Index (RSBI) (*NEJM. 324(21):1445–1450*)
  - RSBI = respiratory rate (bpm)/tidal volume (liters)
  - RSBI >105 predictor for failure of extubation

Example of an SBT
• CPAP ventilator mode with PEEP of 0 cm H_2O, PSV of 5 cm H_2O, FiO_2 of 35%, unchanged for 30 min
• Obtain an RSBI at the end of the 30 min
• SBT termination criteria
• RR >35 for >5 min
• SpO_2 <90% for >2 min
• Development of ectopy
• RSBI ≥105 for 5 min
• HR >140 bpm or ≥20% change from baseline
• SBP >180 or <90 or ≥20% change from baseline
• Excessive use of accessory muscles, excessive diaphoresis, or increased anxiety

Basic ABG Interpretation
• Step 1: Assess the pH (normal 7.35–7.45)
• If <7.35 acidosis, if >7.45 alkalosis
• Step 2: Is this respiratory of metabolic?
• Compare the pH and match with the pCO_2 and the HCO_3
• pCO_2 normal 35–45, >45 acidic, <35 alkalotic
• HCO_3 normal 22–26, <22 acidotic, >26 alkalotic
• Step 3: Are all three the same?
• If all variables are acidotic, then a combined acidosis

- Step 4: Is there compensation?
  - Uncompensated: pH is outside normal range and unmatched variable still in normal range
  - Partially compensated: pH abnormal and unmatched variable outside of normal range in an attempt to compensate for primary problem.
- Step 5: Analyze the pO_2 and the SpO_2

Alveolar–Arterial Gradient

- A-a Gradient = $P_AO_2 - P_aO_2$
- $PAO_2 = (FiO_2 \times (P_{atm} - P_{H_2O})) - (PaCO_2/0.8)$
- P_aO_2 = arterial PO_2 as measured by blood gas
- Normal in healthy patient breathing room air at sea level is 5–10 mm Hg
- Increased with age (~1 mm Hg per decade of life)
  - Estimate (age in years/4) + 4
- Useful in determining the source of hypoxemia
  - Elevated: V/Q mismatch, shunt, alveolar hypoventilation
  - Depressed: hypoventilation (COPD, CNS disorder), low FiO_2

2-5: Common Problems in the ICU

Acute Respiratory Distress Syndrome
Definition (JAMA. 2012; 307(23):2526–2533)
- Acute diffuse, inflammatory lung injury, leading to increased pulmonary vascular permeability, increased lung weight, and loss of aerated lung tissue
- Clinically:
  - Acute onset over 1 week of less
  - Bilateral opacities consistent with pulmonary edema
  - PaO_2/FiO_2 ratio <300 mm Hg with a minimum of 5 cm H_2O PEEP
  - Must not be fully explained by cardiac failure or fluid overload
- Severity:
  - Mild: PaO_2/FiO_2 = 200–300
  - Moderate: PaO_2/FiO_2 = 100–200
  - Severe: PaO_2/FiO_2 = <100
- Causes
  - Direct: pneumonia, aspiration, lung contusion, fat embolism, near drowning, or inhalational injury
  - Indirect: nonpulmonary sepsis, polytrauma, massive transfusion, pancreatitis, or cardiopulmonary bypass

Treatment
- Supportive care and treatment of offending agent
- Mechanical ventilation
  - Low TV—6 cc/kg (NEJM. 2000; 342(18):1301–1308)
  - PEEP
  - Lower oxygenation target: SpO_2 >88% or PaO_2 >55 mm Hg
- Techniques to improve oxygenation
  - Early prone positioning
  - Recruitment maneuvers
  - Inhaled nitric oxide or prostacycline
  - ECMO

Pneumonia
Definition
- Infection that inflames the alveoli causing dense area of inflammation in the lung
- Alveoli may become filled with fluid, purulence, or exudative secretions
- Can be caused by bacteria, viruses, fungi

Diagnosis
- Symptoms: cough, productive sputum, fever, tachypnea, dyspnea, pleuritic chest pain, or abdominal pain
- Signs: rhonchi/decreased breath sounds, tachycardia, and decrease in O_2 saturation
- Elevated white blood cell count in immunocompetent individuals
- Chest x-ray, bronchoscopy, or CT
- Clinical Pulmonary Infection Score (CPIS)
  - Used to assist in the clinical diagnosis of ventilator-associated pneumonia by predicting which patients will benefit from obtaining pulmonary cultures
- Sputum cultures, protected catheter sampling, or bronchoalveolar lavage

- Atypical organisms:
  - Cold agglutinin titers: *Mycoplasma*
  - Urinary *Legionella* antigen: *Legionella*
  - Specific antibody titers

Community-Acquired Pneumonia
Epidemiology
- Acute infection of the pulmonary parenchyma in a patient who has acquired the infection in the community
- Usually single organism

Organisms
- Bacteria: *Streptococcus pneumoniae* (most common organism), *Haemophilus influenza*, *Mycoplasma pneumoniae*, *Chlamydia pneumoniae*, *Legionella*, *Klebsiella pneumoniae*, *Pseudomonas aeruginosa*, *Acinetobacter*, *Moraxella*, or *Staphylococcus aureus*
- Viruses: influenza, parainfluenza, RSV, adenovirus, or rhinovirus
- Fungi: *Cryptococcus*, *Histoplasma*, or *Coccidioides*

Treatment
- Antibiotics and supportive care

Nosocomial Pneumonia (Hospital-Acquired)
Epidemiology
- Pneumonia that was not present at admission and develops in a patient hospitalized for >48 hours

Organisms
- Gram-negative bacteria
- MDR (multidrug-resistant) organisms—MRSA, *Enterobacteria*, *P. aeruginosa*, Acinetobacter, Stenotrophomonas
- Viruses—influenza, RSV, adenovirus, parainfluenza
- Aspergillus
- Legionella
  Gram-negative bacteria, e.g., *Pseudomonas*, *Escherichia coli*, *Serratia*

Treatment
- Broad-spectrum antibiotics for critically ill patients (i.e., piperacillin–tazobactam)
- Pathogen- and sensitivity-directed antibiotics, usually a fluoroquinolone or a second- or third-generation cephalosporin with a Macrolide

Ventilator-Associated Pneumonia
Epidemiology
- Occurs in up to 25% of ventilated patients on a ventilator for >48 hours
- Colonization of the oral cavity and hypopharynx with pathogenic organisms
- Endotracheal tube or tracheostomy tube cuffs prevent macroaspiration but allow for microaspiration of secretions pooled above the cuff

Organisms
- <48 hours in hospital, often community organisms
- 48 hours–5 days community and nosocomial organisms
- >5 days often MDR organisms

Prevention
- Good oral care with chlorhexidine
- Stress ulcer prophylaxis when indicated
- Elevate head of bed >30 degrees
- Subglottic suctioning
- Maintain adequate cuff pressure to avoid macroaspiration
- Minimize duration of mechanical ventilation as possible

Atrial Fibrillation
Background
- Most common cardiac arrhythmia affecting 1–2% of the population where:
  - RR interval shows no repetitive pattern
  - There are no distinct P-wave heart rhythm
- In the ICU will be addressing either new onset atrial fibrillation (AF) or paroxysmal, persistent, or longstanding AF
- Symptoms of new onset AF are generally related to a rapid ventricular response (RVR)

Management
- All patients should be evaluated for precipitating cause and it should be treated/addressed
- Management strategy depends upon stability of patient

Unstable Patient

These patients require urgent or emergent cardioversion:
- Patients with active myocardial ischemia
- Evidence of organ hypoperfusion
- Severe manifestations of heart failure

Stable Patient

- If rate control is needed, consider the use of beta-blocker or calcium channel blocker IV or PO depending on urgency of clinical situation
  - If converts determine the need for anticoagulation based on $CHA_2DS_2-VAS_c$ score and consider long-term rate or rhythm control
- If patient does not require rate control or remains in AF in the above situation
  - If documented in AF for <48 hours, then proceed with cardioversion and if successful, determine need for anticoagulation and consider long-term rate or rhythm control
  - If in AF for >48 hours, then either investigate for intracardiac thrombus by TEE, and if negative, cardiovert as above or delayed cardioversion after 3 weeks of anticoagulation
- If after all of the above patients remain in AF, then consider alternative methods of rhythm or rate control

Venous Thromboembolism (VTE)

Background
- Definition: blood clot that forms in the venous circulation
- Most common presentation of venous thrombosis are deep vein thrombosis (DVT) of the lower extremity and PE

Pathophysiology
- Major theory—Virchow's triad (*NEJM*. 2008;359(9):938–949)
  - Alteration in blood flow (stasis), vascular endothelial injury, and alteration in the constituents of the blood (inherited or acquired hypercoagulable states)
- Inherited thrombophilias: factor V Leiden mutation, prothrombin gene mutation, protein C and S deficiency, and antithrombin deficiency
- Acquired disorders: malignancy, surgery, pregnancy, trauma, oral contraceptives, hormone replacement therapy, prolonged immobilization, antiphospholipid syndrome, myeloproliferative disorders, inflammatory bowel disorders

DVT
- Can be subdivided between distal (calf) and proximal (popliteal, femoral, or iliac)
- 90% of PEs occur as emboli from proximal DVTs
- Can have swelling, pain, and erythema in the affected extremity

Diagnosis
- Impedence plethysmography
- Compression ultrasonography
- D-dimer levels
- All tests are most useful when combined with assessment of pretest probability via score calculator (e.g., Wells score, Hamilton score, or AMUSE score)

Treatment
- Prevention: subcutaneous heparin and pneumatic boots
- Patient with proximal DVT and no cancer: dabigatran, rivaroxaban, apixaban, or edoxaban are the first-line agents.
- Patient with proximal DVT and cancer: LMWH is the first-line agent (*CHEST*. 2016;149(2):315–352)
- IVC filters for patients with a contraindication to anticoagulation

PE
- Obstruction of the main pulmonary artery or one of its branches by material from another region of the body, in this case thrombus
- Clinical signs are variable from complete hemodynamic collapse to shortness of breath to asymptomatic
- Hemodynamically unstable PE is any that results in SBP <90 mm Hg for >15 minutes or requires vasopressors or inotropic support not explained by other causes

Diagnosis
- Calculate Wells score for PE—score >4.0, then PE likely
- CT-based diagnosis
  - If PE likely obtain CT pulmonary angiogram
  - If PE unlikely obtain D-dimer, if >500 ng/mL, then CT-PA if not, observe

- V/Q Scan-based diagnosis
  - If PE likely, then obtain V/Q scan and interpret scan in conjunction with clinical probability
  - If PE unlikely, then obtain D-dimer and proceed with V/Q if >500 ng/mL

Treatment
- Mainstay of treatment is anticoagulation with the same agents as for DVT
- Hemodynamically unstable PE patients must be resuscitated and then evaluated for right heart failure and overload
  - If present and no contraindications, thrombolysis should be attempted
  - If fails, can have repeated systemic thrombolysis, catheter-directed thrombolysis, or embolectomy
  - When thrombolysis is contraindicated should progress directly to embolectomy, either catheter-directed or surgical

Heparin-Induced Thrombocytopenia (HIT)
Pathophysiology
- Life-threatening complication of exposure to heparin
- Autoantibody directed against endogenous platelet factor 4 in complex with heparin
- Activates platelets and can lead to arterial and venous thrombosis

Variants
Type I HIT
- Mild, transient drop in platelet count, platelet count typically returns to normal with continued heparin administration
- May be due to direct effect of heparin on platelets
- Not considered clinically significant
- Frequency 10–20%
- Occurs between days 1–4
- Nadir platelet count 100,000

Type II HIT
- Clinically significant variant, due to antibodies to PF4
- Frequency 1–3%
- Occurs generally 5–10 days after exposure to heparin
- Nadir platelet count usually >20,000 with median 60,000

Subclinical HIT
- Patient who has recovered from HIT and still had antibodies
- High risk if they are re-exposed to heparin

Spontaneous HIT
- Rarely, has been described to occur in patients without exposure to heparin

Heparin-Induced Antibodies
- Patient makes antibodies that cross-react on the lab assays for HIT but do not cause thrombocytopenia or thrombosis

Diagnosis
- Clinical suspicion: new onset thrombocytopenia, drop in platelet count ≥50% from prior value, venous or arterial thrombosis, necrotic skin at SQH injection sites, systemic symptoms after heparin IV bolus
- Calculate "Four T" score to estimate the pretest probability *(Circulation. 2004;110:e454-e458)*
  - Thrombocytopenia: **2 points**—>50% fall to nadir ≥20; **1 point**—30–50% platelet fall or nadir 10–19, or >50% fall secondary to surgery; **0 points**—<30% platelet fall or nadir <10
  - Timing of onset: **2 points**—days 5–10 or ≤1 day with recent heparin (within 30 days); **1 point**—>day 10 or timing unclear or <1 day with recent heparin (within 31–100 days); **0 points**—<4 days with no recent heparin
  - Thrombosis or other sequelae: **2 points**—proven new thrombosis, skin necrosis or systemic reaction after heparin; **1 point**—progressive or recurrent thrombosis, erythematous skin lesions, suspected but not proven thrombosis; **0 points**—none
  - Other causes for platelet fall: **2 points**—none evident; **1 point**—possible; **0 points**—definite
  - Pretest probability score: 6–8 high, 4–5 intermediate, 0–3 low (NPV of 98.1%)
- If result is intermediate or high pretest probability: obtain immunoassay/ELISA
  - If optical density is >2.00, no further testing and treat for HIT
  - If optical density is <0.40, no further testing in majority of patients because <1% chance of HIT

- Functional assay if intermediate or high pretest probability and ELISA optical density between 0.40 and 2.00 or if the pretest probability and ELISA are discordant

Treatment
- Stop all heparin-related products (heparin, heparin IV locks, and removal of heparin-coated catheters)
- Switch to nonheparin-based anticoagulation (Argatroban, Fondaparinux, Bivalirudin, Lepirudin), then transition to warfarin when stable on alternative anticoagulation and platelet count recovers to >150,000

Disseminated Intravascular Coagulation (DIC)
Etiology
- Widespread fibrin thrombi in the circulation from the consumption of platelets and coagulation factors
- Common causes: sepsis, trauma, and shock

Clinical Presentation
- Diffuse bleeding
- Circulatory insufficiency of vital organs
- Less often, arterial and venous thrombosis

Diagnosis
- Elevated PT/PTT
- Decreased platelet count
- Increased fibrin degradation products
- Positive D-dimer
- Low fibrinogen levels

Treatment
- Correct underlying disorder
- General supportive care
- Patient with serious bleeding and platelet count <50,000 transfuse platelets
- Patient with serious bleeding and increased PT or aPTT or fibrinogen level <50 mg/dL should receive the appropriate coagulation factor replacement

Indications for Stress Ulcer Prophylaxis
Indications
- Should be administered to all critically ill patients who are at a high risk for gastrointestinal bleeding
- Definition of high risk is variable but general characteristics are:
  - Coagulopathy (platelet count <50,000, INR >1.5 or PTT >2 times control)
  - Mechanical ventilation >48 hours
  - History of GI ulceration or bleeding within the past year
  - Traumatic brain or spinal cord injury
  - Large surface area burn injury
  - Two or more of: sepsis, ICU stay >7 days, occult GI bleeding for 6 days or more or glucocorticoid therapy

Agent
- Efficacy of PPI, H_2 blockers or antacid seems to be similar
- In patients that are able to tolerate enteral nutrition, an oral PPI or H_2 blocker acceptable coverage
- In patients unable to tolerate enteral nutrition, IV H_2 blocker may be more cost effective
- Patients already taking a class of agent at home, continue treatment with that class of agent

TRAUMA

CHARLES COOK • CAROLINE PARK

3-1: ABCs AND OVERALL PROGNOSIS

Airway

Assessment
- If able to speak clearly, the patient has patent airway
- Signs of compromise: stridor, hoarseness, regurgitation, difficulty with ventilation/oxygenation
- Examine oropharynx for bleeding, foreign bodies, trauma

Etiology of Compromise
- Direct mechanical injury from the trauma
- Depressed sensorium
- Aspiration
- Excessive hemorrhage from nearby structures limiting air passage

Intervention
- Oropharyngeal suctioning
- Chin lift/jaw thrust maneuver (keep cervical spine stabilization)
- Oropharyngeal/nasopharyngeal airways
- Endotracheal intubation
- Cricothyroidotomy—indications (see below)
  - Severe maxillofacial trauma precluding endotracheal intubation
  - Inability to perform successful endotracheal intubation
  - Laryngeal fracture
  - Avoid cricothyrotomy in pediatric population (<12 years)
- Awake tracheostomy

Surgical Technique—Cricothyroidotomy
• Palpate cricothyroid membrane directly inferior to the thyroid cartilage and superior to the cricoid cartilage
• Make a small vertical skin incision over the membrane
• Brief blunt dissection to the cricothyroid membrane
• Incise the membrane transversely and dilate

Breathing

Assessment
- Equal excursion of the chest bilaterally
- Bilateral, equal breath sounds
- Absence of abnormal tympany or dullness
- Adequate arterial oxygenation and ventilation of carbon dioxide: check pulse oximetry and end-tidal CO_2

Etiology of Compromise
- Central nervous system injury
- Pneumothorax
- Hemothorax
- Airway disruption

Intervention
- Bag–mask ventilation
- If suspect tension pneumothorax → needle decompression in the second intercostal space of the affected side
- Tube thoracostomy for pneumothorax or hemothorax

Complications
- Initiation of positive pressure ventilation may exacerbate pre-existing pneumothorax and lead to cardiac arrest

Circulation

Assessment
- Abnormal mental status (agitation, confusion, obtunded, etc.)
- Tachycardia
- Hypotension
- Skin color and turgor
- Capillary refill

Intervention

- Immediate placement of two large bore (16–18 gauge) antecubital IVs
- If peripheral venous access is unobtainable, insert central venous catheter with a large bore trauma catheter in the femoral vein. Consider ultrasound-guided IJ multiaccess catheter if patient has suspected pelvic trauma
- 2L crystalloid bolus
- Give blood if active bleeding, persistent hemodynamic instability, and no response to crystalloid bolus
- Identification and control of hemorrhage site

Disability and Exposure
Assessment

- Glasgow Coma Scale (GCS; see Section 3-2)
- Pupil size and reactivity
- Secondary survey
- Identification of penetrating wounds/external signs of potential injury

3-2: HEAD TRAUMA

Overview
Etiology

- Direct blunt force trauma
- Penetrating trauma
- Secondary to sudden acceleration/deceleration

Diagnosis

- Noncontrast computed tomography (CT)
- GCS: assess level of consciousness, score range 3–15

	1	2	3	4	5	6
Glasgow Coma Scale						
Eyes	Does not open eyes	Opens eyes in response to painful stimuli	Opens eyes in response to voice	Opens eyes spontaneously	N/A	N/A
Verbal	Makes no sounds	Incomprehensible sounds	Utters inappropriate words	Confused, disoriented	Oriented, converses normally	N/A
Motor	Makes no movements	Extension to painful stimuli	Abnormal flexion to painful stimuli	Flexion/ withdrawal to painful stimuli	Localizes painful stimuli	Obeys commands

GCS ≤8, severe; indication for intubation
GCS 9–12, moderate
GCS ≥13, mild

For all head injuries, a central therapeutic tenet is avoidance of hypoxemia and hypotension.

Common Types of Head Trauma
Epidural Hematoma

- Etiology: laceration of middle meningeal artery and dural sinus tear
- Clinical manifestation: lucid interval
- Imaging: lenticular biconcave mass on CT
- Surgery if
  - Neurologic deficit attributable to the mass
  - Midline shift of >5 mm
  - Elevated intracranial pressure (ICP) refractory to medical management
- Prognosis: 20–50% mortality

Subdural Hematoma

- Etiology: tear of bridging veins, laceration of parenchymal and cortical vessels, and linear acceleration
- Imaging
  - Crescent-shaped mass on CT
  - Acute: hyperdense
  - Subacute: isodense

- Surgery if
  - Neurologic deficit attributable to the mass
  - Midline shift of >5 mm
  - Hematoma >1 cm thick
  - Elevated ICP refractory to medical management
- Prognosis: 50–90% mortality

Hemorrhagic Contusion
- Etiology: parenchymal collision with the skull
- Imaging: focal edema on CT
- Treatment: avoid hypotension; at risk for delayed intraparenchymal hemorrhage

Diffuse Axonal Injury
- Etiology: shearing injury to white matter secondary to rotational forces
- Imaging
  - CT: unremarkable to punctuate areas of hemorrhage in deep cerebrum
  - MR: may provide more definitive diagnosis
- Treatment: avoid hypotension
- Prognosis: overall poor

Skull Fracture
- Classification: closed, linear, compound, and depressed
- Treatment: open wound, irrigate, debride devitalized tissue, and close dura
- If <1 cm in depth: manage nonoperatively if no underlying neurologic deficit attributable to the fracture
- **Surgery if angulation > thickness of the skull:** open reduction in the OR

Basilar Skull Fracture
- Clinical manifestations
  - Anterior: anosmia, cavernous fistula (CSF) rhinorrhea, and periorbital ecchymosis "raccoon-eyes"
  - Middle/temporal: hemotympanum, CSF tympanum, CN VII or VIII palsy, and mastoid ecchymosis (Battle's sign)
- Complications
  - Injury: optic nerve or carotid artery
  - Fistula: carotid–CSF
  - Arteriovenous fistula—patient "hears" each heartbeat

ICP Monitoring

Indications for ICP Use
• Patients in whom neurologic examination cannot be followed
• GCS score <8 with abnormal CT scan
• Two or more of:
• >40 yrs old
• Posturing
• Systolic blood pressure <90 mm Hg

Classification
- Parenchymal bolt: fiberoptic/strain gauge catheter measuring surface pressure of brain
- Intraventricular catheter (ventriculostomy)
  - Catheter within the lateral ventricle with tip at the foramen of Monro
  - Allows for drainage of CSF in addition to monitoring of ICP

Treatment of Elevated ICP (Normal Is 7–15 mm Hg)
- Overall goal to decrease cerebral edema
- Elevate head of bed
- Hyperventilate briefly in the acute setting ($PaCO_2$ ~35 mm Hg)
- Mannitol 0.25–1 g/kg every 6 hours to keep serum osm <300; can develop hypernatremia
- Hypertonic saline solution

Spine Fractures
- Most common mechanism (greatest to least): motor vehicle accidents, falls, violence (gun-shot wounds, stabbings, etc.)
- Major types characterized by injury mechanism
  - Vertebral body compression
  - Vertebral burst fractures (stable and unstable)
  - Fracture—dislocations
    - Chance fractures: pure bony injuries extending through spinal column

- Other: laminar, transverse process, spinous process
- Assessment:
  - Spine immobilization, inspect and palpate bony prominence for external trauma, pain, step-offs, weakness (if patient cooperative). Check rectal tone
- Imaging
- Standard three-view series (AP, lateral, open-mouth odontoid—requires cooperative patients have been largely abandoned in favor of CT spine
- Thoracolumbar series if warranted

Facial Trauma
Lacerations
- Irrigate wounds
- Remove all foreign bodies
- Sharply debride any nonviable tissue
- Repair with fine nonabsorbable suture
- Identify salivary, lacrimal duct injuries; these require operative repair over a stent
- Facial nerve injury lateral to the canthus will require operative repair

Fractures
- Imaging: CT with facial reconstruction, Panorex plain films for mandible
- Classification
  - Superior 1/3: supraorbital ridge, orbital roof, frontal sinus, and naso-orbitoethmoid
  - Middle 1/3: maxilla, zygoma, orbit, and nose
  - Lower 1/3: mandible
- Surgical management
  - Superior 1/3: ORIF with ductal repair if necessary (if the posterior table is intact)
  - Nose: closed reduction and splinting
    - Diagnose clinically with palpation
    - Check for septal hematomas—can lead to necrosis if undrained
- Maxilla: ORIF within 1–2 weeks
- LeFort classification
- Zygoma
  - Nondisplaced fractures: no treatment
  - Displaced fracture without comminution: reduction only
  - Displaced fractures with comminution or frontal suture separation: ORIF
- Orbit: ORIF
- Mandible: closed reduction, maxillomandibular fixation, or ORIF

TRAUMA 3-4

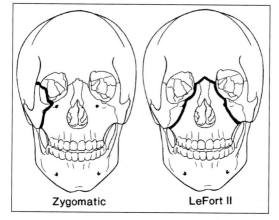

Figure 3-1 LeFort classification of facial fractures. (From Fischer JE, Bland KI. *Mastery of Surgery*, 5th ed. Philadelphia, PA: Lippincott Williams & Wilkins, 2007.)

Zygomatic   LeFort II

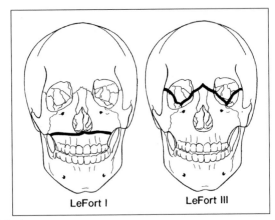

LeFort I

LeFort III

LeFort I: transverse
LeFort II: pyramidal
LeFort III: craniofacial dysjunction

3-3: NECK TRAUMA

Penetrating Trauma

Zone I (Arch Surg. 1995;130(9):971–975)
- Definition: suprasternal notch to cricoid cartilage
- Imaging: CXR, CTA, +/– angiography, laryngoscopy, bronchoscopy, and esophagoscopy
- Surgical management: based on injury
  - Sternotomy: all vascular injuries to the right of the left midclavicular line
  - Left lateral thoracotomy: injuries to the left of the left midclavicular line

Zone II
- Definition: cricoid cartilage to the angle of mandible
- Diagnosis
  - Operative exploration for platysma penetration (conventional)
  - CTA +/– Angiography + laryngoscopy + bronchoscopy + esophagoscopy (select cases)
- Surgical management: based on injury
  - Prep earlobe to umbilicus and upper thigh (saphenous vein harvest)
  - Incision on anterior border of sternocleidomastoid muscle
  - First priority is proximal and distal control of any bleeding vessel
- Esophageal injury (see Chapter 4)
  - <24 hours: washout, repair in two layers, chest tube drainage if thoracic
  - >24 hours: washout, chest tube drainage, may need diverting esophagostomy
- Tracheal injury
  - Primary repair; tracheostomy if severe. Watch for recurrent laryngeal nerve
- Jugular vein injury
  - Repair if possible, can ligate unilaterally
  - Watch for air embolism
- Carotid artery injury
  - Evaluate for hard signs (see below). Repair even if comatose
  - End to end for small defects, saphenous vein graft (SVG) interposition for defects >2 cm
  - Shunt if unstable, ligation if not possible
  - May need to divide omohyoid or digastric muscles for high injuries
  - Postoperative: frequent neurovascular checks, consider systemic anticoagulation

Zone III
- Definition: angle of the mandible to the base of the skull
- Imaging
  Four-vessel angiography if direct evidence of vascular trauma
  Noninvasive imaging in asymptomatic patient

- Surgical management
  - Most difficult open operative exposure (may require mandible dislocation)
  - Consider endovascular techniques

Hard Signs of Injury Mandating Operative Exploration
Penetration in Zone II (controversial)
Subcutaneous or retropharyngeal emphysema
Hoarseness or stridor
Active bleeding
Absent carotid pulse
Bruit or thrill
Neurologic deficit

Blunt Trauma
Laryngeal
- Imaging: CT
- Treatment
  - First secure the airway
  - Minor injury: head of bed elevation and corticosteroids
  - Major injury: operative exploration and repair

Vascular
- Anatomy: common carotid, internal carotid, or vertebral arteries
- Etiology: extreme hyperextension, flexion, or rotation of the neck, direct blunt force
- injury, cervical spine fractures
- Risk factors
  - GCS <6
  - Petrous bone fracture
  - LeFort II or III
  - Diffuse axonal injury
- Imaging: four-vessel arteriography
- Treatment
  - Operative repair if the vessel is accessible
  - Anticoagulation (if not accessible)
- Prognosis: worse than in penetrating injuries

3-4: CHEST TRAUMA

Overview
Blunt Trauma
- Blast: pressure wave causes tissue disruption, tears blood vessels, disrupts alveolar tissue and tracheobronchial tree; can cause traumatic diaphragmatic rupture
- Compression: torso compressed between an object and a hard surface, direct injury of chest wall and internal structures
- Deceleration: body in motion strikes a fixed object
  - Blunt trauma to chest wall
  - Shearing injury to internal structures as they continue in motion (ligamentum arteriosum, 93% of lesions)
- Age factors
  - Extremes of age have a higher mortality and need aggressive monitoring
  - Pediatric thorax: more cartilage, absorbs forces; less fractures, and increased lung contusion
  - Geriatric thorax: calcification and osteoporosis, more fractures; hypoventilation, mortality increased for pneumonia

Penetrating Trauma
- Low energy
  - Etiology: arrows, knives, and handguns
  - Injury: caused by direct contact and cavitation
- High energy
  - Etiology: military, hunting rifles, and high-powered hand guns
  - Injury: extensive due to high-pressure cavitation
  - Can also occur in combination with blast injury (IED, bombs)

ED Thoracotomy
- Indications
  - Loss of vital signs in the trauma bay
  - Loss of vital signs in the field but regained in the trauma bay
- Best results when used for penetrating chest trauma

Figure 3-2 Location for ED thoracotomy. (From Fischer JE, Bland KI. *Mastery of Surgery*, 5th ed. Philadelphia, PA: Lippincott Williams & Wilkins, 2007.)

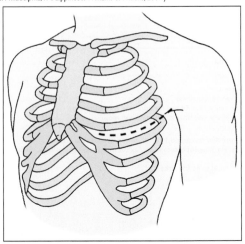

- Left anterolateral incision through fourth or fifth intercostal space
- Cardiac injury: open pericardium longitudinally anterior to phrenic nerve
- Abdominal injury: clamp descending aorta inferior to left pulmonary hilum
- Air embolism: Trendelenburg, clamp pulmonary hilum, aspirate air from left ventricle, and open cardiac massage

---

CXR Findings
- Widened mediastinum (>8 cm)
- Look for associated:
  - Left apical cap
  - Right paratracheal widening
  - Depression of left main bronchus
  - Absence of aortic arch definition/obliteration of aortic knob
  - Obliterated aortopulmonary window
  - Tracheal or esophageal deviation
- Causes: major deceleration
- Associated injuries
  - Scapular fracture, first and second rib fracture
  - Traumatic rupture aorta (usually at takeoff of left subclavian artery) or
  - Traumatic rupture of root of innominate artery near its takeoff
  - Rib and sternal fractures
  - Hemothorax

Surgical Management
- Place a chest tube in the case of
  - Absence of breath sounds
  - Penetrating injury
- Indications for OR thoracotomy
  - 1,500 cc output initially
  - 200 cc/h chest tube output for 4 consecutive hours

- Large air leak with hypoxemia
- Esophageal injury
- Left subclavian or descending aorta injury
- Indications for OR median sternotomy
  - Left supraclavicular stab wound
  - Suspect great vessel, right innominate, or subclavian injury
  - Distal tracheal injury
  - Cardiac injury

Chest Wall Injuries

Contusion

- Etiology: most commonly results from blunt injury
- Physical examination: erythema, ecchymosis, dyspnea, limited breath sounds, hypoventilation, crepitus, and paradoxical chest wall motion

Rib Fractures

- Etiology: compressional forces flex and fracture ribs at weakest points
- Ribs 1–3: require great force to fracture, possible underlying lung injury
- Ribs 4–9: most commonly fractured
- Ribs 9–12: less likely to be fractured; suspect liver and spleen injury

Sternal Fracture and Dislocation

- Etiology: direct blow (i.e., steering wheel)
- Associated with severe blunt anterior trauma: incidence, 5–8%
- Mortality: 25–45% from associated injuries
  - Myocardial contusion, pericardial tamponade, cardiac rupture, and pulmonary contusion

Flail Chest

- Definition: three or more adjacent ribs fractured in two or more places causing paradoxical chest wall motion
- Pathophysiology
  - Segment of chest is free to move with the pressure changes of ventilation
  - Reduction in volume of ventilation
- Treatment
  - Look for underlying pulmonary injury
  - Positive pressure ventilation (underlying pulmonary contusion and abnormal ABG)
  - Aggressive pulmonary toilet
  - Pain control; consider epidural catheter

Lung Injuries

Closed Pneumothorax

- Etiology: lung tissue disrupted and air leaks into the pleural space
- Pathophysiology
  - Air accumulates in pleural space, lung collapses, atelectasis
  - Reduced oxygen and carbon dioxide exchange
- Ventilation/perfusion mismatch
  - Increased ventilation but no alveolar perfusion
  - Reduced respiratory efficiency results in hypoxia

Open Pneumothorax

- Etiology: more common with penetrating trauma
- Pathophysiology
  - Free passage of air between atmosphere and pleural space
  - Air replaces lung tissue
  - Air will be drawn through wound if ≥2/3 diameter of the trachea
- Clinical manifestations: mediastinal shift to uninjured side, sucking chest wound, frothy blood at wound site, severe dyspnea, and hypovolemia

Tension Pneumothorax

- Etiology: progression of simple or open pneumothorax
- Pathophysiology
  - Buildup of air under pressure in the thorax
  - Excessive pressure reduces effectiveness of respiration
  - Air is unable to escape from inside the pleural space
  - Hemodynamic compromise and collapse ensues from poor diastolic filling

Massive Hemothorax

- Accumulation of blood in the pleural space
  - Initial drainage
  - >1,500 mL of blood or
  - >200 cc/h for 4 hours

- Etiology
  - Mediastinal vascular injury
  - Hemoperitoneum with ruptured diaphragm
- Each side of thorax may hold up to 3,000 mL
- Surgical management: thoracotomy
- Complications
  - Blood loss in thorax causes a decrease in tidal volume
  - Ventilation/perfusion mismatch and shock
- Prognosis: mortality rate as high as 75%

Pulmonary Contusion: Parenchymal Contusion of the Lung
- Epidemiology: up to 75% of patients with significant blunt trauma; associated rib fracture
- Etiology
  - Deceleration with chest impact on steering wheel
  - Bullet cavitation from high-velocity ammunition
  - Clinical manifestations: progressive deterioration of ventilatory status and hemoptysis

Cardiovascular Injuries
Blunt Myocardial Injury
- Epidemiology
  - Occurs in 75% of patients with severe blunt chest trauma. Often have concurrent sternal fractures
  - Right atrium and ventricle most commonly injured (43%)
- Pathophysiology
  - Reduces strength of cardiac contractions
  - Reduces cardiac output
  - Electrical disturbances due to irritability of damaged myocardial cells
- Treatment: admit for observation, continuous telemetry. Echocardiogram if patient has dysrhythmias. Cardiac enzymes are neither diagnostic nor prognostic
- Complications: hematoma, hemoperitoneum, myocardial necrosis, dysrhythmias, CHF and/or cardiogenic shock, valvular rupture (9%): aortic > mitral > tricuspid, late ventricular aneurysm

Pericardial Tamponade
- Definition: restriction of cardiac filling from blood or fluid within pericardium
- Etiology
  - Occurs in <2% of all serious chest trauma
  - Laceration of the coronary artery
  - Penetration of myocardium
  - Blunt rupture of myocardium
- Pathophysiology
  - Blood in pericardium—fixed space
  - 200–300 mL of blood can restrict effectiveness of cardiac contractions
- Clinical manifestations
  Beck triad: hypotension, elevated JVP, distant heart sounds (positive only in 40% of patients)
- Diagnostic Imaging: FAST exam, subxyhpoid or parasternal view
- Treatment
  - Pericardiocentesis (conventional) with removal of as little as 20 mL can provide relief
  - May require ED or OR thoracotomy with digital control of disruption

Aortic Injuries
- Classification: traumatic aneurysm or aortic rupture
- Etiology: most common injury is penetrating, but aorta can also be injured with severe blunt trauma. For blunt injuries often confined to areas of aorta attachment
- Prognosis—most blunt injuries die immediately from exsanguination
  - For those surviving the initial injury for 1 hour that remain untreated
  - Mortality rates:
    - 85–95% overall
    - 30% mortality in 6 hours
    - 50% mortality in 24 hours
    - 70% mortality in 1 week
- Clinical manifestations
  - Rapid deterioration of vitals
  - Pulse deficit between right and left upper or lower extremities

Other Vascular Injuries
- Rupture or laceration: superior vena cava, inferior vena cava, and thoracic vasculature
- Complications
  - Blood collects in mediastinum
  - Compression of great vessels, myocardium, and esophagus
- Clinical manifestations
  - Hypovolemia and shock
  - Hemothorax or hemomediastinum

Tracheal and Esophageal Injury
Esophageal Injury
- Pathophysiology: contents in esophagus/stomach contaminate mediastinum
- Physical examination: subcutaneous emphysema
- Complications: mediastinitis, pneumomediastinum, chemical irritation
- Prognosis: 30% mortality

Tracheobronchial Injury
- Etiology: disruption can occur anywhere in tracheobronchial tree
- Clinical manifestations: dyspnea, cyanosis, hemoptysis, and massive subcutaneous emphysema, large air leak in chest tube
- Prognosis: 50% of patients die within 1 h of injury

3-5: ABDOMINAL TRAUMA

Overview
Etiology
- Penetrating: nipples to groin creases
- Blunt: direct contusion, severe deceleration, or falls

Unstable Patients in Shock
• 1st: ABC's (with rapid sequence intubation, assessment of ventilation, proper IV access, and inspection of the back)
• If chest trauma and hypotension: Bilateral needle decompression Followed with bilateral chest tubes If clinical signs and FAST confirmation of tamponade: pericardiocentesis
• **OR for laparotomy** **Patients arriving with no palpable pulses but witnessed recent or current signs of life** **Penetrating trauma** **Positive DPL (50 cc of blood)** **Positive FAST**

Stable Patients
- Perform complete primary and secondary survey in trauma bay
- FAST
- CT scan (IV contrast)
  - Very sensitive for solid organ injury
  - Decreased sensitivity for hollow viscous injury
  - Intra-abdominal fluid without solid organ injury: suspect bowel injury
- Follow with serial physical examinations
- Laparotomy is indicated for:
  - Exposed bowel in an open wound
  - Peritoneal signs
  - Significant blood on rectal exam or in NGT

Diagnostic Modalities
Focused Abdominal Sonography for Trauma (FAST)
- Sensitivity, 83.3%; specificity, 99.7% (Surgery. 1998;228(4):557–567)
- Highest in precordial or transthoracic wounds and hypotensive patients with blunt abdominal trauma
- Technique: four quadrants
  - Precordial
  - Right upper quadrant (Morrison's pouch or hepato-renal)
  - Left upper quadrant
  - Pelvis (pouch of Douglas, or spleno-renal)

- Advantages: can detect as little as 200 cc of fluid; easy to learn, cost-effective, noninvasive, and quick
- Limitations: poor ability to depict parenchymal injuries, operator dependent, not reliable for hollow visceral injury, and difficult in obese patients. Does not evaluate injuries to retroperitoneum

Diagnostic Peritoneal Lavage (DPL)

Surgical Technique—Diagnostic Peritoneal Lavage
• Make a small midline incision below the umbilicus
• If pelvic trauma is suspected or confirmed, incise above umbilicus
• Access peritoneum via a Seldinger or open technique; advance catheter toward pelvis
• Aspirate with a 20-cc syringe
• If <10 cc obtained, introduce 1,000 cc of normal saline into peritoneum (the fluid is drained by gravity after gentle movements of the abdomen)

- "Positive" test (for blunt trauma)
  - If more than 10 cc are initially obtained
  - Introduced fluid is observed via the Foley or chest tubes
  - If the patient is unstable, blood or dark red fluid is obtained
  - Pink or clear fluid analysis:
    - RBC more than 100,000/mm^3
    - WBC more than 500/mm^3
    - Bile
    - Bacteria
    - Feces/intestinal content
- Limitations
  - Oversensitive for solid organs
  - Not sensitive in retroperitoneal injury unless the peritoneum is open
  - Pelvic fractures can produce false positives
  - It does not detect central parenchymal solid organ injuries

Chest Radiography
- CXR: all trauma patients
- Pneumoperitoneum mandates laparotomy in patients with blunt trauma

CT
- Advantages
  - Noninvasive
  - Assess abdominal and pelvic cavities, retroperitoneum, soft tissues, and bones
  - Very high sensitivity (92–97.6%) and specificity (98.7%) in blunt trauma
  - NPV >99%, so a negative CT can rule out an immediate laparotomy
- Usage
  - Evaluation of the abdomen for hemodynamically stable patients
  - Unreliable exam (GCS <10, spine trauma, drug or alcohol abuse, multiple extra-abdominal injuries)
  - Nonoperative management of solid viscera
  - FAST positive for fluid in stable patients
  - Macroscopic hematuria
- Signs of bowel or mesenteric injuries
  - Pneumoperitoneum
  - Leak of the contrast into the peritoneal cavity
  - Thickening of bowel wall
  - Thickening of the mesentery
  - Free fluid without solid visceral injury

3-6: OPERATIVE STRATEGIES FOR ABDOMINAL TRAUMA

Nonoperative Management
- Blunt trauma and a stable patient are prerequisites
- Clinical scenarios
  - Isolated grade I–III liver injuries
  - Isolated grade I–III splenic injuries
  - Most kidney injuries
  - Select grade IV–V liver and spleen injuries
- Management: serial HCTs and possible angiography

Abdomen Filled With Blood

- **Pack all four quadrants**
- Place a surgical clamp on subdiaphragmatic aorta by entering the lesser sac if the diaphragmatic hiatus is free of hematoma
- Systemically search all four quadrants in turn for source of bleeding
- Can move the aortic clamp infrarenal if bleeding limited to inframesocolic or iliac vessels

Vascular Injuries
- Supramesocolic aorta and major branches
  - Maintain aortic clamp at hiatus
  - Mattox maneuver: left medial visceral rotation
    - Free descending colon, spleen, tail of pancreas, and retract medially
- Celiac and IMA: can ligate in an emergency, consider shunt for celiac
- SMA: in general cannot ligate—shunt for damage control
  - Hematoma at base of transverse mesocolon
- Inframesocolic aorta/iliac or IVC and iliac veins
  - Free ascending colon and hepatic flexure, retract medially along with small bowel
  - Mandatory exploration of all midline inframesocolic hematomas
- Suprarenal IVC: cannot ligate
- Infrarenal IVC: best tolerated ligated major vessel
- Retrohepatic vena cava: pack
  - Do not explore stable nonexpanding hematoma in this area

Liver Trauma
- Classification: CT based

Liver Injury Grades

- Grade 1: capsular tear <1 cm deep
- Grade 2: capsular tear 1–3 cm deep
- Grade 3: capsular tear >3 cm deep
- Grade 4: parenchymal disruption 25–75% or
- Grade 5: >75% parenchymal disruption or
- Grade 6: hepatic avulsion

- Surgical technique
  - Pack all four quadrants
  - Mobilize the liver by dividing the falciform, triangular, and coronary ligaments and place more packs anterior and posterior
  - Pringle maneuver to stop hepatic artery, portal vein massive hemorrhage
  - Repair hepatic artery if possible but ligate if necessary
  - If persistent venous ooze from outflow bleeding (hepatic veins, IVC), clamp the IVC above and below the liver
- Surgical management of specific injuries
  - Simple laceration: pressure, topical agents, and argon beam
  - Deep laceration: ligate individual vessels and pack laceration with omentum
  - Biliary duct laceration: repair over stent (T-tube) or choledocho/hepaticojejunostomy
  - Extensive injuries: damage control with packing, drains, and temporary closure
  - Repair end to end if possible

Splenic Trauma (J Am Coll Surg. 2005;201:179–187)
- #1 predictor of successful nonoperative management is hemodynamic stability
- Increased use of interventional/angiographic embolization with decreased morbidity
- Operative management
  - Indications
    - Penetrating injuries
    - Grade V lacerations (avulsion of pedicle)
    - Failed nonoperative management
  - Splenorrhaphy possible but uncommon: fibrin glue, mattress pledgeted sutures, and dexon/vicryl mesh wrap
- Do not forget vaccines: Pneumovax, HIB, Meningococcal

Duodenal Trauma

- Surgical technique
  - Wide Kocher maneuver extended to ligament of Treitz
  - Always carefully inspect the pancreas
- Surgical management of specific injuries
  - Simple laceration: debride, approximate, close in two layers, omental patch, and drain
  - Larger injuries to first, third, and fourth part: resection with primary anastomosis
  - Larger injury to second portion: Roux-en-Y duodenojejunostomy
  - Multiple injuries: duodenal diversion via pyloric exclusion, diverting gastrojejunostomy, tube duodenostomy and external drainage
- Always leave drains and NGT postoperatively
- Consider J-tube for enteral feeds
- Duodenal hematoma
  If found on CT, can observe in a stable patient with a negative swallow study
  If found intraoperatively, should explore to rule out duodenal wall laceration or leak
  If not resolved after 2 weeks, OR for exploration

Colon and Rectal Trauma

- Primary repair: localized, stable patient, not on mesenteric border, and no other severe associated injuries
- Diverting sigmoid colostomy: all open pelvic fractures, peritonitis, and shock
- Consider colonic diversion when concomitant urologic or pancreatic injuries
- Presacral drainage of rectal injury: high-energy blunt trauma or pelvic fracture
  - 3-cm curvilinear incision between coccyx and rectum with posterior dissection up to level of injury

Retroperitoneal Hematoma

- Explore all penetrating trauma except for stable subhepatic hematoma
- Can observe blunt trauma in a stable patient if not expanding

Pelvic Fractures

- Classified by force vectors
  - Anterior–posterior, lateral compression, vertical shear, and combined vector injury
- Important ED steps
  - FAST/diagnostic peritoneal lavage (above umbilicus)
  - Inspect the meatus before placing a Foley catheter
  - Blood at meatus: urethrogram, then Foley and cystogram if negative
  - Urethrogram positive: suprapubic catheter
  - Rectal examination
  - Consider stabilization of unstable pelvic fractures (controversial)
- Surgical management
  - Proctosigmoidoscopy in operating room
  - Diverting sigmoid colostomy in the case of rectal injury or open fracture
  - If active bleeding, clamp distal aorta and try to identify and stop bleeders, pack
  - Nonruptured or nonexpanding hematoma is observed
    - Angiography and embolization
    - Internal or external fixation
    - If explored, ligate internal iliac arteries, pack, and angiography
    - Imaging: contrast CT to evaluate vascular pedicle, collecting system, and parenchyma

---

3-7: GENITOURINARY TRAUMA

Renal Trauma

Renal Injury Classification
• Grade I: contusion or nonexpanding perinephric hematoma
• Grade II: nonexpanding subcapsular hematoma or <1 cm parenchymal laceration without urinary extravasation
• Grade III: >1 cm parenchymal laceration without collecting system involvement
• Grade IV: parenchymal laceration with collecting system involvement
• Grade V: shattered parenchyma or major vascular injury

Treatment

- Minor and Grade I–III blunt renal injuries
  - Nonoperative
  - Foley catheterization and hydration

- Grade IV injuries: dependent upon contralateral renal function
- Grade V injuries, expanding hematomas, and incompletely staged injuries
  - Operative exploration
  - Renorrhaphy or partial nephrectomy are options but unusual for trauma

Ureter
Etiology
- Penetrating trauma
- 15% of pelvic fractures have associated ureteral injury
  - Imaging: contrast CT to look for urinary extravasation, ureteral deviation, or proximal ureteral dilation

Treatment
- Lower third: surgical
  - Bladder re-implantation +/− psoas hitch
- Middle third injuries: surgical
  - Ureteroureterostomy: bring proximal ureter through retroperitoneum to contralateral ureter and sew end to side over a stent with absorbable interrupted sutures; drain
- Proximal third: nephrostomy tube in ipsilateral kidney
- Always drain repair site
- For damage control acceptable to drain only

Bladder
Etiology and Classification
- Blunt or penetrating trauma
- 7% of pelvic fractures have associated bladder injury
- Intraperitoneal vs. extraperitoneal
  Imaging: CT scan or cystography

Treatment
- Extraperitoneal: nonoperative with Foley catheter for 10–14 days, follow-up cystography
- Intraperitoneal injury: operative exploration, primary repair

Urethra
Etiology
- Secondary to pelvic fractures in blunt direct penetrating trauma

Physical Examination
- Blood at urethral meatus, "boggy or high-riding prostate" in males
- Scrotum is edematous
- Ecchymosis

Treatment
- Do not place Foley catheter until retrograde urethrography (RUG) is performed
- Partial urethral disruption: Foley catheter for 14–21 days may be attempted
- Complete disruptions: primary endoscopic realignment or bladder diversion with delayed repair

---

3-8: THERMAL INJURY/TRAUMA

Flame/Scald
Classification
- Based on depth
  - First degree: "superficial" limited to epidermis; skin is dry, erythematous, and tender
  - Second degree: "partial thickness" partial dermal involvement; skin is blistered and tender
  - Third degree: "full thickness" full dermal involvement; skin is dry, leathery, and insensate
  - Fourth degree: involvement of underlying fascia, muscle, or bone
- Based on size (percentage of body surface area [% BSA])

Figure 3-3 Extent of Burn Damage: Rule of 9's. (From Fischer JE, Bland KI. *Mastery of Surgery*, 5th ed. Philadelphia, PA: Lippincott Williams & Wilkins, 2007.)

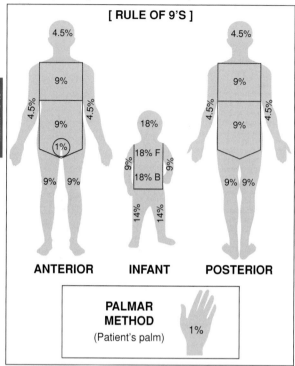

[RULE OF 9'S]

ANTERIOR

4.5%
9%
9%
1%
4.5% 4.5%
9% 9%

INFANT

18%
18% F
18% B
9% 9%
14% 14%

POSTERIOR

4.5%
9%
9%
4.5% 4.5%
9% 9%

PALMAR METHOD
(Patient's palm)   1%

Treatment
- ABCs followed by full body exposure
- Fluid resuscitation: based on the Parkland formula for burns second-degree and higher
  - Lactated Ringers solution, 4 cc/kg x %BSA involved
  - 50% of the volume over the first 8 hours from the time of injury
  - Remaining 50% of calculated volume over the following 16 hours
  - Give maintenance fluid volume in addition to resuscitation volume
  - Volume may need to be adjusted based on urine output
- Apply cool NS pads to burned areas
- Give Tetanus shot
- Topical antimicrobials (second and third degree)
  - Silvadene: not on face, may cause reversible leukopenia, and ineffective against *Pseudomonas* and *Enterobacter*
- Sulfamylon: can be used on face, painful, good eschar penetration, but worsens acidosis
- Nutrition
- Antibiotics: only for proven infections

Surgical Interventions
- Early grafting decreases inflammatory response
- Escharotomy: to prevent compartment syndrome and impedance of venous return
  - Incision: biaxial for extremities, uniaxial for fingers, bilateral midaxial and midclavicular for chest

- Excision and grafting: some partial thickness and all full thickness burns as early as possible
  - Surgery magnitude as patient will tolerate with goal of early excision and coverage to minimize risk of burn wound sepsis
  - Cover with autograft, allograft, or Biobrane (infected)

Chemical
Etiology
- Acid burns: induces coagulative necrosis
- Alkali burns: induces liquefactive necrosis

Treatment
- Remove chemical agent
- Brushing or suction for dry agents or copious irrigation with NS
  - 1 hour for acid burns; three hours for alkaline burns
- Avoid neutralization
- Keep room temperature around 85–90°F

Electrical
Etiology
- Alternating current: household items and power lines
- Direct current: lightning and batteries

Clinical Manifestations
- Tissue injury from thermal necrosis and thrombosis
- Spinal cord injury and fractures secondary to severe muscle contraction
- Rhabdomyolysis may result in acute renal failure, hyperkalemic acidosis

Treatment
- Local wound care for entry and exit points of current (often are minor)
- Cardiac monitoring for the development of dysrhythmia
- Prompt debridement/amputation to dead injured limbs
- Neurovascular monitoring for the development of compartment syndrome
- Fluids: generous fluid to keep urine output >100 cc/h
- Renal
  - Check serum CK and urine frequently for myoglobin/hemoglobin for signs of muscle damage
  - Bicarb, keep urine pH around 7
  - Mannitol 1–2 g/kg (controversial)

Complications
- Initial mortality: cardiac arrest secondary to current through the brain or heart

Inhalational
Etiology and Pathophysiology
- Thermal injury is generally limited to the upper airway, suspect in any facial burn
- Distal airway injury secondary to inflammation from noxious chemical stimuli
- Mechanism: high-pressure steam and confinement

Physical Examination
- Singed facial hair
- Wheezing or hoarseness

Diagnostic Studies
- Bronchoscopy for severity (controversial)

Treatment
- Airway
  - 100% humidified oxygen (displaces carbon monoxide) and racemic epinephrine–hyperbaric treatment is no more efficacious than oxygen for carbon monoxide toxicity
  - Lower airway injuries: bronchoscopy and carboxyhemoglobin level (>10% sig)
- Aggressive pulmonary toilet
- Monitor for pulmonary edema
- Criteria for transfer to burn unit: 15% total body surface area burn, hands, and pediatrics

3-9: ENVIRONMENTAL INJURIES AND BITES

Hypothermia

Definition
- Mild: core temperature 32°–35°C
- Moderate: 27°–32°C
- Severe: <27°C

Clinical Manifestation
- Altered mental status
- Cardiac dysrhythmia (ultimately ventricular fibrillation)
- Coagulopathy
- Apnea

Treatment
- Initial rewarming: remove wet clothing, limit exposure, direct warm air convection, mechanical ventilation with warmed gas, warm IV fluid
- Secondary methods in severe cases: peritoneal or thoracic-pleural lavage with warm crystalloid, hemodialysis, or cardiopulmonary bypass
- Serial monitoring of acid-base status

Frostbite

Definition
- First degree: hyperemia, edema, and absence of necrosis
- Second degree: hyperemia, edema, partial thickness skin necrosis, and superficial vesicular formation
- Third degree: full thickness skin necrosis and hemorrhagic bullae formation
- Fourth degree: gangrenous involvement of skin, muscle, and bone

Treatment
- Extremity elevation
- Conductive re-warming with 40°C water (painful)
- Dry dressings
- Early surgical debridement or amputation should be avoided. Degree of injury may not manifest for up to 4 weeks and viable tissue may be unnecessarily removed

Bites

Initial Management
- Irrigation and debridement of devitalized tissues

Human Bites
- Organisms: *Staphylococcus*, *Streptococcus*, anaerobes, *Eikenella corrodens*, and anaerobic gram-negative rods
- Antibiotics: ampicillin + B-lactamase inhibitor or Cefoxitin
- Wounds over joint spaces may require operative debridement and IV antibiotics

Mammalian Animal Bites
- Organisms
  Domestic canines: *Streptococci viridans*, *Pasteurella multocida*, *Bacteroides*, *Fusobacterium*, and *Capnocytophaga*
  Domestic felines: *Pasteurella multocida* and *Staphylococcus*
- Antibiotics: ampicillin + B-lactamase inhibitor
- Think about rabies

Snake Bites
- Classification
  - Nonvenomous snakes: U-shaped bite
  - Venomous snakes: two puncture wounds
- History and physical examination:
  - Identify the wound, timing of injury, and snake speciation
  - Evaluate local and systemic signs of toxicity
- Organisms: *Pseudomonas*, *Enterobacter*, *Staphylococcus*, and *Clostridium* species
- Treatment
  - Place extremity in a neutral position, immobilize, and cover with compressive dressing
  - Do not use suction tourniquets
  - Empiric antibiotics
  - Support with respiratory, circulatory, and IV fluid resuscitation
  - Administer polyvalent antivenin
  - Monitor for anaphylaxis and serum sickness
  - Monitor for compartment syndrome
- Complications: pulmonary edema, hypotension secondary to systemic vasodilation, acute renal failure, and coagulopathy (i.e., DIC)

TOVY HABER KAMINE • JONATHAN CRITCHLOW

This chapter is a revision and update of that included in the previous version of *Pocket Surgery* written by Andrew H. Stephen.

4-1: DYSPHAGIA

Physiology of Swallowing
- Definitions:
  - **Dysphagia**—difficulty swallowing
  - **Odynophagia**—pain upon swallowing
- Oral phase: the only voluntary phase of swallowing
- Pharyngeal phase: delivers food to the upper esophageal sphincter (UES) and esophagus key steps include cricopharyngeal relaxation, opening of UES
- Esophageal phase: peristaltic contractions of the esophagus to deliver food to the stomach
  - Lower esophageal sphincter (LES): concept and not a single entity
  - Length: 3–5 cm; tonically contracted
  - Resting pressure: 10–30 mm Hg

Esophageal Anatomy
- Esophageal body: 20–25 cm muscular conduit
- Arterial supply depends on segment, but there is a longitudinal network within the submucosa that connects all these branches
  - Cervical esophagus: inferior thyroid artery
  - Thoracic esophagus: aorta and bronchial arteries
  - Abdominal esophagus: left gastric and inferior phrenic arteries
- **Striated muscle: proximal 30–40%** with vagal excitatory stimulation
- **Smooth muscle: distal 60–70%** also with vagal innervations

Clinical Presentation (History)
- Dysphagia characteristics:
  - Solids, liquids, or both
  - Gradual but worsening or severity unchanged but intermittent
  - Regurgitation and burning
  - Frank emesis, blood, or streaks
- Weight loss, anorexia, and alcohol, tobacco, diet, environmental and occupational exposures

Imaging and Studies
- **Barium swallow:** requires radiation; locates and delineates lesions
  - If there is a high concern for perforation, always use water-soluble contrast unless at risk for aspiration
- **Upper endoscopy:** perform after contrast studies in case of perforation; can obtain biopsies, perform interventions, access for endoscopic ultrasound (EUS)
- **Manometry:** diagnose and characterize motility disorder—achalasia, diffuse esophageal spasm (DES), scleroderma, and nutcracker esophagus

Mechanical/Obstructive Etiologies	Functional/Motility Etiologies

• Symptoms: **initially with solid food,** progresses gradually to liquids
• Most frequent lesions:
  Malignancy: squamous cell carcinoma (SCC), adenocarcinoma
  Strictures: chronic reflux, esophagitis, caustic exposures
  Diverticula: Zenker, epiphrenic
  Esophageal webs: Plummer–Vinson syndrome (iron-deficiency anemia, epithelial atrophy)
  Schatzki rings: mucosal, near GE junction
  Infectious ulcers or inflammation: Candida, CMV, HSV, HIV
  Foreign bodies
	• Symptoms: **with solids or liquids,** intermittent or progressive
	• Most frequent disorders:
	  Achalasia: aperistalsis, failure of LES relaxation
	  DES: concurrent uncoordinated contractions, normal LES pressure
	  Scleroderma: LES with low resting pressure, decreased or absent peristaltic amplitude

4-2: GASTROESOPHAGEAL REFLUX DISEASE

Pathophysiology
- Imbalance between esophageal exposure to acid and compensatory mechanisms

LES Insufficiency
- **Normal resting pressure 12–30 mm Hg**
- Normally relaxes in response to peristalsis to accept incoming food/liquid bolus
- Reflux: transient relaxation of the LES

Hiatal Crura and Hiatal Hernia
- **Hiatal crura** are the other major antireflux barriers along with LES
- **Additional barriers**
  - **Length of intra-abdominal esophagus: ideally >2 cm**
  - **Phrenoesophageal membrane**
  - **Angle of His**
- Hiatal hernias (see below) magnify the degree of GERD symptoms

Evaluation
Clinical Presentation
- Symptoms: substernal burning in the chest, regurgitation, acid taste in mouth, dysphagia, hoarseness, cough, wheezing, and aspiration
  - Exacerbating factors: worse with food or certain types of food; worse when lying flat or at night; or stressful situations
  - Relieving factors: proton pump inhibitors (PPI), H_2 blockers; use of pillows, sitting up at night
  - Duration/progression of symptoms
- Signs: often few, may have loss of dental enamel

Imaging
- Barium swallow: delineates anatomy, presence of hiatal hernias, location of GE junction in relation to hiatus, and some assessment of peristaltic function
- Endoscopy: evaluate for the presence of esophageal erosions, strictures, hiatal hernias.
  - Barrett's esophagus: salmon-colored mucosa—must be biopsied as it is a premalignant lesion. See below for the treatment of Barrett's.
- **24-hour pH monitoring: confirms GERD** (sensitivity 80–90%)
  - Details number and duration of episodes of reflux
  - Correlates subjective symptoms with events
  - **Positive test: >6% of the time with a pH <4 (1.5 hours), Demeester score >14.7**
  - Note: H_2 blockers need to be held for at least 3 days prior and PPIs for at least 1 week prior to test due to irreversible parietal cell inhibition
- **Manometry:** assesses location, length, pressure of LES, ability of LES to relax with swallowing, and amplitude of peristalsis of esophageal body
  - With disordered peristalsis some will not perform a Nissen fundoplication, but will do a partial wrap instead.
  - Aperistalsis suggests achalasia or scleroderma—reconsider operation
  - Look for LES <6 mm Hg, LES length <2 cm, and intra-abdominal LES length <1 cm, though many with true reflux have normal values.
- Gastric emptying: assess with nuclear medicine scintigraphy; useful in GERD with significant nausea, emesis, or bloating, as may indicated gastroparesis.
- Impedance monitoring: if atypical symptoms; can detect normal pH or alkaline reflux which may be just as damaging to mucosa

Complication of GERD: Barrett's Esophagus
- Intestinal, columnar metaplasia of the distal esophagus
- Followed with serial endoscopies and biopsies; up to 10% of GERD patients
- 30–40× risk for adenocarcinoma of esophagus compared to general population when high-grade dysplasia is present within Barrett's
- Medical and surgical treatments of GERD **do not** cause significant Barrett's regression; they may prevent/slow the degree of progression of metaplasia
- Radiofrequency ablation (RFA) or cryotherapy can be used to treat Barrett's esophagus

Treatment
Medical Treatment
- Two goals: increase pH of reflux contents and decrease frequency of episodes
- **PPIs and histamine blockers:** lessen symptoms, especially heartburn but do not decrease the amount of nonacid reflux

- Lifestyle/dietary modification: **weight loss**; avoidance of chocolate, caffeine, tobacco/nicotine, especially before bedtime; elevate head of bed when supine with pillows/propping bed, and avoid food before bedtime

Operative Indications
- Symptoms: worsening, no longer alleviated by or need excessive medication doses
- Stricture and esophagitis
- Recurrent aspirations/pneumonias
- Hiatal hernia with anatomic symptoms

Surgical Results
- **Patient satisfaction rates: 85% at 5 years**
- Atypical/respiratory/extraesophageal symptoms less reliably respond to surgery
- Complications (Fig. 4-1)
  - **Dysphagia: 5–10%**
  - Wrap migration through hiatus
  - **Wrap migrations downwards onto stomach, "slipped Nissen"**
  - General anatomic failure: 5–10%

Figure 4-1 A: Disrupted wrap. **B:** Sliding hiatal hernia with wrap in abdomen. **C:** "Slipped" fundoplication onto proximal stomach. **D:** Intrathoracic migration of fundoplication. (From Fischer JE, Bland KI. *Mastery of Surgery.* 5th ed. Philadelphia, PA: Lippincott Williams & Wilkins; 2007.)

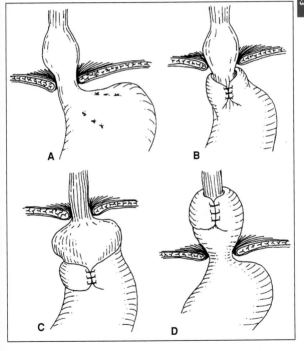

GERD—Operative Management

Nissen Fundoplication

Figure 4-2 Intraoperative anatomy of Nissan fundoplication. (From Fischer JE, Bland KI. *Mastery of Surgery.* 5th ed. Philadelphia, PA: Lippincott Williams & Wilkins; 2007.)

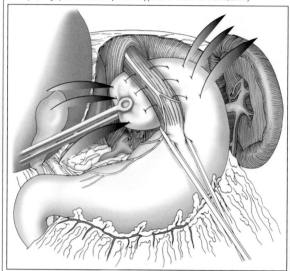

Laparoscopic: five to six ports, lithotomy or supine position
⇩
Divide gastrohepatic ligament
⇩
Dissect distal esophagus and GE junction
⇩
Identify anterior and posterior vagus nerves
⇩
Mobilize gastric fundus
⇩
Divide short gastric arteries down one-third of the greater curvature
⇩
Reapproximate diaphragmatic crura with sizing Bougie (48–60 Fr)
⇩
Wrap lateral border of fundus around esophagus posteriorly (around right vagus and esophagus)
⇩
Fundoplication done over sizing Bougie
⇩
If shortened esophagus, add Collis gastroplasty: create neoesophagus by stapling on stomach parallel to lesser curve

Toupet fundoplication: 270-degree posterior wrap; most common partial fundoplication performed. Used if there are motility issues, or during Heller myotomy for achalasia

Dor fundoplication: 180-degree anterior wrap. Used in the same circumstances as Toupet

Hill repair: upper lesser curvature plicated to right aspect of esophagus, esophagogastropexy to median arcuate ligament, and requires intraoperative manometry

Belsey mark IV: anterior 270-degree fundoplication performed via left thoracotomy or VATS and diaphragmatic crural buttress

Types
- Type I: "sliding" hernia
- Type II: paraesophageal hernia with the gastro-esophageal junction (GEJ) in the abdomen, but the fundus of the stomach in the chest
- Type III: paraesophageal hernia with both fundus of stomach and GEJ in the chest
- Type IV: paraesophageal hernia with another organ (usually colon) in the chest

Evaluation
Clinical Presentation
- ~20% of the population have type I hiatal hernias which are asymptomatic
- Most common symptoms are reflux symptoms, but may include more atypical symptoms:
  - Chest pain, nausea, dyspnea, and postprandial fullness
  - More severe: worsening chest pain, emesis, weight loss, and dysphagia

Complications
- Bleeding: most frequent complication of Type II and III hernias (>30%); chronic blood loss leads to iron-deficiency anemia
- Cameron ulcers: hiatal ring causing vascular congestion
- Obstruction: twisting of greater curvature in chest
- Volvulus/incarceration
  - Organoaxial: stomach twists around anatomic axis with paraesophageal hernia
  - Mesenteroaxial: line of volvulus is horizontal
  - Borchardt triad: severe epigastric pain, retching but inability to vomit, inability to place NG tube

Imaging
- **CXR: air–fluid level in chest and in abdomen**
- Barium swallow: confirms hernia and determines anatomy (Fig. 4-3)

Figure 4-3 A: Sliding hiatal hernia (Type I). **B:** (upper right): Mixed hiatal hernia (Type III). **C:** (lower left): Paraesophageal hiatal hernia (Type II). **D:** (lower right): Complex mixed hiatal hernia (Type IV). (Illustrations reprinted with permission from Atlas of Minimally Invasive Surgery (Jones et al. Cine-Med, 2006). Copyright of the book and illustrations are retained by Cine-Med.)

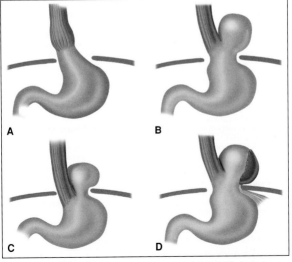

- Manometry: excludes motility disorders and determines degree of fundoplication
- Endoscopy: further defines anatomy; assess for Barrett, esophagitis, malignancy, ulcerations, and diverticula

Treatment

- Operative indications
  - **Emergency: volvulus or obstruction: (increased mortality, up to 5%)**
  - **Elective: most Type II and symptomatic Type III and Type IV hernias**
- **Addition of antireflux procedure**
  - If no motility disorder: most perform a Nissen fundoplication
    - If a severe motility disorder is present, may perform a partial wrap or a gastropexy
  - Hiatal dissection/reduction may harm antireflux mechanisms
- Acute incarceration
  - Attempt NG stomach decompression: decreases acute symptoms, allows for pre-operative resuscitation, and further workup
  - Goal: turn a potentially emergent operation into an elective one

---

4-4: ESOPHAGEAL PERFORATION

Pathophysiology

- Esophagus does not have serosa, so is more prone to perforation
- Cervical perforation: more localized in spread of infection/abscess
  - Iatrogenic (from Esophagogastroduodenoscopy [EGD]) most common reason
- Thoracic perforation: negative thoracic pressure tends to spread mediastinal contamination and rapid polymicrobial infection—Boerhaave syndrome

  Mid-esophageal perforation: right pleural effusion

  Distal perforation: left effusion

  Mortality: rates more than triple if >24 hours between perforation and diagnosis

  Signs: vitals, SQ emphysema, and diminished breath sounds in the left chest

Imaging

- **Start with STAT PA/lateral CXR, upright abdomen**

  Pleural effusion (can take several hours to develop, generally left-sided), pneumomediastinum, subcutaneous emphysema, and hydrothorax
- Esophagram with **water soluble** first followed by thin barium if no perforation identified: upright, supine, and lateral
- CT scan: with water-soluble contrast; assess for mediastinal air, abscess, and extravasation of contrast **only if the patient is stable**

Etiology of Perforation	
Iatrogenic	**Boerhaave syndrome**
• **Endoscopy** (48%): rigid > flexible, #1 at level of cricopharyngeus If dilation, was performed, usually at stricture site May occur after variceal sclerotherapy, thermal therapies, and laser therapy Esophageal stenting: up to 5–25% **Medications:** Tetracyclines, KCl, NSAIDs	• Postemetic • Location of perforation: distal 1/3 • **Tear usually longitudinal** • **Mucosal tear usually longer than muscularis tear** **Infection:** Candida, HSV, CMV

Treatment

Nonsurgical Management

- **Criteria: no signs of sepsis, perforation contained, and drains into esophagus**
- **NPO and NGT**
- **IV antibiotics: broad spectrum covering anaerobes, gram negatives/positives:**
- Surveillance: thin barium esophagogram or CT scan at 6–7 days or if clinical change

Surgical Approach to Esophageal Perforation
Key Principles
• NPO, NGT, and broad spectrum antibiotics • Establish nutrition plan, TPN vs. enteral access with feeding tube—post pyloric if the perforation is not cervical • Debride/resect all necrotic, nonviable material • Wide drainage with 2–3 chest tubes, cervical JP if appropriate • Resect if carcinoma or extensive necrosis; likely two-staged procedure
Incision: Dependent on Location of Perforation
• Cervical: left oblique neck incision—drainage alone is most often sufficient • Upper 2/3 thoracic: right posterolateral thoracotomy or VATS • Lower 1/3 thoracic: left posterolateral thoracotomy or VATS • Abdominal: upper midline incision

Within 24 hours and Stable: Attempt Primary Repair
- Debride all necrotic, nonviable material
- Incise muscularis to reveal the length of mucosal defect
- Close mucosa two layers over NGT; test with NGT air instillation
- Reinforce the closure
  - Flap options: pleural, intercostal muscle, and pericardial flap
  - SCM, pectoralis for cervical reinforcement
  - Diaphragm and fundoplication (Thal patch) if lower 1/3

Greater Than 24 hours and Unstable: Esophageal Exclusion
- Segmental esophagectomy
- Cervical esophagostomy and gastrostomy

Patients Who Will Not Tolerate Surgery: Endoscopic Options
- Endoscopic covered stents may be placed in conjunction with large bore chest tubes for drainage. Also an option for a post-operative leak.

Special Considerations
- Perforation during Heller myotomy for achalasia: do myotomy on side opposite the perforation and close perforation
- Perforation with malignancy: perform esophagectomy
- Perforation with hiatal hernia: repair hiatal hernia in addition

4-5: MALLORY–WEISS TEAR

Etiology
- Repeated emesis + increased intragastric pressures
- Mucosal laceration leads to an upper GI bleed
- Occurs just below GE junction

Clinical Presentation
- **Retching immediately before an upper GI bleed**
- Risk factors: alcohol use, especially binging, NSAIDs, portal hypertension, hiatal hernia, and bouts of coughing

Treatment
Initial Resuscitation
- NPO, establish adequate access
- Type and cross packed red blood cells (PRBC)
- Transfuse blood products as needed
- Lavage, decompress stomach

Endoscopy
- Locate proximal source of bleeding; assess for mucosal tears, exclude varices
- **Predictors of need for operation: visible vessel, adherent clot, and active bleeding**
- Possible interventions: epinephrine injection, heater probe coagulation, multipolar electric coagulation, endoscopic hemoclipping, and band ligation

Angiography
- Embolization
- Vasopressin

Surgery
- Indications: transfusion >6 units PRBC, failure of endoscopy, and/or angiography
- Procedure: gastrotomy + oversew mucosal tears, bleeding areas

4-6: ACHALASIA

Epidemiology
- Etiology: Unknown—autoimmune, infectious hypothesized; some congenital noted in pediatrics; Chagas disease

Pathophysiology
- Disorder of peristalsis: aperistalsis, "incoordination of contraction"
  - Loss of vagal cholinergics
  - Loss of propulsion of food or liquid boluses
- LES: fails to relax
  - Lymphocyte, eosinophil, and mast cell infiltration into myenteric plexus
  - Fibrosis of inner circular > outer longitudinal muscle layers
  - Possible result of loss of NOS-directed inhibition

Evaluation
Clinical Presentation
- Gradual onset of dysphagia, initially worse with solids but progresses to liquids
- Other symptoms: substernal burning (40%), regurgitation, and weight loss—often confused with GERD

Imaging
- **Barium swallow**
  - **Bird's beak** deformity: dilatation proximally with smooth tapering distally
- Endoscopy: dilated esophageal body, tightened LES that scope can usually easily pass
- Rule out esophageal tumors, extrinsic compression: biopsy, EGD, CT, or EUS
- **Manometry: Gold standard**
  - Absent peristalsis, incomplete LES relaxation
  - Elevated LES pressures: >30 mm Hg
  - Sometimes with spasm in type 3 (vigorous)

Treatment
Nonoperative Therapy
- Botulin toxin: injected into LES to decrease LES tone
  - Response is transient—need repeated injections which can lead to LES scarring, stricture
  - Response to Botox predicts favorable response to surgical myotomy
- Balloon dilation: disrupts LES fibers and decreases LES tone
  - Response rates 60–80% but high rate of recurrence, need for multiple sessions
  - Risk of esophageal perforation (~5%)
  - Less effective in patients <40 years old
  - Useful for postmyotomy recurrences

Surgical Treatment
- **Myotomy: 95% effective;** preferred for young patients
- Antireflux procedure: lower GERD incidence; need incomplete wrap
- **Peroral endoscopic myotomy (POEM):** Endoscopic procedure making a subserosal tunnel by cutting the mucosa well above the LES, dissecting this plane to the LES, dividing muscle fibers, closing mucosal defect with clips
  - Successful by highly trained operators
  - Concerns over perforation, high rates of reflux/esophagitis (no fundoplication), and learning curve have limited its use
  - Potential indications: reoperation/morbid obesity, type 3 achalasia/DES

Achalasia: Operative Management—Heller Myotomy

Laparoscopic/abdominal approach

⇩

Dissect and expose hiatus

⇩

Identify vagal branches

⇩

Excise GE fat pad

⇩

Longitudinal myotomy: **5 cm proximal from GE junction to 1–2 cm onto gastric cardia**

⇩

Endoscopy helps ensure completion of myotomy, reveals unseen perforation

⇩

Dor or Toupet fundoplication antireflux procedure

4-7: MOTILITY DISORDERS

Pathophysiology
- DES
  - **Repeated simultaneous, high amplitude, nonperistaltic contractions**
  - Substernal chest pain is the most common presenting symptom
  - Treat with calcium channel blockers, nitrates, phosphodiesterase inhibitors
  - May require a long myotomy or POEM
- Nutcracker esophagus:
  - Very high amplitude of distal esophageal contractions (>180 mm Hg), prolonged contractions

- LES hypertension
  - Normal esophageal body peristalsis
  - Elevated LES resting pressures
  - Treat with CCB, nitrates, PDE inhibitors, or myotomy
  - pH study should be done to exclude reflux
- Scleroderma
  - Progressive sclerosis leading to poor esophageal contraction: symptoms of GERD > dysphagia
  - Low to absent LES pressures, hypomotile esophageal body and normal UES
  - Poor candidates for fundoplication

Evaluation
- Symptoms: dysphagia, chest pain, substernal burning, and regurgitation
- **Manometry: gold standard**

4-8: ESOPHAGEAL DIVERTICULA

Zenker Pharyngoesophageal Diverticula
- Most common esophageal diverticulum
- Incidence increases with age: mostly occurs in elderly men, in the seventh and eighth decades
- **Acquired, pulsion-type, false diverticulum: mucosal and submucosal layers only**
- **Occurs in Killian triangle: between horizontal fibers of cricopharyngeus and oblique fibers of thyropharyngeus; posterior wall and left side**
- Leading etiological hypothesis: increased UES pressures
  - Early UES closure during swallowing + poorly coordinated pharyngeal contraction and sphincter relaxation

Epiphrenic Diverticula
- Typically in distal one-third of esophagus
- Acquired, pulsion type
- Usually associated with a motility disorder and impaired LES relaxation

Clinical Presentation
- Zenker
  - Symptoms: dysphagia, **regurgitation of food or pills, halitosis, aspiration** events, and gurgling sounds with swallowing
  - Signs: can have visible neck swelling
  - Frequently have concurrent GERD and esophagitis
- Epiphrenic diverticula
  - Symptoms: more a result of an underlying motility disorder

Imaging
- **Barium esophagram: gold standard; initial test for suspected Zenker's**
- Endoscopy can be done after barium study to rule out concurrent malignancy, but extreme care is necessary to avoid perforation
- Manometry, pH monitoring, video swallow to assess for underlying/associated pathology (optional)

Surgical complications: hematoma, salivary fistula, neck abscess, thoracic duct injury, recurrent laryngeal nerve injury, hoarseness

Nonoperative management
- Endoscopic stapled diverticulotomy can be performed with large diverticula which completes the myotomy as well as drains the diverticulum—limited use in small and very large diverticula.

Esophageal Diverticula—Operative Management

Zenker Diverticula
- Diverticulectomy and diverticulopexy

  Left-sided neck incision over anterior border of SCM
  ⇩
  Dissect down to neck of diverticulum (between carotid sheath and trachea)
  Myotomy—Always! Cricopharyngeus and cervical striated muscle continued on to esophagus
- Staple across neck of the diverticulum with a bougie (34–38 Fr) in esophagus for large diverticulum

- Turn pouch upside down for small diverticula
  Attach to prevertebral fascia
- Endoscopy (optional)
- POEM: used in select cases in specialized centers

Epiphrenic Diverticula

- Myotomy: from diverticular neck down to gastric cardia, technique similar to myotomy for achalasia
- Consider diverticulectomy if there have been aspiration events, significant dysphagia, or a very large pouch—high leak rate.

4-9: BENIGN ESOPHAGEAL TUMORS

Epidemiology

- Epithelial tumors (30–35%): cysts >> polyps > papillomas > adenomas
- Nonepithelial tumors
  Myomas including leiomyomas (60+% of the benign tumors), intramural fibromas, lipomyomas, hemangiomas, and lipomas
  Giant cell tumors and neurofibromas
  Heterotopic: gastric mucosal tumors, pancreatic, and sebaceous gland tumors

Evaluation

- Clinical presentation: dysphagia, odynophagia, retrosternal/epigastric pain, and halitosis
- Barium swallow: smooth intraluminal filling defect; convex mass
- Angle at junction of tumor and normal mucosa
- CT scan: space-occupying lesions; lesion in posterior mediastinum
- Endoscopy/EUS: submucosal mass, usually fairly mobile
  - Do not biopsy if mucosa intact (if leiomyoma, could prohibit extramucosal excision)
  - Endoscopic ultrasound: leiomyoma as hypoechoic, homogeneous submucosal lesion

Treatment

- Asymptomatic and small leiomyomas: follow with barium swallows, endoscopies
- Symptomatic or lesions >5 cm: extramucosal excision and enucleation
  - Separate leiomyoma from submucosa
  - Approach via VATS, thoracotomy, laparoscopy, or midline laparotomy
  - Intraoperative frozen section should be done to ensure benign pathology
  - Certain lesions require segmental esophageal resection (i.e., giant leiomyomas)
- Complications: mucosal tears during enucleation should be repaired; close longitudinal muscle

---

4-10: MALIGNANT ESOPHAGEAL TUMORS

Epidemiology

- Most patients present with locally advanced disease
- **Significant rise in adenocarcinoma (distal one-third) prevalence in the last three decades in US: Most common in US**
- **SCC most common worldwide, 90+% of esophageal cancers**

Risk Factors

- SCC: alcohol abuse, smoking, nitrosamines, achalasia, HIV, EBV, African American race; Males 5× vs. females
- Adenocarcinoma: **Barrett 30**× with high grade dysplasia, obesity chronic reflux, White; males 7–8× vs. females

Clinical Presentation

- Symptoms: dysphagia, weight loss, chest pain, and regurgitation
- Less typical symptoms: odynophagia, hoarseness, cough, and shortness of breath

Imaging

- Barium studies: intraluminal filling defect, convex, and irregular masses
- Endoscopy: defines location, biopsies, and brush cytology for diagnosis
- **Endoscopic ultrasound: assess tumor depth, nodal metastases;** guide FNA
- CT scan: assess metastases and tumor spread
- PET scan: assess occult metastases

Staging: Standard AJCC TNM Classification

- Tumor
  - T_{is}, high-grade dysplasia
  - T_{1a}, invasion lamina propria or muscularis mucosa

- T_{1b}, invasion of submucosa
- T_2, invasion of muscularis propria
- T_3, invasion of adventitia
- T_{4a}, invasion of pleura, pericardium, diaphragm, but resectable
- T_{4b}, invasion of aorta, vertebral body, trachea, unresectable
- Node
  - N_1, 1–2 regional nodal mets
  - N_2, 3–6 regional nodal mets
  - N_3, 7+ regional nodal mets
- M1 distant metastases

Surgical Treatment

- Barretts esophagus may be treated with RFA or endoscopic mucosal resection (EMR)
- Treatment of Tis lesions includes EMR: requires accurate staging, treatment if limited
- T_{1b} or higher lesions require esophagectomy: 15–20% lymph node metastasis rate in T_{1b} lesions.
  - T_{1a} lesions may be treated by EMR in some centers
- **Contraindications for esophageal resection**
  - **Metastatic disease**
  - **Enlarged mediastinal/paratracheal/celiac lymph nodes not in field of resection**
  - **Bronchoesophageal fistula**
- Colon interposition can also be used
- Complication with most morbidity: leak
  - Risk factors: poor nutritional status, preoperative radiation, and tension of anastomosis
  - Leak management
    - Cervical leaks usually close with conservative management: drain
    - Thoracic leaks can be treated with covered endoluminal stent if contained, may require reoperation.

Neoadjuvant Treatment

- Indication: locally advanced tumors: $\geq T_3$, N_{1-3}; T_2 controversial
  - Goal to downstage, enable R0 resection, improved survival over postoperative treatment
  - Combined chemoradiation therapy most common
  - PET/CT necessary after neoadjuvant treatment to rule out progression
  - Consider placing a feeding J-tube prior to treatment

Adjuvant Treatment

- Radiotherapy: palliates symptoms, decreases tumor size
  - Lengthy treatments over 1–2 months, 40–50 Gy
  - Adenocarcinoma less responsive
- Chemotherapy: Platinum based
  - Regimens usually 2–3 months in duration
- Further palliation to limit dysphagia:
  - Esophageal stenting (metal self-expanding stents)
  - Laser
  - Photodynamic therapy
  - Cryotherapy

Esophageal Cancer—Operative Management

Ivor Lewis Esophagectomy: intrathoracic anastomosis usually near azygous vein (divided)

⇩

Advantage: improved nodal resection

⇩

Disadvantage: difficult to manage a leak which has a high mortality; more pain, respiratory compromise with thoracotomy

⇩

Upper midline laparotomy first

⇩

Right posterolateral thoracotomy: fifth or sixth intercostal space (more proximal lesions may require left cervical incision; more distal third lesions may need left thoracotomy)

⇩

En bloc resection of esophagus, lymphatics

⇩

Preserve right gastric and gastroepiploic arteries

⇩

Pyloroplasty/pyloromyotomy (optional)

Transhiatal Esophagectomy

Advantage: avoids thoracotomy, **easier to manage cervical anastomotic leak**

⇩

Disadvantage: does not provide a complete node dissection

⇩

Upper midline laparotomy: assess for celiac nodes, remove left gastric nodes

⇩

Fasion the gastric conduit: **save right gastric and gastroepiploic arteries**

⇩

Mobilize esophagus through upper midline laparotomy

⇩

Dissect under vision and bluntly through esophageal hiatus and left cervical incision

⇩

Cervical esophagogastric anastomosis—check frozen section margin first

⇩

Drain near cervical anastomosis

⇩

Feeding jejunostomy

McKeown Esophagectomy: 3-hole approach, neck anastomosis

⇩

Advantage: nodal resection of an Ivor Lewis, cervical anastomosis

⇩

Disadvantage: requires three incisions: laparotomy, thoracotomy, neck incision

⇩

Right thoracotomy first to perform the intrathoracic dissection

⇩

Upper midline laparotomy to perform abdominal dissection

⇩

Cervical incision to pull the esophagus and stomach out and perform anastomosis

Minimally Invasive:

VATS mobilization of esophagus, with laparoscopic mobilization of the stomach; transhiatal, Ivor Lewis, or McKeown possible

⇩

Entirely laparoscopic transhiatal approach

⇩

Combination of laparotomy with VATS or thoracotomy with laparoscopic mobilization

ROGER EDUARDO • BENJAMIN E. SCHNEIDER

5-1: ANATOMY

Vascular and Lymphatics

Arterial Supply

Lesser Curvature
- Left gastric artery: the largest arterial supply to the stomach (90% from celiac axis)
- Right gastric artery: branch from common hepatic artery (35% from left hepatic artery)

Greater Curvature
- Left gastroepiploic: from splenic artery
- Right gastroepiploic: from gastroduodenal artery (GDA) off the hepatic artery
- Other vessels: short gastric (from splenic), posterior gastric, left inferior phrenic

Pylorus
- GDA
  - NB: Right gastroepiploic artery is sufficient to maintain viability of stomach and is preserved on stomach conduit when doing esophagectomy.

Venous Drainage Parallels Arterial Supply
- Left gastric vein (Coronary): communicates with azygos (**site of esophageal varices**)
- Right gastric vein: drains distal gastric unit

Lymphatics
- Intrinsic (submucosal level): Upward invasive spread of gastric cancer to the esophagus is more common than downward invasion of duodenum.
- Extrinsic nodule basins: There are 16 nodal stations, generally separated into 4 groups based on their resection location for gastric cancer.
  - D1 dissection—removal of perigastric nodes directly attached along the lesser curvature and greater curvatures of the stomach (stations 1–6)
  - D2 dissection—add the removal of nodes along the left gastric artery (station 7), common hepatic artery (station 8), celiac trunk (station 9), splenic hilum, and splenic artery (stations 10 and 11)
  - D3 dissection—adds dissection of lymph nodes along the hepatoduodenal ligament and the root of the mesentery (stations 12 through 14)
  - D4 dissection—add the para-aortic and the paracolic region (stations 15 and 16).

Neurological Innervation
- **Right vagus (posterior vagal trunk):** divides into celiac and posterior gastric
  - Criminal nerve of Grassi: usually the first branch from posterior vagal trunk (can lead to recurrent ulcers if not ligated during vagotomy)
- **Left vagus (anterior vagal trunk):** divides into hepatic and anterior gastric
  - Anterior nerve of Latarjet: terminal branch; 90% are afferent fibers to CNS

Histology

Proximal Stomach (Fundus and Body)
- Parietal cells: produce acid and intrinsic factor
  - Stimulated by acetylcholine, gastrin, and histamine
  - Inhibited by somatostatin, secretin, CCK, and prostaglandin
    - H_2 blockers (histamine receptor antagonists)—block histamine signaling (but parietal cell still stimulated by gastrin and acetylcholine)
    - Proton pump inhibitors—blocks H/K ATPase pump in parietal cell membrane (the final mechanism for release of H+)
  - Intrinsic factor—binds B12 in acid environment and the compound is absorbed in terminal ileum
- Chief cells: release pepsinogen (first enzyme in proteolysis)

Distal Stomach (Antrum and Pylorus)
- Mucus cells: secrete mucus and bicarbonate to protect stomach lining
- G-cells: secrete gastrin to stimulate parietal cells
  - Inhibited by H+ in duodenum
  - Stimulated by acetylcholine and amino acids in stomach
- D-cells: secrete somatostatins (inhibits both acid and gastrin secretion)
  - Released with acidification of antrum and duodenum

5-2: Peptic Ulcer Disease

Epidemiology
- Incidence: peak between 55 and 65 years of age
  - Non–*Helicobacter pylori*-infected individuals: 0.1% per year
  - ***H. pylori*-infected** individuals: 1% per year **(10-fold higher)**
- Risks factors *(Semin Gastrointest Dis. 1993;4:2)*
  - ***H. pylori*: 80% of ulcers;** secretes toxin, stimulates immune response, and upregulates gastrin production; inverse relationship between infection and socioeconomic status
  - **NSAIDs: 55% of non-*H. pylori* ulcers**
  - Family history of hypersecretory states: gastrinoma, Zollinger–Ellison syndrome
  - Smoking and alcohol
  - Stress ulcer: multiple, superficial fundic ulcers secondary to mucosal ischemia shock, hemorrhage, malnutrition, Cushing (CNS), and Curlings (burn)

Helicobacter pylori Diagnosis

- Serology—IgM, IgG to *H. pylori*
- Urease breath test (CLO test—detects urease released by *H. pylori*)
- Endoscopic biopsy (must be from the antrum)
- Culture

Helicobacter pylori Treatment

Gold standard: quadruple therapy (14 days—PPI + Clarithromycin + Amoxicillin + Bismuth)
- First line is triple therapy without bismuth
Repeat EGD/biopsy at 6–8 wk up to two times; surgery if intractable *(N Eng J Med. 1998;339:1869–1874)*

Antisecretory Therapy
- Antacids: magnesium and aluminum complexes
- H_2 receptor antagonists: low cost and good safety profile. Block histamine signaling (but parietal cell still stimulated by gastrin and acetylcholine)
- Proton pump inhibitors: require acid environment for activation. Blocks H/K ATPase pump in parietal cell membrane (the final mechanism for release of H+) *(N Eng J Med. 2000;343:310–316)*
- Sucralfate: polymerizes to form a protective coating of stomach
- Bismuth: Suppresses *H. pylori*
- Prostaglandins: inhibits parietal cells

Anatomic Locations of Peptic Ulcers

- Type I: lesser curvature, majority of gastric ulcers (70–80%)
  - No excess acid secretion; due to decreased mucosal protection
  - Type A blood type
- Type II: two ulcers—duodenal and lesser curvature
  - Excess acid secretion, type O blood
- Type III: antrum (prepyloric), second most common gastric ulcer
  - Excess acid secretion, type O blood
- Type IV: lesser curvature close to GE junction, less than 10% of ulcers
  - No excess acid secretion; due to decreased mucosal protection
  - Type O blood
- Type V: diffuse; ulcers associated with NSAID use.

Complications/Indications for Surgery
- *Perforation*
  - **Most common indication for operative repair of *gastric* ulcers**

Perforation Algorithm
- Diagnosis: upright AXR showing free air (generally gastric or anterior duodenal)
- Treatment: contained perforated duodenal ulcer in stable patient: nonoperative, intravenous fluids + antibiotics + nasogastric decompression + *H. pylori* treatment
- Surgery: biopsy base of ulcer (for cancer and *H. pylori*), Graham patch (omental patch placed over perforation). Start patient on Omeprazole.

- High-risk or unstable patient: biopsy base of ulcer (for cancer and *H. pylori*), Graham patch (omental patch placed over perforation). Start patient on Omeprazole.
- Low-risk patient (<24-hour sxs): omental patch and parietal cell vagotomy.
- If patient already on PPI—consider truncal vagotomy and pyloroplasty or highly selective vagotomy or antrectomy and vagotomy.

Bleeding

- **Most common indication for operative repair of *duodenal* ulcers**
  - **Anterior duodenal ulcers perforate. Posterior ones bleed (GDA)**

Bleeding Ulcer Algorithm (Duodenal > Gastric)

- Initial Rx—transfusions. PPI drip
  - Major bleed (>6u in 24 hours) or hypotension despite transfusion requires intervention.
- Diagnosis: endoscopy, which can also be treated with cauterization, sclerotherapy, vasopressin
  - Predictors of rebleeding: active bleed, pulsatile vessel, or visible clot
- Surgery: duodenostomy and GDA suture ligation
  - Three-point ligation—proximal GDA + distal GDA + transverse pancreatic artery
- Low-risk patient, acid-producing, never been medically treated: Only three-point ligation, biopsy for *H. pylori*, postoperative medical therapy with PPI.
- If patient is high risk, already on PPI—consider adding truncal vagotomy and pyloroplasty or highly selective vagotomy. Pyloroplasty: longitudinal myotomy and close transversely.
- If large (>2 cm) ulcer, in antrum/prepyloric—consider antrectomy + vagotomy

Obstruction

- **Least common complication**—usually in patients with chronic ulcer disease and often near antrum, pylorus, or duodenal.

Obstruction Algorithm

- Diagnosis: UGI or CT scan
- Treatment: NGT decompression, H_2 blocker, or PPI
- Surgery: endoscopic serial dilations. If unable—options based on ulcer location.
- If in antrum—antrectomy (including the ulcer), with Billroth II reconstruction and truncal vagotomy.
- If removal of polyp difficult (duodenal)—Billroth II (gastrojejunostomy)—to bypass the obstruction, with antrectomy and truncal vagotomy.
- Recurrent ulcerations
  - Most likely due to inadequate previous ulcer operation
  - Evaluate for retained antrum, incomplete vagotomy, Zollinger–Ellison syndrome, *H. pylori*, and neoplasm

Elective Surgery for Gastric Ulcers

- Indications: Large ulcers (>2.0 cm), chronic ulcer or ulcer complications, NSAID dependence, *H. pylori* treatment failure or *H. pylori* negative patients, and young patients (<40) who would otherwise have an intractable course
- Type I ulcers: Antrectomy/distal gastrectomy to include ulcer with BI or BII reconstruction
- Type II and III: Antrectomy/distal gastrectomy with ulcer, BI/BII, and truncal vagotomy
- Type IV: Ulcer excision or Distal gastrectomy with Roux-en-Y anastomosis

PUD—Operative Management
• Truncal vagotomy: abolishes the cephalic phase of gastrin secretion. 10% recur, 10% dumping syndrome.
⇩
• Mobilize esophagus and expose vagus trunks with blunt dissection. NGT as guide
⇩
• Identify the anterior vagal trunk about 2–4 cm above the GE junction
⇩
• Divide just above the branch of hepatic and cephalic division along the intra-abdominal esophagus; send a 2-cm portion for pathology confirmation

- NB: Posterior vagal trunk is larger than the anterior vagus; inability to correctly identify this nerve is the most common reason for recurrence

⇩

- Highly selective vagotomy (parietal cell vagotomy): (Fig. 5-1). Preserves anatomy and function of the antrum and decreases parietal cell secretion; liquids empty faster, the same with solids; 10% recur, 1% dumping syndrome

Figure 5-1 Highly selective vagotomy. (From Fischer JE, Bland KI. *Mastery of Surgery*, 5th ed. Philadelphia, PA: Lippincott Williams & Wilkins, 2007.)

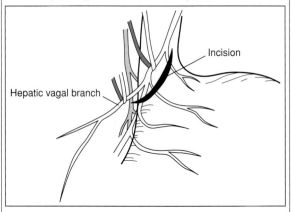

- Identify anterior portion of nerve of Latarjet "crow's foot" along lesser curvature; divide one to two branches

⇩

- Enter lesser sac; divide one to two branches of posterior "crow's feet," **including the criminal nerve of Grassi**

⇩

- Skeletonize 5–7 cm of esophagus

⇩

- Approximate the anterior to posterior serosal surface

⇩

- Sphincter-preserving pyloromyotomy

⇩

- **Antrectomy**
  - Usually preserves the left gastric and left gastroepiploic artery

⇩

  - Incise the gastrocolic ligament to expose the greater curvature

⇩

  - Perform a Kocher maneuver to expose duodenum

⇩

  - **Billroth I anastomosis: stomach to duodenum**

⇩

- Preserves passage of contents through duodenum and its endocrine response

SaD 5-4

- **Billroth II anastomosis: stomach to jejunum** (Fig. 5-2)

Figure 5-2 Billroth II anatomy. (From Fischer JE, Bland KI. *Mastery of Surgery*, 5th ed. Philadelphia, PA: Lippincott Williams & Wilkins, 2007.)

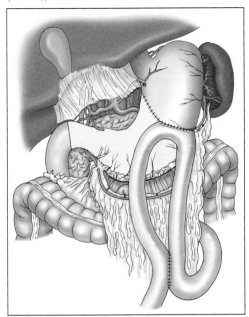

- Mobilize at least a 30-cm proximal jejunum to prevent bile reflux, place retrocolic

Mallory Weiss Tear
- Etiology
  - Often secondary to forceful vomiting that causes mucosal laceration
- Symptoms
  - Hematemesis **after** severe retching
- Diagnosis
  - EGD. Mucosal tear is usually on lesser curvature of stomach (near GE junction).
- Treatment
  - Transfusion, PPI. If continued bleeding, may need gastrostomy and oversew of vessel

5-3: GASTRIC NEOPLASMS

Epidemiology
- Adenocarcinomas account for 95% of gastric cancer (40% are located in antrum)
- Incidence: declining since 1930s, but increases with age; >7× more in Japan/Korea

Risk Factors for Gastric Cancer
Diet high in salt and nitrates (raw vegetables, citrus fruits, and high-fiber lower risk)
Low socioeconomic status (except in Japan)
Family history
Tobacco
Male gender
Blood groups A and O

H. pylori infection
Any gastric ulcer (10% malignancy rate)
Pernicious anemia
Chronic gastritis
Gastric remnant from prior gastric surgery
Gastric polyps (villous)
Adenomatous polyps >2 cm (10–20% malignancy rate)

Gastric Polyps
- Risk factor: gastritis
- Types: tubular, tubulovillous, or villous
- Treatment
  - Polypectomy sufficient if no invasive cancer
  - Further excision if sessile lesions >2 cm, invasion, symptomatic pain, and bleeding

Adenocarcinoma
Preoperative Planning
- Physical examination
  - **Virchow's node (supraclavicular), Sister Mary Joseph's node (umbilical)**
- Chest x-ray, CT scan abdomen (+/–chest), and labs (CBC, Chem7, T&C, and LFTs)
- **Endoscopic ultrasound with biopsy:** most sensitive method for determining the T-stage and assessing regional nodes (ANZ J Surg. 2004;74:108–111)
- +/–Staging laparoscopy
  - Upstages 25% of patients
  - Feeding jejunostomy tube can be performed during the same procedure

TNM Staging—Adenocarcinoma (Minimum 15 Nodes Required)

Primary Tumor (T)
T_x: Primary tumor cannot be assessed
T_0: No evidence of primary tumor
T_{is}: Carcinoma in situ: intraepithelial tumor without invasion of the lamina propria
T_1: Lamina propria, muscularis mucosa or submucosa
    T1a: Tumor invades lamina propria or muscularis mucosa
    T1b: Tumor invades submucosa
T_2: Muscularis propria or subserosa
    T_{2a}: Muscularis propria
    T_{2b}: Subserosa
T_3: Serosa (visceral peritoneum), no invasion of adjacent structures
T_4: Adjacent structures or organs

Regional Lymph Nodes (N)
N_x: Regional lymph nodes cannot be assessed
N_0: No regional lymph node metastasis
N_1: 1–2 lymph nodes
N_2: 3–6 lymph nodes
N_3: >7 lymph nodes

Distant Metastasis (M)
M_x: Distant metastasis cannot be assessed
M_0: No distant metastasis
M_1: Distant metastasis

Staging Group
Stage 0: T_{is}, N_0, M_0
Stage I: $T_{1–2b}$, $N_{0–1}$, M_0
Stage II: $T_{1–3}$, $N_{1–2}$, M_0
Stage III: $T_{2a–4}$, $N_{0–2}$, M_0
Stage IV: $T_{0–4}$, $N_{1–3}$, M_1

Surgery
- Extent based on location and extent of the primary tumor
- **Distal gastric tumors: radical subtotal gastrectomy** (similar survival vs. total gastrectomy)—5–6 cm margins, includes first 3-cm duodenum, hepatogastric + greater omentum; D_1 lymphadenectomy; leaves an adequate gastric remnant
- **More proximal tumors: total gastrectomy with Roux-en-Y for an R_0 resection**

- Unresectable for cure if—peritoneal metastases, liver mets, and lymph nodes high in porta or remote. Total gastrectomy for palliation (when indicated).
- Lymphadenectomy *(J Clin Oncol. 2004;22:2069; Br J Surg. 2004;91:283–287)*
  Extended ($D_2 + D_3$) is controversial, has not been shown to improve survival
  D_1, perigastric nodes (stations 1–6)
  D_2, common hepatic, left gastric, celiac, and splenic arteries (stations 7–11)
  D_3, porta hepatis and adjacent to the aorta (stations 12–16)

Adjuvant Therapy *(N Engl J Med. 2001;345:725)*
- **Resectable: postoperative chemoradiation (T2, T3, and N+ disease)—5-FU, cisplatin**

Gastric Cancer—Operative Management
Subtotal Gastrectomy: 80% resected with gastric remnant en bloc
⇩
Mobilize greater curvature; divide left and right gastroepiploics, leave proximal short gastrics
⇩
Perform an infrapyloric and suprapyloric D_1 dissection
⇩
Divide the stomach 2 cm distal to GE junction (always check margins by frozen section)
⇩
Omentectomy
⇩
Fashion a Billroth II anastomosis
Total Gastrectomy
Similar dissection as subtotal
⇩
Divide the short gastrics and fashion a Roux-en-Y reconstruction

---

Palliative Considerations *(World J Surg. 2006;30:21–27)*
- 20–30% present with stage IV disease
- Management options
  - Endoscopic laser fulguration
  - Dilation
  - Stenting
  - Surgery
  - Chemotherapy

Other Neoplasms
Gastric Lymphoma
- Usually non-Hodgkin's lymphoma
- 90% *H. pylori* positive
- Precursor lesion: mucosal-associated lymphoid tissue (MALT)
- Symptoms: usually ulcer symptoms
- Diagnosis: EGD with deep biopsy and CT scan
- Treatment
  - Stage I (tumor confined to mucosa)—surgery and then chemoradiation
  - Stages II–IV: chemotherapy and XRT

Gastrointestinal Stromal Tumors (GIST)
- Etiology: originates from interstitial cells of Cajal, CKIT+, and CD34+
- Symptoms: usually asymptomatic; may obstruct or bleed
- Diagnosis: extrinsic bulge on endoscopy, characteristic CT findings
- Malignancy ("high risk"): based on mitotic figures (>5–10 mitoses/HPF) and size (>5 cm)
- Treatment
  - Surgical resection with 1-cm margins
  - Chemotherapy-tyrosine kinase inhibitor (Gleevac) for "high risk" or recurrence

Gastrinoma (Zollinger–Ellison Syndrome)
- Epidemiology: 50–60% malignant and 50% multiple tumors;
  - High degree of suspicion for MEN1 syndrome
- Symptoms: abdominal pain, GERD, and secretory diarrhea
- **Location: gastrinoma triangle**
  - **Junction of cystic duct and common bile duct**
  - **Junction of head and neck of pancreas**
  - **Junction of second and third portions of duodenum**

- Laboratory diagnosis
  1. Serum gastrin levels >1000 pg/mL is diagnostic; >150 pg/mL suspicious
  2. Secretin-stimulated levels—a 2U/kg bolus of secretin—increase in serum gastrin >200 pg/mL
  3. Basal acid output greater than 15 mEq/h is highly suggestive
  4. Gastric volume >140 mL and pH of less than 2.0 are highly suggestive of gastrinoma
  5. Calcium level (elevated serum calcium levels should prompt workup for MEN1)
- Treatment: surgery (pancreatic tumors <2 cm can be enucleated)

Differential Diagnosis of Elevated Gastrin Level
- Retained gastric antrum - Atrophic gastritis - Chronic renal failure (gastrin metabolized by kidney) - Short gut syndrome - Vagal denervation (chronic alkaline release leads to G-cell hyperplasia) - PPI therapy

---

5-4: MORBID OBESITY

Definitions
- Overweight: BMI 25–29.9 kg/m^2
- Obesity: BMI 30–34.9 kg/m^2
- Moderate obesity: BMI 35–39.9 kg/m^2
- Morbid obesity: BMI 40–59.9 kg/m^2
- Super obesity: BMI >60 kg/m^2

Epidemiology
- Two-thirds of US adults and 20% children are overweight or obese.
- Comorbidities: type 2 diabetes, hyperlipidemia, coronary artery disease, hypertension, obstructive sleep apnea, GERD, depression, pseudotumor cerebri, endocrine (polycystic ovary disease, gynecomastia, and hirsutism), stress urinary incontinence, venous stasis disease, degenerative joint disease, steatohepatitis, stroke, endometrial cancer, and abdominal wall hernias.

Treatment
Medical
- Typically unsuccessful
- Lifestyle changes: diet, exercise, and behavior modifications (ineffective long term)
- Pharmacotherapy: second-line therapy
  - Sibutramine and orlistat approved by FDA; 5 kg weight loss over 6 months

Surgical (Fig. 5-3) (JAMA. 2004;292(14):1724)

Figure 5-3 A: Roux-en-Y gastric bypass. **B:** Laparoscopic adjustable gastric band. **C:** Laparoscopic gastric sleeve. (From Fischer JE, Bland KI. *Mastery of Surgery*, 5th ed. Philadelphia, PA: Lippincott Williams & Wilkins, 2007.)

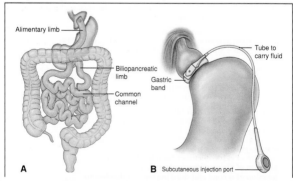

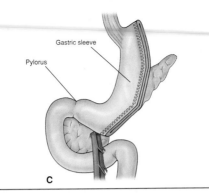

- **Criteria: BMI >40 kg/m^2 or BMI >35 kg/m^2 + comorbidities and failed medical therapy**
- Laparoscopic adjustable gastric band: restrictive procedure
  - Adjustable band placed to create a proximal pouch
  - Excess weight loss (30–40%), and low mortality
  - Not routinely done anymore
  - Complications: slipped band/prolapse, stomal obstruction, band erosion, device malfunction/leak, and pouch or esophageal dilation
- Sleeve gastrectomy: **restrictive procedure**
  - Leaves antrum and pylorus intact
  - Excess weight loss (60–70%), and low mortality
  - Creates a narrow gastric tube using laparoscopic linear stapler and excising remainder of the stomach (use a 36 Fr Bougie)
  - Complications: staple line leak, stricture
- Biliopancreatic diversion and duodenal switch: **malabsorptive procedures**
  - Considered in patients with higher BMI (>50 kg/m^2)
  - Excess weight loss (70–90%), higher mortality than with other procedures
  - Greater incidence of protein malnutrition
  - Risk of cirrhosis with BP diversion
- RYGB (Roux-en-Y gastric bypass): mix of restrictive and malabsorptive

Laparoscopic Roux-en-Y Gastric Bypass
Excess weight loss (60–80%)
⇩
Divide a 30–50 cm length of jejunum with its mesentery distal to ligament of Treitz to create a 75–150 cm Roux limb
⇩
Fashion a side-to-side jejunojejunostomy by making two adjacent enterotomies and closing the remaining enterotomy with a linear stapler
⇩
Fashion a small gastric pouch using linear staplers
⇩
Create a gastrojejunal anastomosis (either stapled or sutured)
⇩
Close mesenteric defects to avoid hernias
Complications: Internal hernias (2–5%), anastomotic strictures, fistulas, pulmonary embolus, staple line leaks, metabolic derangements, marginal ulcer

5-5: COMPLICATIONS OF GASTRIC SURGERY

Dumping Syndrome
Early
- Timing: **occurs minutes after a meal**
- Etiology: rapid gastric emptying of hyperosmolar chyme into small bowel causes rapid fluid shifts
- Symptoms: postprandial tachycardia, diaphoresis, abdominal pain, and diarrhea
- **Incidence: occurs in 75% of patients after gastric surgery,** more common after BII vs. BI

Late
- Timing: **occurs hours after a meal**
- Etiology: hyperosmolar chyme causes hyperglycemia → insulin hypersecretion → hypoglycemia.
- Symptoms: palpitations, weakness, sweating, and dizziness

Diagnosis
- UGI contrast study

Treatment
- **Majority of cases resolved with conservative dietary and medical management**
- Dietary: small meals, no liquids with food, and limit sugars
- Somatostatin: inhibits vasoactive peptides and slows transit time
- Surgery: convert BI or BII to Roux-en-Y; used for serious dumping syndrome; increase gastric reservoir with a jejunal pouch or increase emptying time (reversed jejunal loop)

Afferent Loop Syndrome (Incidence of ~1%)
Etiology
- Only occurs with Billroth II or Roux-Y operations—increased intraluminal distention due to accumulation of enteric secretions in a partially or completely obstructed afferent limb; secondary bacterial stasis.
- Differential: internal hernia, adhesions, anastomotic stricture, ulceration, and carcinoma

Symptoms
- Acute: can cause obstructive jaundice, ascending cholangitis, and pancreatitis due to high pressures in biliopancreatic ductal system. Abdominal pain, nausea, vomiting.
- Chronic: stasis and bacterial overgrowth—deconjugate bile acids—can cause steatorrhea, malnutrition, and B12 deficiency.

Treatment
- Endoscopic decompression or dilatation; surgical revision of afferent limb to relieve obstruction or make shorter (<40 cm)

Alkaline Reflux Gastritis (5% of Patients After Billroth I or II and Pyloroplasty)
1. Etiology: prolonged exposure to bile salts leads to loss of gastric mucosa protection
2. Symptoms: bilious vomiting

Treatment
- Medical: metoclopramide and sucralfate
- Surgery: convert to Roux-en-Y with jejunal limb >60 cm

Postvagotomy Diarrhea
1. Etiology: sustained postprandial MMCs results in non-conjugated bile salts in colon
2. Symptoms: diarrhea

Treatment
- Medical: octreotide, cholestyramine
- Surgery: reversed interposition jejunal limb

Metabolic Derangements
- Megaloblastic anemia: loss of intrinsic factor leads to decreased vitamin B12 absorption
- Microcytic anemia: secondary to iron deficiency
- Vitamin D and calcium malabsorption

JORDAN PYDA • STEPHEN ODOM

First edition authored by Stephen Odom, David Odell, and Christopher Boyd

6-1: ANATOMY

Gross Anatomy

Blood Supply
- SMA (midgut): all but the proximal duodenum (celiac → foregut)
- Venous drainage parallels the arterial supply
- SMV joins the splenic vein behind the pancreas to form the portal vein

Nerve Innervations
- Parasympathetic fibers from vagus nerve: control motility and secretion
- Sympathetic fibers form three sets of splanchnic nerves: motor nerves affect vessel diameter, gut secretion, and motility; afferent fibers carry pain sensation

Orientation
- Bowel undergoes a 270-degree (extra-abdominal) counterclockwise rotation about SMA at 10 weeks of gestation, fixing cecum in right upper quadrant by 3–5 months, then develops caudally to rest in right lower quadrant
- Incomplete rotation may result in compression and obstruction of the duodenum by Ladd's bands (peritoneal cecal attachments)

Histologic Layers (Outer to Inner)
- Serosa
- Muscularis: innervated by myenteric (Auerbach) nerve plexus
  - Thin outer longitudinal layer
  - Thick inner circular layer
- Submucosa: **strength layer (important in small bowel anastomosis)**; fibroelastic connective tissue with nerves (Meissner plexus), lymphatics, and blood vessels
- Mucosa: forms complete rings, called plicae circularis or folds of Kerckring (except in duodenum and distal ileum)
  - Muscularis mucosa
  - Lamina propria: base of the epithelium; forms structure of crypts of Lieberkühn; noncellular connective tissue with plasma cells, lymphocytes, mast cells, eosinophils, macrophages, fibroblasts, and smooth muscle
  - Epithelial cell types
    - Villous cells: digestion and absorption
    - Crypt cells: generation of new epithelium
    - Goblet cells: secretion of mucus
    - Enteroendocrine cells: secretion of gastrin, secretin, cholecystokinin (CCK), somatostatin, enteroglucagon, motilin, neurotensin, and GIP
    - Paneth cells: mucosal defense
    - Undifferentiated epithelial cells: cell renewal
    - Glycocalyx: fuzzy coat of glycoproteins
    - Microvilli: contain enzymes for digestion and some cells have specialized receptors (e.g., distal ileal cells with B12 receptors)

6-2: GI PHYSIOLOGY

Motility
- Pacesetter potentials: originate in duodenum
- Migrating motor complex (MMC): mediated by motilin, somatostatin, enkephalins, and neural input during the fasting state
  - Vagal fibers: cholinergic input = excitatory, peptidergic input = inhibitory
  - Sympathetic fibers: modulate intrinsic nerve function
  - Gut peptides
    - Motilin: modulates MMC
    - Gastrin, CCK, motilin: modulate muscle contraction
    - Secretin, glucagon: inhibits muscle contraction

Digestion

Fat
- Triglycerides are broken down by pancreatic lipase into two single fatty acids and glycerol (β-monoglyceride)
- These combine with bile salts to form micelles that are passively transported through the diffusion barriers

- They disaggregate in mucous coat; bile salts are returned to the lumen where they form additional micelles and are almost completely resorbed in the distal ileum (5 g total pool, recirculated six times, and 0.5 g lost per day in stool)
- Triglycerides are reformed, combined with cholesterol and phospholipids to form chylomicrons that are absorbed across basal membrane into lymphatics
- A few small chain fatty acids are absorbed directly into the portal vein

Protein
- Stomach acid begins to denature proteins
- Pancreatic trypsinogen is converted by enterokinase to trypsin that in turn activates other pancreatic proteases
- The endopeptidases (trypsin, elastase, and chymotrypsin) act on internal peptide bonds and exopeptidases remove single amino acids (AA) or dipeptides from the terminal ends
- Single AA and short-chain peptides are transported into the cell
- Most of the remaining peptides are converted to single AA by cytosolic peptidases
- These are then transported across the basal cell membrane into the portal vein

Carbohydrate
- Starch is converted by α-amylase to maltose, maltotriose, and α-limit dextrins
- The enzymes maltase, alpha dextrinase, sucrase, and lactase break down these molecules to glucose at the brush border
- Glucose is actively absorbed into the cell
- Fructose is absorbed by facilitated diffusion
- Sucrose is broken down to glucose and fructose in the brush border by sucrase
- Lactose is broken down to glucose and galactose in the brush border and absorbed by active transport

Water and Electrolytes
- Water: the majority is absorbed proximal to the ileocecal valve
- Sodium and chloride: absorbed by active transport and coupled to organic solutes (most commonly) by co-transporters
- Bicarbonate: absorbed by sodium–hydrogen exchange
- Calcium: active transport in the duodenum and proximal jejunum
- Potassium: passive diffusion
- Folate and iron: absorbed in proximal bowel
- Vitamin B12: specific receptors in the distal bowel

Endocrine Function
Secretin
- Released from S cells in duodenum in response to acid, bile, and fat
- Function
  - Release of water and bicarbonate from ductal cells of the pancreas
  - Stimulates the flow of bile and inhibits the release of gastrin, gastric acid, and gastrointestinal motility
- Can also cause release of gastrin from gastrinomas: diagnostic test in Z–E syndrome

Cholecystokinin (CCK)
- Released from small bowel mucosa in response to certain AAs and fats
- Release is inhibited by trypsin and bile acids
- Function (similar to gastrin)
  - Stimulates gallbladder contraction
  - Relaxes sphincter of Oddi
  - Stimulates growth of small bowel mucosa and pancreas
  - Stimulates small bowel motility and the release of insulin

Vasoactive Inhibitory Peptide (VIP)
- Causes vasodilation
- Stimulates pancreatic and intestinal secretion
- Inhibits gastric acid secretion
- Responsible for watery diarrhea in certain neuroendocrine tumors of the pancreas

Others
- Gastric inhibitory peptide
  - Released by fat and stimulates insulin release; mechanism responsible for higher insulin response to oral glucose compared to an equivalent IV dose
- Enteroglucagon: inhibits bowel motility
- Motilin: stimulates smooth muscle contractions and modulates the MMC
- Bombesin: generalized "on" switch for the bowel
- Somatostatin: paracrine "off" switch for gut hormones and secretion

- Neurotensin: stimulates water and bicarbonate secretion from the pancreas, inhibits gastric acid secretion, and has trophic effects on the small and large bowel mucosa
- Peptide YY: released from the distal ileum and colon in response to fat in the blood; inhibits gastric and pancreatic secretions and has trophic effects on the small bowel

Immune Function

Antibody-Mediated Immunity

- Antigen is presented to M cells overlying Peyer patches (lymphoid aggregations in the ileum) and transported to lymphoblasts that release IgA
- This is circulated and stimulates lymphoblasts in lamina propria, which differentiate into plasma cells that can produce specific IgA in response to similar antigen

Cell-Mediated Immunity

- M cells process antigen that stimulates lymphocytes and macrophages
- These in turn produce IL-1 that stimulates helper T cells that release IL-2 and gamma interferon that stimulate MHC II on epithelial cells

Translocation of Bacteria

- Unclear of the importance in human illness
- Gastrin, neurotensin, bombesin, and epidermal growth factor all have trophic effects on small bowel mucosa and may modulate permeability in sepsis and shock states

6-3: APPENDICITIS AND MECKEL'S DIVERTICULUM

Appendicitis

- Epidemiology
  - Lifetime prevalence 7%
  - **Most common in second to fourth decade but can occur at any age**
- Etiology: viral illness (especially kids) > appendicolith > idiopathic > appendiceal tumor
- Pathophysiology
  - Blockage of appendiceal ostium prevents drainage of appendiceal fluid
  - Increased pressure within appendix is transmitted to appendiceal wall, causing venous congestion
  - Venous infarction leads to appendiceal wall perforation within 72 h
- Organisms: *Escherichia coli*, *Bacteroides* spp., and *Pseudomonas*
- Perforation **(12%)**
  - Most common: younger than 10 and older than 50
  - Atypical to perforate within 24 hours of onset of symptoms

Clinical Presentation

- Symptoms: (in "classic" order of presentation) **vague periumbilical pain migrating to right lower quadrant,** subsequently nausea, vomiting, **anorexia,** abdominal or pelvic tenderness and then subjective fevers
- Physical examination
  - Rectal examination may demonstrate pelvic phlegmon or tenderness
  - Testicular pain on either or both sides is common in men
- Laboratory: mild WBC elevation **(between 10 and 18 K with left shift)** but can be normal in up to 10% of patients; classically appears after above sequence of symptoms; urinalysis has few RBC and some WBC

Differential Diagnosis of Appendicitis	
Meckel's diverticulitis	Mesenteric adenitis
Perforated malignancy	Peptic ulcer
Cholecystitis	Diverticulitis
Epiploic appendicitis	Spontaneous bacterial peritonitis
Infectious: yersiniosis and gastroenteritis	
Renal: pyelonephritis, UTI, and kidney stones	
Urologic: testicular torsion or epididymitis	
Gynecologic: pelvic inflammatory disease, ectopic pregnancy, ovarian cyst, middlesmertz, and ovarian torsion	
Typhlitis (inflammation of the cecum, most common in neutropenic patients)	

"Signs" in Appendicitis
- McBurney's point: site of maximal tenderness one-third distance from right anterior superior iliac spine in straight line towards umbilicus where base of appendix may lie
- Rovsing's sign: right lower quadrant pain when pressure applied in left lower quadrant
- Psoas sign: right lower quadrant pain with hyperextension of right hip
- Obturator sign: right lower quadrant pain with internal rotation of flexed right thigh

Imaging
- Abdominal x-rays: normal, loss of psoas stripe, decreased gas in RLQ, and fecalith
- Ultrasound: useful examination for children or slim adults; shows inflamed appendix or pelvic fluid
- **CT scan: fat stranding, dilated appendix and/or thickened wall, perforation, pelvic fluid, and fecalith**

Treatment
- Standard of care for **both** acute complicated and uncomplicated appendicitis: **Perioperative antibiotics** to cover skin/colonic flora + **appendectomy (lap vs. open)**
- Complicated (i.e., perforated or associated with abscess)
  - Stable (nonperitoneal): antibiotics, IR drainage abscess, delayed appendectomy
  - **Frank peritonitis: surgical exploration and washout**
  - Ileocecal resection if appendiceal base too inflamed to divide safely
- Uncomplicated (i.e., nonperforated and without abscess): (*JAMA.* 2015;16:313)
  - Recent short-term data prompted discussion of nonoperative management of uncomplicated appendicitis with antibiotics; significant recurrence rate ultimately requires surgical management in ~25% of patients at 1 year after initial episode

Appendectomy—Operative Management
Open Appendectomy
Incision: in the RLQ over the point of maximal tenderness (McBurney incision is made perpendicularly and extended inferiorly from McBurney's point. More common is the Rocky–Davis transverse incision from McBurney's point along a skin crease.)
⇩
Divide anterior fascia along external oblique fibers
⇩
Bluntly spread abdominal wall muscles and sharply enter abdomen
⇩
Identify and deliver cecum through wound and track taenia to appendix
⇩
Ligate the vessels of the mesoappendix and then divide the appendix at its base
⇩
Irrigate abdomen and close wound in layers
Laparoscopic Appendectomy
Three ports: umbilical, left lower quadrant, and suprapubic or right mid-abdomen
⇩
Identify and grasp the appendix
⇩
Create window through mesentery at base of appendix
⇩
Endo-GIA stapler for appendiceal base and vascular load for mesoappendix
⇩
Irrigate pelvis and paracolic gutters; ensure hemostasis

Meckel's Diverticulum

Etiology
- Persistent vitelline duct remnant
- Usually found **on antimesenteric border of ileum 60 cm from ileocecal valve**

Clinical Presentation
- Bleeding (22%): painless; ulceration of adjacent tissue due to acid production from ectopic gastric tissue
- Obstruction (13%)
- Inflammation (2%), can mimic appendicitis
- Intussusception (1%)

Rule of 2's
• 2% of the population
• 2% asymptomatic
• 2 feet from the ileocecal valve
• 2 inches long
• 2 types of mucosa (gastric/pancreatic)
• 2:1 Male:Female

Diagnosis
- Requires a high clinical index of suspicion
- Meckel scan: technetium-99 pertechnetate uptake in ectopic **gastric** tissue (H_2 blockers held prior to test to avoid a possible false-negative result)

Treatment
- Symptomatic
  - Segmental resection with primary end-to-end anastomosis
  - Wedge resection of diverticulum
  - Should perform appendectomy as well
- Incidental discovery: resect if patient <18 years or if ectopic tissue is felt; may leave alone if in an adult and otherwise asymptomatic

6-4: INFLAMMATORY AND INFECTIOUS DISEASES

Crohn's Disease

Epidemiology
- Etiology: unknown (infectious, immunologic, environmental, and genetic)
- Bimodal distribution: teens–20s and 50s–70s; slightly favors females
- Likely increased risk of colorectal CA (less than with UC) and small bowel CA
  (World J Gastroenterol. 2008;14:1810)

Pathology
- Transmural involvement with cyclic inflammation and subsequent fibrosis
- Can occur anywhere along GI tract from mouth to anus
- Most common location: terminal ileum, 10–20 cm proximal to ileocecal valve
- "Skip lesions": discontinuous areas of inflammation/stricture

Clinical Presentation
- Symptoms: crampy pain (# 1), nonbloody diarrhea, fever (30%), weight loss, fatigue, and malaise
- Complications: bowel obstruction, perforation, fistula, abscess, and colitis
- Can present with perianal disease (~30%); perioral (~10%)
- **Extra-intestinal symptoms (30%): arthritis/arthralgias, uveitis, iritis, hepatitis, cholangitis (PSC), erythema nodosum, and pyoderma gangrenosum**

Imaging
- CTAP with IV and PO contrast: wall thickening, abscess, and fistula
- Barium contrast series: nodularity, strictures, linear ulcerations, and sinuses

Treatment (Nat Rev Gastroenterol Hepatol. 2013;10:345)
- Acute exacerbations: sulfasalazine, steroids, antibiotics
- Maintenance and refractory disease: 5-ASA (e.g., mesalamine); 6-mercaptopurine, azathioprine, and biologics
- Biologics: anti-TNF (e.g., Adalimumab and Infliximab) for induction and maintenance of remission; novel agents include anti-Integrin
- Surgical principles: **operate for symptomatic disease not for cure and avoid resection if possible;** preserve functional intestinal length and absorptive capacity; resection of diseased segments can improve extra-intestinal symptoms

---

Crohn's Disease—Operative Management

- **Heineke–Mikulicz strictureplasty:** appropriate for strictures 2–3 cm in length
  Place stay sutures 1 cm proximal and distal to the stricture
  ⇩
  Incise bowel longitudinally along antimesenteric border; extend into normal bowel
  ⇩
  Close transversely in one or two layers

- **Finney strictureplasty:** for strictures up to 15 cm in length
  Fold strictured segment onto itself into "U" configuration and sew together with seromuscular suture (Lambert suture)
  ⇩
  Make U-shaped enterotomy; close sides together anteriorly with full-thickness sutures
  ⇩
  Increased risk for bacterial overgrowth in "diverticulum"

- **Side-to-side iso-peristaltic strictureplasty:** for long or clustered segments
  Divide bowel and mesentery at the midpoint of the stricture
  ⇩
  Bring proximal divided end side-to-side with distal extent of the stricture
  ⇩
  Make longitudinal enterotomy; sew together with full thickness sutures

- **Resection:** for focal point of obstruction

Radiation Enteritis (Ther Adv Chronic Dis. 2014;5:15)

Etiology
- Transmural intestinal injury due to oxidative damage from high doses of radiation
- **Dose dependent: >4,500 cGy**
- Risk factors: thin, elderly female, prior surgery, certain chemotherapy, pre-existing comorbidities of heart failure, DM, HTN, and PVD

Clinical Presentation
- Acute (2nd–4th week XRT): diarrhea, bloating, malabsorption, colic
- Late (1–6 years post-XRT): strictures, obstruction, and fistula
- Prevalence: 50–90% of XRT patients
- Diagnosis: history of radiation and clinical symptoms

Imaging
- Enteroclysis: good for evaluation of stricture and fistula formation
- CT: visualizes bowel wall thickening, may show areas of stricture, abscess

Treatment
- Dietary: NPO acutely, then low residue, low fat, lactose free; TPN if not tolerated
- Medications: probiotics, octreotide, 5-ASA, loperamide, antibiotics, steroids (acute), antispasmodics, narcotics, and glutamine +/– bombesin; cholestyramine for bile acid malabsorption
- Hyperbaric oxygen: increases oxygen tension in poorly perfused tissue; may accelerate healing
- Surgery: **AVOID if at all possible**; stricturoplasty if necessary to retain intestinal length or bypass if segment inaccessible; fistulas must be resected

Prevention
- Localization markers to minimize radiation field
  - Mesh slings, reperitonization, or omental transposition to keep bowel from pelvis
  - Statins and ACE inhibitors significantly decreased XRT associated GI symptoms

Gastroenteritis

Typhoid (Salmonella typhus)
- Clinical presentation: hemorrhage (10–20%) and perforation (2%) (typically at terminal ileum due to concentration of Peyer's patches; see *Immune Function* above)
- Treatment: Bactrim or Amoxicillin; may need operation if perforated

Traveler's diarrhea
- Etiology: 70%—enterotoxic E. coli > Salmonella (nontyphoid), *Shigella, Giardia*; spread by fecal–oral route
- Treatment: symptomatic, re-hydration; if fever or hematochezia, Bactrim or Ciprofloxacin

Food Poisoning
- Etiology: *Salmonella, Staphylococcus aureus, Clostridium perfringens, Yersinia enterocolitica, Giardia, Helicobacter,* and viral; often no identifiable cause
- Clinical presentation: symptoms begin 6–8 hours after ingestion and last 1–3 days; fever is rare; Yersinia can cause pharyngitis in kids (50%) and adults (10%)
- Treatment: antibiotics only if fulminant

Tuberculosis
- Epidemiology: disease of poverty, disproportionately afflicts developing world, inmates, HIV/AIDS, immunosuppressed, and transplant pts
- Primary disease (less than 10%): bovine strain
- Secondary disease: pulmonary disease with swallowed bacteria (25%) that usually cause growth in the ileocecal region. Hypertrophic TB leads to obstruction. Ulcerative TB leads to pain, diarrhea, and constipation. Surgery for perforation, obstruction, or hemorrhage.

Chronic Diarrhea (>2 Weeks)
- *Yersinia, Clostridium, Cryptosporidium,* or other parasites

Viral
- Rotavirus: usually children age 6–24 months
- Norwalk virus: Older children and adults

Etiology of Mechanical Small Bowel Obstruction
• Adhesions: most common cause in adults
• Incarcerated hernia: most common cause in children, #2 in adults
• Neoplasm
• Strictures: postoperative, postischemic, and postradiation
• Crohn's disease
• Intussusception
• Volvulus
• Gallstone ileus (stone passes via biliary–enteric fistula and typically obstructs ileum)
• External compression: annular pancreas, pancreatic pseudocyst, abscess, carcinomatosis, abdominal compartment syndrome, and pregnancy
• Foreign bodies

Pathophysiology
- Early: increased peristalsis throughout the bowel
- Late: bowel fatigues and becomes dilated
  - "Third spacing" of fluid in the distended bowel with loss of electrolytes and fluid
  - Fluid loss and dehydration can cause hypotension with diminished blood flow to the bowel and subsequent shock
  - Mucosal ischemia with translocation of bacteria and eventually full thickness ischemia and perforation
- Proximal obstruction: additional loss of hydrogen, potassium, and chloride in vomitus, leading to metabolic alkalosis
- Distal obstruction: water loss more pronounced with less dramatic electrolyte disturbances

Clinical Presentation
- Signs and symptoms: **nausea and vomiting + abdominal distention + intolerance of oral intake + decreased flatus/bowel function**; blood in the stool or vomitus is a cause for concern for ischemia or strangulation
  - **Proximal: prominent vomiting and less distention**
  - **Distal: obstipation and more prominent distention**
- Physical examination: fever, tachycardia, abdominal distention—check for abdominal scars, masses, hernias—**digital rectal examination**
- Laboratory: elevated WBC, BUN/Cr, and Hct/Hgb; electrolyte derangements

Imaging
- Abdominal x-ray (upright): decreased colonic gas, air–fluid levels; closed-loop obstructions may show tapering of air to a "birds beak"; upright chest x-ray can demonstrate free air if perforation has occurred; small bowel becomes secretory organ which contributes to dilation, obstruction, and subsequent ileus
- Small bowel follows through: if diagnosis is in doubt and partial obstruction is likely
- **CT abd/pelvis with IV and PO contrast; test of choice:** look for proximal dilation, distal collapse (i.e., transition point), dosed pool, thickening of wall or fat stranding are evidence of inflammation/ischemia; pneumatosis intestinalis (finding of circumferential air within bowel wall) usually portends necrosis

Treatment (Arch Surg. 1993;128:765)
- Partial obstruction: 70% resolve without surgical intervention
  - NPO, bowel rest, IVF resuscitation, NGT decompression, avoid ileus-producing drugs, and pulmonary toilet
  - **If fever, increased abdominal pain, rising WBC, or other sign or concern for ischemia develop, exploration is indicated**
- **Complete obstruction: exploration after fluid and electrolyte resuscitation**
- Paralytic Ileus: delayed intestinal transit caused by poor intestinal motility
- Most common: postoperative laparotomy
- Other etiologies
  - Drugs: opiates, anticholinergics, and antipsychotics
  - Electrolyte derangements: hypokalemia, hyponatremia, hypomagnesemia, and uremia
  - Chronic diabetes from enteric neuropathy
  - Infections: pneumonia, UTI in elderly, and systemic sepsis
  - Ischemia
  - Retroperitoneal process: abscess and inflammation
- Treatment: bowel rest, correct electrolyte and fluid derangements, stop causative medications, and treatment for constipation, ambulation, gum chewing

6-6: ENTEROCUTANEOUS (EC) FISTULA AND SHORT GUT SYNDROME

EC Fistula

Etiology (J Am Coll Surg. 2009;209(4):484–491)

- Definition: abnormal communication between two epithelialized surfaces
- Most common: postoperative after surgery for inflammatory bowel disease, cancer, or lysis of adhesions
- Usually iatrogenic and the result of surgical misadventure (85–90%)
  - Anastomotic leak (50%)
  - Inadvertent enterotomy
- About 15–25% occur spontaneously (Crohn's disease, neoplasm, infectious, and radiation)

Classification

- Low output: <200 mL/day
- High output: >500 mL/day
- "Likely to close": pancreaticobiliary, jejunal, and esophageal
- "Unlikely to close": gastric, duodenal, and ileal

Etiology and Persistence of EC Fistulas
Friends
Foreign body
Radiation
Inflammatory process (Crohn's disease)
Infections (diverticulitis, tuberculosis, and actinomycosis)
Epithelialization
Neoplasm and **N**utrition
Distal obstruction
Sepsis and **S**teroids

Imaging

- Fistulogram: delineate fistula tract and rule out distal obstruction
- **CT abd/pelvis:** localize inflammatory or infectious processes, neoplasms, and distal obstruction

Treatment

- Initial conservative management: 80–90% will close spontaneously; varied success
  - Fluid replacement, NPO, and control sepsis
  - Optimize nutrition (TPN or enteral via Dobhoff catheter, PO, or via catheter inserted distally into fistula)
  - Control drainage and protect skin; consider VAC dressing
  - Consider octreotide to decrease output
- Surgical repair: best delayed at least 4–6 months in stable patients; requires meticulous entry into the abdomen and prolonged adhesiolysis with resection of involved segment of bowel and re-establishment of GI continuity

Short Bowel Syndrome

Etiology (Curr Gastroenterol Rep. 2016;18:40)

- Intestinal malabsorption following large segment resection of small intestine, usually for Crohn's disease, malignancy, vascular insufficiency, or radiation enteritis
- Definition: approx. <200 cm of small bowel whereas normal length is 300–850 cm
- Clinical presentation: intolerance of oral feeds and diarrhea
- Bowel attempts adaptation by a glucagon like peptide-2 (GLP-2) mediated process which increases gut length and diameter (increasing villi and absorptive area)

Region of Resected Bowel Determines Symptoms		
Jejunum	**Ileum**	**Ileocecal Valve**
• Impaired absorption: protein, carbohydrate, fat • Deficiencies: iron, calcium, folate • Best-tolerated resection	• **B12 deficiency if resect >60 cm** • **Bile salt loss if resect >100 cm** • **Fat malabsorption; loss of fat-soluble vitamins** • "Ileal brake": loss of receptors for peptide YY in terminal ileum—increased motility	• Resection results in bacterial reflux/overgrowth in the distal small bowel • If preserved, increases transit time and allows survival with less small bowel • Malabsorption: fat-soluble vitamins, B12, bile salts

Treatment (Gut 2006; 55(Suppl 4))
- Early: TPN for nutritional support and repletion of fluid and electrolyte losses
  - Fluids: must contain Na, KCl, and Mg
  - H_2 blocker to suppress gastric hypersecretion
  - Monitor Se, Ca, Mg, Zn, and fat-soluble vitamins (A, D, E, and K) every 3 months
- Late: slow introduction of enteral feeding
  - Continuous or small frequent meals of complex diets
  - Medications: Octreotide may slow transit time. Growth hormone may speed intestinal adaptation.
  - GLP-2 analogue, teduglutide, helps increase absorptive area and wean TPN
  End-stage
  - Small bowel transplant: if contraindications to or complications from TPN
  - Interposition: reversed segment of small intestine or colon; may slow transit through shortened small intestine and increase time for absorption
  - STEP procedure: laddering technique to increase bowel length

Small Intestinal Bacterial Overgrowth (SIBO) Syndrome
Etiology
- Definition: bacterial overgrowth of a stagnant loop of small bowel
- Cause: stricture, fistula, bypassed or defunctionalized segment, and diverticulum
- Intestinal motility disorders, irritable bowel syndrome (IBS), and chronic pancreatitis may contribute in up to 90% of cases
- Pathophysiology: **vitamin B12 is consumed by the bacteria leading to megaloblastic anemia and B12 deficiency; bile salts are deconjugated by the bacteria and steatorrhea develops; other nutrients are lost secondary to direct mucosal injury from bacteria and their metabolic products**

Diagnosis
- Jejunal aspirate and culture: nonpractical diagnostic standard ($>10^3$–10^5 organisms/mL)
- Carbohydrate breath test (e.g., lactulose or glucose test): administer carbohydrate load and measure hydrogen/methane in breath in absolute terms and peak patterns

Treatment
- Fluid and electrolyte repletion
- Treatment of overgrowth with antibiotics: prokinetics, octreotide
- Surgical resection of "blind" segment

6-7: VASCULAR ENTITIES

Acute Mesenteric Ischemia
Etiology
- Arterial embolus (40–50%)
  - Cardiac source: **atrial fibrillation** >> endocarditis or ventricular clot
  - **Most clots (85%) lodge 6–8 cm past the SMA origin,** 15% at origin (due to the oblique angle of SMA); **clinically spares proximal jejunum**
- Arterial thrombosis (20–30%)
  - Requires disease in more than one vessel; plaque near the origin of the vessel
- Non-occlusive mesenteric ischemia (20%): splanchnic hypoperfusion
  - Older, ill patients with episode of decreased cardiac output (e.g., after MI, on pressor therapy, hypovolemia, acute valvular insufficiency, or aortic dissection); also described as low flow state
- Venous thrombosis (10%)
  - Hypercoagulable state (90%): factor V Leiden, lupus anticoagulant, protein C or S deficiency, and antithrombin III deficiency
  - Other risk factors (10%): obesity, previous DVTs, hepatosplenomegaly, hepatic disease, malignancies, pancreatitis, polycythemia, sickle cell disease, postoperative

Clinical Presentation
- **Pain out of proportion to exam**
- Arterial embolus: **classically, acute onset with pain out of proportion to examination in patient with atrial fibrillation;** watery diarrhea and nausea are common; bloody diarrhea and peritoneal signs are late findings associated with ischemia
- Arterial thrombosis: may occur in patients with previous attacks of mesenteric insufficiency ("abdominal angina") or may occur as an initial event
- Nonocclusive mesenteric ischemia: critically ill patient with abdominal pain, diarrhea, or lactic acidosis; requires high degree of suspicion
- Venous thrombosis: presentation varies based on degree of thrombosis and necrosis

- Labs: generally evidence of hypovolemia with elevated hematocrit and BUN/Cr; metabolic acidosis with elevated serum lactate and base deficit is common; may have elevation of potassium, phosphorus, AST, ALT, amylase, LDH, CPK, and alkaline phosphatase; leukocytosis with a left shift is common

Imaging
- Mesenteric duplex ultrasound: little use in the acute setting; limited by body habitus, bowel gas, and operator experience
- CT angiogram: can demonstrate atherosclerotic disease; 64% specificity and 92% sensitivity in acute setting; test of choice if venous disease suspected
- MR angiogram: better for disease at SMA origin
- Angiogram: "gold standard" in acute setting; may be contraindicated in severely ill patients or those with renal dysfunction; +/– therapeutic in certain situations

Nonsurgical Treatment
- Resuscitation
  - **All patients will likely require fluid and electrolyte resuscitation**
  - **Broad-spectrum antibiotics**
  - **Vasopressors as needed, preferably agents that increase splanchnic blood flow, such as dobutamine, low-dose dopamine, or milrinone**
  - Systemic anticoagulation if no contraindication exists
- Percutaneous treatment options: may be attempted for acute arterial occlusions. Infusions of tissue plasminogen activator can dissolve some clots and intra-arterial papaverine can benefit some patients with nonocclusive disease; sheath can be left in place for repeat procedures

Surgical Treatment
- Prep leg into field to have access to saphenous vein
- Key points: exposure, proximal, and distal control, consider second look in 12–24 hours (see Chapter 14)
- Arterial embolus: **transverse arteriotomy distal to occlusion,** embolectomy catheters proximally and distally, and primary closure
- Arterial thrombus: **longitudinal arteriotomy,** thrombectomy, and vein patch angioplasty or bypass of affected segment; can use synthetic graft unless necrotic bowel; can consider endovascular stenting if no concern for necrotic bowel
- Nonocclusive mesenteric ischemia: surgical resection of necrotic bowel; usually add arterial papaverine + heparin
- Venous thrombosis: systemic heparinization and avoid low cardiac output; identify primary clotting disorder

Chronic Mesenteric Ischemia
Etiology
- **Requires >70% stenosis of two or three vessels (Celiac, SMA, and IMA)**
- Most patients are smokers with DM, HTN, PVD, or CAD

Clinical Presentation
- Symptoms: dull, crampy, **postprandial pain, within 30–60 minutes of eating**
- **Food aversion** develops leading to **weight loss**
- Signs: abdominal bruit (50%)

Imaging
- US: screening
- **CT abdomen/pelvis with IV contrast initial study of choice**
- Angiography: "gold standard"

Treatment
- Angioplasty (PTA): preferred in most patients
  - Similar outcomes as open approach: 80% with <50% residual angiographic stenosis at 3 years, 50% have weight gain
  - Complications: reperfusion syndrome (depends on severity of lesion)
  - Delayed re-stenosis: managed with repeat angioplasty
- Angioplasty with stent: may improve primary patency, but similar long-term patency compared with PTA
- Surgical reconstruction
  - Bypass from abdominal aorta to occluded mesenteric vessel
  - Conduit: greater saphenous vein preferred
  - Mesenteric endarterectomy or re-implantation of vessel

Median Arcuate Ligament (Dunbar) Syndrome
Epidemiology
- Compression of celiac artery by median arcuate ligament of the diaphragm
- Rare and controversial disease, four times more common in women

Clinical Presentation
- Symptoms: vague pain that typically progresses slowly over years, variable in timing, no "food fear"
- Signs: epigastric bruit increased with expiration (50%)

Treatment
- Surgery: expose root of vessel, divide the arcuate ligament and overlying nerves

SMA (Wilkie) Syndrome
Etiology
- Compression of the third portion of the duodenum by the SMA or one of its branches after abrupt loss of fat pad between the SMA and the aorta
- Risk factors: eating disorders causing acute weight loss or after surgery (disruption of anatomy)

Clinical Presentation
- Symptoms: proximal bowel obstruction with early satiety, postprandial bloating, epigastric pain, and relief with vomiting

Imaging
- Angiography: gold standard
- UGI, CTA: shows abrupt stop of oral contrast at third portion of duodenum

Treatment
- Conservative: fluid and electrolyte resuscitation, correct contributing factors, nutrition with small frequent meals; psychiatry evaluation if underlying eating disorder
- Surgical—three classic options:
  - Division of ligament of Treitz and mobilize duodenum with placement of duodenum to the left of the SMA
  - Division of and anterior transposition of third part of duodenum in front of SMA
  - Duodenojejunal bypass

6-8: NEOPLASMS
Benign Lesions
Clinical Presentation
- Usually vague, asymptomatic
- Symptoms: bleeding, anemia, and obstruction

Classification
- Adenoma (35% overall): 20% occur in the duodenum, 30% jejunum, and 50% ileum
  - Brunner gland adenoma: no malignant potential
  - True adenomas: malignant potential
  - Villous adenomas: 35–50% harbor malignancy
- Hamartoma (Peutz–Jeghers syndrome)
  - Autosomal dominant lesion with high penetrance
  - Often multiple perioral and buccal hyper-pigmented lesions
  - Jejunum and ileum most commonly affected
  - **50% have additional lesions in colon or rectum, 25% gastric polyps**
  - **No malignant potential**
  - Resect for intussusception or bleeding
- Leiomyoma: firm submucosal mass of well-differentiated smooth muscle tissue
  - Must be differentiated from leiomyosarcoma by tissue biopsy
  - **Most common benign lesion to cause symptoms** (bleeding and anemia)
- Lipoma: most commonly small submucosal lesion in ileum
  - Low attenuation on CT
  - Excised only if symptomatic
- Hemangioma: submucosal proliferation of blood vessels, 60% are multiple, most common in jejunum
  - **Can be seen in Osler-Weber-Rendu syndrome and Turner syndrome**
  - Diagnosis: angiography
  - Treatment: angiographic ablation or surgical resection

Malignant Lesions

Carcinoma (50%) (Ann Surg. 2009;249:63; World J Gastroint Oncol. 2011;3:33)
- Epidemiology
  - Average age: 50 years
  - Genetic risk factors: HNPCC, FAP, celiac sprue, and Crohn's
  - **Location: mostly occurs in the duodenum or proximal jejunum**
- Clinical presentation: symptoms depend on location
- Treatment
  - **Wide oncologic local resection**
  - **Whipple procedure if mass in the first or second portion of duodenum**
  - If advanced disease: palliative resection or bypass may be indicated to prevent obstruction or ongoing bleeding
  - Adjuvant therapy has little benefit
- Prognosis
  - Duodenal lesions
    - Stage I, 100%; Stage II, 52%; Stage III, 45%; Stage IV, 0%
  - Distal small bowel: survival correlates with lymph node status
    - 60–70% 5-year survival in node-negative disease
    - 12–14% 5-year survival with positive nodes

Carcinoid Tumor (40%)
- Etiology
  - Originates from Kulchitsky (enterochromaffin) cells in the crypts of Lieberkühn
    Vast majority found in appendix (46%), ileum (28%), and rectum (17%)
- **Search entire small bowel because up to 30% patients have multiple tumors**
- Clinical presentation: most asymptomatic
  - Vague abdominal pain, diarrhea or bowel obstruction
- Diagnosis: 24-hour urine for 5'-HIAA (serotonin metabolite), pentagastrin stimulation
- Imaging: octreotide scan, cardiac echo (right-sided valvular fibrosis)
- Treatment
  - Small bowel: <1 cm and negative LN: local resection; >1 cm or + LN: wide resection
  - Appendix
    - 2 cm at tip: simple appendectomy
    - 2 cm, involves the base, or evidence of +LN: right hemicolectomy
  - Rectal
    - 2 cm or fixed: abdominoperineal resection
    - Metastases: debulk + streptozocin and 5-FU; hepatic lesions—RFA or resection

Carcinoid Syndrome (<5%)
Only Once Metastasizes to Liver
Episodic
• Watery diarrhea
• Flushing
• Sweating
• Dyspnea
• Abdominal pain
• Rarely, right heart failure
Treatment
• Somatostatin (relieve symptoms)

Sarcoma (10–15%)
- Treatment
  - En-bloc resection if possible (50% unresectable at the time of diagnosis)
  - Adjuvant treatment has no clear benefit
- Prognosis: based on histologic grade

Lymphoma (15–20%)
- Epidemiology
  - 10% of all GI tract malignancies
  - Age: sixth or seventh decade; in children <10 it is the most common bowel tumor
  - Histology: predominantly B-cell lymphoma (except in celiac sprue, then T cell)
- Prognosis
  - Worse if high grade, extra-intestinal disease, increased number of lesions, perforation, or post-operative residual disease
- Treatment: CHOP (cyclophosphamide, doxorubicin, vincristine, prednisone) + XRT

KATHRYN A. STACKHOUSE • JENNIFER F. TSENG

7-1: BILIARY STONES AND ASSOCIATED COMPLICATIONS

Biliary Stones
Incidence
- General population: 10–20% within a lifetime, risk increases with age, women > men
- Select groups with increased incidence: transplant recipients (30–40%), hemoglobinopathies: hereditary spherocytosis (85%), sickle cell (70%), thalassemias (25%); prolonged TPN (35%), and rapid weight loss (30–40%)
- **Female, fat, fertile, and 40:** three times as likely due to estrogen effect
- **Most are asymptomatic;** <20% develop biliary colic; 4% will develop cholecystitis, obstructive jaundice, or gallstone pancreatitis

Etiology
- Homeostatic imbalance of the three major constituents of bile: bile salts, cholesterol, and phospholipids (90% lecithin)

Types of Stones
Nonpigmented Stones
• 75% of stones found in Western countries
Pigmented Stones
• Insolubilization of unconjugated bilirubin + precipitation of calcium bilirubinate
Brown stones

Complications of Biliary Stone Disease
• Symptomatic cholelithiasis
• Choledocholithiasis (common bile duct [CBD] stones)
• Cholecystitis
• Cholangitis
• Gallstone pancreatitis
• Gallstone ileus
• Mirizzi syndrome

Symptomatic Cholelithiasis and Biliary Colic
Etiology
- Transient obstruction of the cystic duct (CD) or common bile duct (CBD) by stones or sludge, causing GB distension

Clinical Presentation
- Symptoms
  - Nausea
  - **Biliary colic pain: abrupt onset, constant, localized to the RUQ, or epigastrium with rare radiation to the back or R scapula**
  - Lasting hours and usually occurring after meals
- Exam
  - Tenderness in the RUQ and epigastrium *without* fever or signs of peritonitis
- Labs: all normal except for possible nonspecific elevation in alkaline phosphatase

Imaging
- Plain films: only 10% of stones are radiopaque, making plain films of little value
- RUQ US: initial study of choice
  - **95% sensitivity in detecting GB stones**
  - Echogenic, mobile structures with posterior acoustic shadowing within the GB
    - Treatment = cholecystectomy

Choledocholithiasis (CBD Stones)
Etiology
- 5–10% of patients with symptomatic cholelithiasis will have concurrent CBD stones
- Complications: cholangitis, pancreatitis, and, rarely, benign biliary strictures

Clinical Presentation
- Symptoms
  - **Similar to symptomatic cholelithiasis but with hyperbilirubinemia**
  - +/– transient dark urine and acolic stools

- Examination: similar to symptomatic cholelithiasis +/– icterus and jaundice
- Labs
  - **Elevation of alkaline phosphatase and GGT +/– indirect and direct bilirubin**
  - CBC, amylase, and lipase are normal

Imaging
- RUQ US: operator-dependent and poor sensitivity for CBD stones
  - Highly sensitive in detecting bile duct dilatation: **normal CBD diameter is 6 mm** (baseline diameters up to 8 mm in elderly)
- MRCP and endoscopic US: high sensitivity; no therapeutic intervention *(Endosc Ultrasound. 2016;5(2):118–128.)*
- Endoscopic retrograde cholangiopancreatography (**ERCP**): **diagnostic and therapeutic**
- Intraoperative cholangiography (IOC) and US: high sensitivity for CBD stones

Treatment
- Prompt removal of stones is necessary to avoid progression to cholangitis
- ERCP: sphincterotomy and stone extraction
  - Performed preoperative or postoperative in institutions where CBD exploration (CBDE) is not performed OR when complete CBD clearance is not obtained after intraoperative exploration
  - Failure rates (4–10% range, <1% mortality, and 10% morbidity risk)
  - **Complications: # 1 pancreatitis (up to 10–15%)**
- CBDE via transcystic and transductal approaches
- Transduodenal sphincteroplasty

Complications of ERCP
• #1: Pancreatitis
• Bleeding
• Duodenal perforation
• Cholangitis

Cholecystitis
Etiology
- Infectious
  - Obstruction of the CD by gallstones or biliary sludge causes GB distension and bile stasis, leading to bacterial overgrowth and eventual infection
  - Positive bile cultures in 50–75% of patients
  - **# 1 → gram-negative bacteria (*Escherichia coli*, *Klebsiella*, and *Enterobacter*)**
  - Also *Enterococcus* and anaerobes
- Sterile
  - GB distends with continued mucous secretion leading to venous congestion
  - Progresses to decreased arterial inflow and eventual inflammation and ischemia
  - Recurrent, transient episodes may lead to chronic inflammation
- Acalculous: risk factors
  - Critically ill patients (i.e., trauma and burn) with bile stasis
  - Following episodes of global hypoperfusion
  - Prolonged TPN

Clinical Presentation
- Symptoms: RUQ/epigastric pain, fever, +/– nausea/vomiting, and anorexia
  - **Pain is constant and may radiate to the R shoulder or scapula and does not resolve with time, persisting beyond a few hours and escalating**
- Physical examination: low-grade fever, tachycardia, and RUQ tenderness to palpation
  - **Positive Murphy sign: halt in inspiration with deep RUQ palpation** (irritation of diaphragm as it descends during inspiration)
- Labs: mild leukocytosis
  - High leukocytosis: gangrenous gallbladder, cholangitis, or pancreatitis
  - Alkaline phosphatase and GGT are frequently elevated

Ultrasound Characteristics of Cholecystitis
• Gallbladder wall thickening (normal <4 mm)
• Pericholecystic fluid
• **Sonographic Murphy sign (has the highest sensitivity)**
• +/– Stones or sludge

Diagnosis
- RUQ US: **initial study of choice in most centers**
  - Operator-dependent with a sensitivity of only 60–70% in some studies
- HIDA scan: 95% sensitivity and specificity
  - Use when US is negative but clinical suspicion is high
  - Radionucleotide injected IV, taken up by hepatocytes, eventually excreted in bile
  - **CD obstruction/cholecystitis are confirmed if GB does not fill in 4 hours**

Treatment
- Antibiotics
  - **Start promptly once the diagnosis is made; stop postoperative unless gangrenous**
  - **Broad spectrum** (ampicillin–sulbactam [Unasyn] or quinolone/metronidazole)
- Cholecystectomy
  - **Perform within 72 hours of initial onset of symptoms, "golden window"**
- Percutaneous cholecystostomy (PTC)
  - Patients too unstable to undergo an operation or have significant comorbidities
  - Allows for decompression of the gallbladder via an external drain
  - Cholecystectomy can ultimately be undertaken at a later time if appropriate
- Cut-down cholecystostomy
  - Critically ill patients; can usually be undertaken at the bedside in an ICU setting

Cholangitis
Etiology
- Obstruction of the biliary tree and bile stasis that inhibits the normal clearance of ascending bacteria from the duodenum, leading to eventual infection (most common)
- Seeding of the biliary system from hematogenous spread of bacteria
- Iatrogenic
  - Strictures: traumatic, ischemic, and anastomotic
  - Foreign bodies: obstructed stents/endoprostheses
  - Biliary tract instrumentation
- Noniatrogenic
  - Choledocholithiasis (most common)
  - Pancreatitis and its complications (chronic or acute inflammation, and pseudocysts)
  - Mirizzi syndrome
  - Choledochal cysts
  - Biliary or pancreatic neoplasms
  - Oriental cholangiohepatitis

Clinical Presentation
- Signs and symptoms
  - **Charcot triad: fever (90%), RUQ abdominal pain and tenderness (70%), jaundice (60%) → all three (50–75%)**
  - **Reynold pentad (suggestive of systemic sepsis):**
    Charcot's triad + mental status changes + hypotension +/– Murphy sign or diffuse peritonitis, and tachycardia
- Labs
  - Leukocytosis with left shift, +/– coagulopathy
  - Elevated alkaline phosphatase, GGT, and bilirubin
  - Elevated transaminases: severe ascending infection and possible hepatic microabscess

Treatment
- **Drain biliary system**
- **Aggressive fluid resuscitation**
- **Reverse coagulopathy with Vitamin K and FFP**
- **IV empiric antibiotics**
  - Polymicrobial infection with gram-negative bacteria
  - Anaerobes more common than in cholecystitis, especially in patients with prior manipulation of the biliary tree
  - Metronidazole + fluoroquinolone or ampicillin–sulbactam (Unasyn)

Biliary System Drainage
- **ERCP: cornerstone of treatment**
  - Cholangiography, sphincterotomy, and removal of CBD stones
  - Change out and culture obstructed stents and biopsy any masses

- PTC: if ERCP fails or is unavailable
  - Higher associated morbidity, including bleeding and biloma
  - Externalized drains should be opened to gravity drainage
- Operative decompression: mortality is high and should be used as a last resort at high volume centers
  - No attempt to remove stones, treat strictures, or remove the GB should be made
  - Perform CBD ductotomy, extract immediately visible stones, and place T-tube for decompression, using absorbable sutures in CBD closure
  - Other options: choledochoduodenostomy or jejunostomy, sphincteroplasty
  - If porta hepatitis scarred down, make a transverse incision in the second part of duodenum at level of ampulla, sphincteroplasty, and remove stone
- **Definite treatment with cholecystectomy once the patient has stabilized and obstruction relieved either during that hospitalization or at a later date**

Gallstone Ileus
Etiology—Rare
- Large gallstone, usually >2.5 cm, passes into the GI tract causing mechanical obstruction in bowel
- Stone is initially impacted in the GB, causing localized pressure necrosis
- **Inflammatory adhesions between the GB and surrounding structures (transverse colon, duodenum, and antrum), with eventual fistulization and passage into GI tract**

Clinical Presentation
- Typical signs of GI obstruction (nausea, vomiting, distension, and constipation)
- Bouveret syndrome: gastric outlet obstruction with proximal GI fistulization
  - Stone obstructs in the pylorus or duodenal bulb
- Small bowel obstruction: most common presentation
  - Stone passes more distally and most frequently obstructs at the ileocecal valve

Imaging
- Plain films: **"Rigler triad": pneumobilia, small bowel air–fluid levels, and gallstone**
- CT scan: air or oral contrast in gall bladder or biliary tree with bowel obstruction

Treatment
- Stone extraction
  - Longitudinal enterotomy proximal to palpable stone, "milk" stone back for extraction, and transverse closure of the enterotomy in two layers
  - Bowel resection with primary anastomosis if full-thickness bowel wall necrosis
- Cholecystenteric fistula
  - Cholecystectomy with takedown of the fistula and closure of bowel—reasonable if patient stable and can be safely performed through same incision

Mirizzi Syndrome
Etiology
- **Impaction of multiple small stones or a single large stone in the infundibulum or the CD leading to inflammation, CBD obstruction, and jaundice**
- Inflammation can cause adherence of the CD to the CBD, with subsequent stricturing
- External compression of CBD can lead to pressure necrosis and cholecystobiliary fistula

Clinical Presentation
- Abdominal pain
- Hyperbilirubinemia
- Usually jaundice
- +/– Symptoms consistent with cholecystitis and cholangitis

Diagnosis
- CT or MRCP: when malignancy is suspected as the cause of obstruction
- ERCP or PTC: helpful in determining the cause and level of obstruction
  - Identify a fistula as well as external compression laterally and duct narrowing
  - Stent placement can help control jaundice and facilitate operative repair
- Intraoperative: shrunken GB, severe inflammation and a fibrotic mass in the triangle of Calot, and dense adhesions in the subhepatic space

Classification
- Type I: hepatic duct compressed by large stone impacted in CD
- Type II–IV: based on extent of compromise of the common hepatic and bile duct
  - Type II: <1/3 of bile duct involved by the fistula
  - Type III: 1/3–2/3 of the bile duct involved by the fistula
  - Type IV: >2/3 of the bile duct involved by the fistula

Treatment
- **Open cholecystectomy**
- Type I: subtotal cholecystectomy, remove stones, and leave adherent portion of the GB
- Type II–IV: **subtotal cholecystectomy**
  - Identify fistula when bile is seen leaking from the remnant GB
  - **Place T-tube through fistula defect and close remnant GB around it**
  - Use the remnant GB neck as a flap to close the defect
  - If the remnant GB tissue is too friable or the defect is large, bring up a loop of bowel and perform a biliary–enteric bypass and remove diseased tissue; hepaticojejunostomy may be necessary in severe cases.
- Biliary decompression
  - ERCP stent placement and stone extraction or PTC drain in patients unable to tolerate surgical correction

---

7-2: Congenital Abnormalities

Choledochal Cysts
Etiology
- Congenital malunion of the pancreaticobiliary ducts, leading to reflux of pancreatic enzymes and damage to the bile duct epithelium, duct dilation, and cyst formation
- **Sequelae: increased risk of jaundice, recurrent cholangitis, acute pancreatitis, biliary strictures, choledocholithiasis, and cholangiocarcinoma**

Todani Modification of Alonso–Lej System for Classification of Choledochal Cysts
Type I (85%): saccular, cystic, or fusiform dilation of extrahepatic biliary tree
Type II (3%): true, single diverticulum of the extrahepatic biliary tree
Type III (1%): choledochocele: cystic dilation of the distal CBD that protrudes into the lumen of the duodenum
Type IV (10%): multifocal cystic disease of both intra- and extrahepatic biliary tree
Type V (1%): Caroli disease: single or multifocal cystic disease confined to the intrahepatic biliary tree

Clinical Presentation
- Children
  - **Triad: RUQ pain, jaundice, palpable abdominal mass +/– nausea, vomiting, and fever**
  - Normal labs except for elevated bilirubin
- Adults
  - RUQ or epigastric pain and jaundice, palpable mass is rare +/– nausea, vomiting, and fever
  - Diagnosed after recurrent bouts of pancreatitis or RUQ pain after cholecystectomy
  - Elevated bilirubin, alkaline phosphatase, and GGT
  - Signs of cirrhosis if longstanding partial biliary obstruction
- Complications
  - Peritonitis: if cyst ruptures and creates bilious ascites (rare)
  - Cholangitis: biliary obstruction with sludge

Imaging
- RUQ US: **study of choice in children;** biliary tree patency can rule out biliary atresia
- CT scan: **first study in older populations**
- MRCP: preoperative planning
- PTC: **invasive study of choice** and possibility of transhepatic stents
- HIDA scan: neonates with a prenatal diagnosis of a biliary abnormality
  - **If the biliary system is not patent, the patient is treated for biliary atresia**

Treatment

- **All suitable operative candidates must undergo resection given the cyst's malignant potential and the number of other possible complications**
- Type I and IV
  - Cyst resection with an excision of the entire lining and all abnormal ducts
  - Re-establish biliary drainage with an end-to-side choledochojejunostomy (type I) or hepaticojejunostomy (type IV) with a standard Roux-en-Y drainage limb
- Type II: simple cyst excision with transverse closure of the CBD
- Type III (choledochocele): transduodenal cyst excision and sphincteroplasty
- Type V (Caroli disease)
  - If disease localized to one-half of the biliary tree, perform a hepatic resection
  - If extensive hepatic fibrosis or bilateral intrahepatic duct involvement: transplant

---

7-3: BILIARY TRACT MALIGNANCIES

Gallbladder Cancer

Epidemiology

- Risk factors
  - **Chronic cholelithiasis (# 1, stones >2.5 cm)**
  - Porcelain GB (calcification of the GB wall)
  - Primary sclerosing cholangitis (recommend annual ultrasound screening)
  - Chronic infection (salmonella, helicobacter)
  - Anomalous pancreaticobiliary duct junction
  - Medications (methyldopa, isoniazid)
  - Obesity
- **Overall 5-year survival <5%**
- About 80–95% adenocarcinomas (papillary, tubular, mucinous, or signet-cell type)

Metastasis

- Direct invasion
- Lymphatic
- Hematogenous: #1 lung and brain
- Can seed the peritoneum, port sites, and wounds

Clinical Presentation

- Incidental: most found incidentally in 1–2% of all cholecystectomies
  - Mucosal-based lesions (T1a)
  - Five-year survival: 85–100% for T1a disease
  - Can seed peritoneum or trocar-site after spillage
- Symptomatic: pain (colic) and jaundice
- Labs: occasional elevations in alkaline phosphatase, transaminases, CEA, and CA19-9

Imaging

- RUQ US: 38% accuracy; 50% sensitivity for liver infiltration or nodal metastasis
- EUS: Sensitivity 92%, specificity 88%; useful for staging and for obtaining bile for cytologic analysis
- ERCP: Mid-bile duct obstruction is GB cancer until proven otherwise
- CT or MRCP: depth of liver invasion, lymph nodes, vasculature involvement, invasion of the hepatoduodenal ligament, and lungs
- PET scan: staging; not useful to determine need for further resection after cholecystectomy (often positive in absence of disease after surgery)

Treatment

- Basic principles
  - **Surgical treatment is the only chance of cure**
  - **Staging laparoscopy to rule out advanced disease**
  - Survival benefit is seen only in those with R0 resection, not debulking
  - Positive margins or lesions extending beyond the lamina propria found on routine cholecystectomy require re-exploration when resectable disease is identified
- Unresectable lesions
  - Peritoneal and distant metastases
  - Locally unresectable: vascular invasion, involvement of multiple adjacent organs
- Limited to lamina propria: TIS or T1a lesions *(Ann Surg. 2008;247(5):835–838.)*
  - **Cholecystectomy with negative margins is curative in >85% of patients**
  - **Open cholecystectomy to decrease risk of bile spillage and peritoneal seeding**
- Muscle layer involvement: T1b or T2 lesions *(J Am Coll Surg. 2008; 207(3):371–382.)*
  - More likely to have regional lymph node spread

- **Radical cholecystectomy: gallbladder + 2 cm of hepatic parenchyma of GB fossa + lymphadenectomy (porta hepatis, gastroduodenal and gastrohepatic ligaments, and retroduodenal nodes)**
- Main bile duct involvement requires excision and biliary reconstruction
- Invasion of visceral peritoneum, adjacent structures, or vascular structures: T3 or T4
  (Ann Surg. 2005;241(3):385–394.)
  - If distant disease or peritoneal seeding is not present, resection may be attempted with diagnostic laparoscopy to decrease unnecessary laparotomy
  - En bloc resection of involved adjacent organs, including pancreas in highly selected cases
  - Liver resection ranges from wedge to trisegmentectomy with central portal nodes
  - Median survival time 17 months; mortality 2%
- Palliation
- **If unresectable disease found during laparotomy, do biliary–enteric bypass**
- If known preoperatively, relieve biliary obstruction with ERCP stenting or PTC drain placement for decompression, followed by internal stenting
- Locoregionally advanced unresectable disease: FU-based chemo + radiation
- Systemic chemotherapy: gemcitabine + cisplatin and radiation for local control
  - No randomized trials to define optimal regimen

Cholangiocarcinoma

Definition: bile duct cancer arising in the intrahepatic, perihilar, or extrahepatic biliary tree, exclusive of gallbladder and ampulla of Vater

Epidemiology
- Risk factors: primary sclerosing cholangitis, choledochal cysts, intrahepatic stones, and infection with the liver fluke *Clonorchis sinensis*, HBV/HCV, cirrhosis, Lynch syndrome, obesity/metabolic syndrome

Classification *(Nat Rev Gastroenterol Hepatol. 2011;8(9):512–522)*
- Proximal (intrahepatic and hilar)
- Central extrahepatic
- Distal intrahepatic (intrapancreatic)
- Hilar carcinoma = Klatskin tumors bridge both the left- and right-sided systems

Clinical Presentation
- Symptoms
  - Nonspecific findings: anorexia, weight loss, malaise, and fatigue
  - Intrahepatic lesions: abdominal pain
  - Hilar and distal bile duct lesions: biliary obstruction and jaundice
- Labs
  - Elevation of tumor markers: CEA, CA19-9, AFP—nonspecific
  - Elevation of alkaline phosphatase and GGT
  - Extrahepatic lesions causing biliary obstruction will have an elevated bilirubin

Imaging
- US and CT: first
- MRCP: define biliary tract anatomy and examines liver parenchyma
- PTC or ERCP: decompression if biliary obstruction, bile duct brushings, and FNA
- CTA: assess involvement of major vasculature
- PET: changes surgical management in 25% of cases, usually by detecting distant disease

Treatment
- **Resection is the only hope for cure (30–50% of patients)**
  - Elective after optimization of comorbidities
  - **Exhaustive search for metastatic disease with staging laparoscopy +/– intraoperative ultrasound (IOUS)**
  - Preoperative stenting in patients with biliary sepsis or markedly elevated bilirubin (preoperative manipulation increases infectious complications—avoid if possible)
  - **Must leave at least 25% of normal functioning liver** that has adequate arterial inflow, venous outflow, and biliary drainage
    - Portal vein embolization: on side of proposed resection and contralateral hypertrophies

- Criteria for resectability:
  - Absence of retropancreatic and paraceliac nodal metastases or distant liver metastases
  - Absence of invasion of the main portal vein or main hepatic artery (some centers will do en bloc resection with vascular reconstruction)
  - Absence of extrahepatic adjacent organ invasion
  - Absence of disseminated disease
- Intrahepatic lesions
  - Nonanatomic wedge resection for peripheral lesions
  - Anatomic hepatectomies for more extensive disease
  - Lymphadenectomy does not provide therapeutic benefit
- Hilar lesions
  - Resect entire extrahepatic biliary tree, including the GB and bile duct bifurcation
  - Roux-en-Y hepaticojejunostomy
  - Perform extensive hilar lymphadenectomy
- Distal extrahepatic
  - Pancreaticoduodenectomy
  - Curable resection is far more likely (metastatic disease must be absent)
  - Portal vein and SMV involvement is a relative contraindication
- Adjuvant therapy (nccn.org)
  - Acceptable options include gemcitabine or FU-based chemotherapy
  - May consider radiation after noncurative resection

Palliation
- **Biliary decompression with ERCP-placed self-expanding (metal) stent**
  - Stent occlusions are frequent and can be replaced
  - PTC drain placement can reestablish bile drainage into the duodenum once an internalized stent is placed
  - Biliary–enteric bypass above the hilum (i.e., segment III ductal drainage)

7-4: OPERATIVE TECHNIQUES AND BILE DUCT INJURIES

Contraindications for Laparoscopic Cholecystectomy
Absolute
• Inability to tolerate general anesthesia
• "Frozen abdomen" due to prior surgery or peritonitis
Relative
• Prior RUQ abdominal surgery
• Portal hypertension
• Uncorrected coagulopathy
• Cholecystenteric fistulas
• First or third trimester of pregnancy
• Gallbladder cancer

Laparoscopic Cholecystectomy
Technique
- Positioning
  - Monitors at 10 and 2 o'clock position relative to patient's head
  - Surgeon stands to the patient's left and assistant stands to patient's right
  - Reverse Trendelenburg once the abdomen is accessed
- Pneumoperitoneum: Veress needle or Hasson (open) periumbilical trocar
- Trocar placement
  - 10–12 mm in periumbilical incision
  - 5 or 10–12 mm epigastric, entering the peritoneum to the right of the falciform ligament, depending on surgeon preference
  - 5 mm as laterally as possible under the right costal margin
  - 5 mm in the midclavicular line a few centimeters below the costal margin
- Exposure
  - Retract the GB fundus over the liver via the lateral port
  - Retract the infundibulum laterally via the other 5-mm port
  - Take down adhesions with gentle traction and obtain critical view of safety

Figure 7-1 Critical view of laparoscopic cholecystectomy. (Illustrations reprinted with permission from Jones et al. *Atlas of Minimally Invasive Surgery*. Cine-Med, 2006. Copyright of the book and illustrations are retained by Cine-Med.)

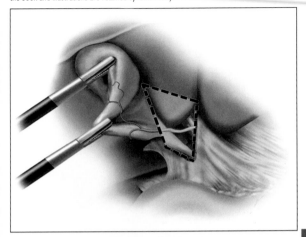

Dissection/Critical View

- Score the peritoneum with hook cautery; free the gallbladder from the peritoneal attachments to the liver proximally for a few centimeters on both sides
- **Dissect free the anterior and posterior aspects of Calot triangle to expose the "Critical View": only two structures (cystic duct [CD] and cystic artery) are seen traversing the triangle of Calot with only the liver posteriorly** (Fig. 7-1)
- Perform cholangiography if desired prior to division of the CD (see "Complications of Laparoscopic Cholecystectomy")
- Double-clip the CD and artery and then divide
- Use the hook cautery to free the GB from the hepatic bed in a retrograde fashion
- Assure hemostasis of liver bed with cautery or argon laser, remove any dropped stones, and irrigate the RUQ
- Gallbladder removal
  - Move camera to epigastric port. Place an endoscopic retrieval bag through the umbilical port. Place gallbladder in bag, close, and cut string. Remove along with umbilical port.

Complications of Laparoscopic Cholecystectomy

- Wound infection
- Abscess from spillage of infected bile or stones
- Retained CBD stones
- Bile leak from CD stump, ducts of Luschka, or major bile duct injuries
- Trocar or Veress needle injury (bowel or major vascular)
- Bleeding (cystic artery and liver bed)
- Late incisional hernias at port sites

(*Hepatogastroenterology*. 2012;59(113):47–50)

Intraoperative Cholangiography (IOC)

Indications (*J Gastrointest Surg*. 2013;17(3):434–442)

- No evidence that routine IOC in every patient prevents common duct injury
- Patients with CBD stones identified on preoperative imaging, not addressed by ERCP
- Hyperbilirubinemia due to suspected CBD stones
- Difficult cases in order to clearly identify central structures
- IOUS is a suitable alternative, which is cheaper and can be faster, operator-dependent

Technique (Fig. 7-2)

Figure 7-2 Intraoperative cholangiography. (Illustrations reprinted with permission from Jones et al. *Atlas of Minimally Invasive Surgery*. Cine-Med, 2006. Copyright of the book and illustrations are retained by Cine-Med.)

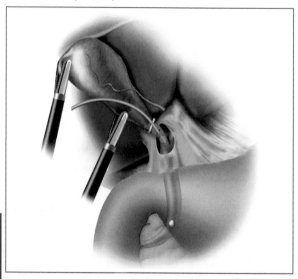

- Percutaneous
  - Puncture the abdominal wall with a 2-in 14G needle over the CD after a cystic ductotomy has been made
  - Pass a 5F catheter through the needle; guide it into the duct with a grasper via the epigastric port
  - Secure the catheter in place with a clip distal to the ductotomy
- Olsen cholangiogram clamp
  - Pass the specialized clamp into the abdomen via the subcostal port
  - Pass a 60-in 5F catheter through the clamp into the cystic ductotomy
  - To secure the catheter, close the clamp around the distal CD
- Milk out any CD stones or sludge via the ductotomy site
- After IOC is completed, place clips proximally and distally on the CD and divide the CD at the ductotomy site

Cholangiogram Findings
1. Contrast passes easily into the duodenum
• Failure of the duodenum to fill may also indicate complete CBD obstruction
2. Visualize the proximal biliary tree, including right and left hepatic duct systems
3. No filling defects in the bile ducts (stones)
• Do not confuse air bubbles with filling defects
• Assure that there is no extravasation of contrast

Laparoscopic Common Bile Duct Exploration (CBDE)
Technique for Transcystic Exploration
- Performed through the cystic ductotomy made for IOC
- Use if
  - Stones <8 mm
  - Less than eight stones are present
  - Stones are distal to CD entrance
  - CBD >3 mm in diameter

- Multiple, small stones (<2–3 mm)
  - Flush the duct and allow the stones to pass distally into the duodenum
  - Administer 1–2 mg of glucagon to relax the sphincter of Oddi
  - Can pass a balloon catheter (4–6 mm) over a wire to dilate the duct and ampulla
- Medium or large stones (or those that don't pass by flushing)
  - Balloon dilate the CBD to 8 mm (if needed)
  - Insert an angiocatheter and a helical stone basket (medium stones) or flat-wire Segura basket (large stones) using the modified Seldinger technique
  - Ensnared stones removed in a retrograde fashion through the ductotomy
  - Can also try pushing stones distally into duodenum
- Electrohydraulic lithotripsy
- Confirm CBD clearance with a completion cholangiogram

Technique for Transductal Exploration
- Use if
  - Failure of transcystic approach
  - Small (<4 mm diameter) or tortuous CD
  - Stones >8 mm
  - Stones proximal to the CD–CBD junction
- Make a longitudinal 1–2 cm incision on well-visualized CBD with laparoscopic scissors
- To clear the duct attempt irrigation and Fogarty catheters, basket techniques, and lithotripsy
- Confirm CBD clearance by choledochoscopy or IOC
- Close ductotomy primarily or over a T-tube (10–14 F), C-tube, or internalized biliary catheter

Impacted Stones
- Anterograde sphincterotomy
  - Pass a guidewire beyond the stone, then an endoscopic sphincterotome over the wire to the sphincter of Oddi
  - Perform concurrent endoscopy to the duodenum to ensure that the sphincterotomy is made at the 11 or 12 o'clock position
  - Push the stone into the duodenum with a choledochoscope
- In difficult situations, close over a T-tube to drain the proximal biliary tree and refer to ERCP for stone removal
- Convert to an open procedure with a transduodenal approach and sphincteroplasty or extensive Kocher maneuver with exposure of the retroduodenal and intrapancreatic bile duct

Bile Duct Injuries (Fig. 7-3) (Surg Clin North Am. 2014;94(2):297–310.)

Figure 7-3 Strasberg classification: Bile duct injuries. **A:** Leaks at cystic duct stump or gallbladder bed (do not require reconstruction). **B:** Occlusion of aberrant right hepatic duct. **C:** Transection of aberrant right hepatic duct. **D:** Partial (<50%) transection of major bile duct. **E:** Circumferential injury or stenosis of the main bile duct. **E1:** >2 cm from confluence of R and L bile ducts. **E2:** <2 cm from confluence of R and L bile ducts. **E3:** Confluence preserved but no remaining main hepatic duct. **E4:** No communication between right and left bile ducts. **E5:** Common hepatic duct and aberrant right hepatic duct injured simultaneously. (From Fischer JE, Bland KI. *Mastery of Surgery.* 5th ed. Philadelphia, PA: Lippincott Williams & Wilkins, 2007.)

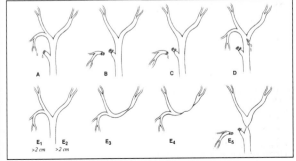

Risk Factors for Injury

- Failure to obtain the "Critical View" prior to division of structures
- Inflammation: distorts the normal anatomy
- Aberrant anatomy: most common abnormality is aberrant posterior R hepatic duct
- Improper technique
  - Failure to occlude the CD securely leading to CD stump leak
  - Errant deep dissection when removing the GB from the hepatic bed, leading to leaking from transected ducts of Luschka
  - Tenting injuries of the CBD due to improper (excessive lateral) retraction of GB
  - Thermal injuries to CBD from excessive use of electrocautery, leading to stricture or necrosis of the major ducts later in the postoperative course
- Failure to convert from a laparoscopic to open procedure if difficulty encountered

Classification Systems of Bile Duct Injuries

Strasburg Classification

- Modified Bismuth classification: reflects common injuries in laparoscopic era
- Type A: bile leak from a minor duct (duct of Luschka or CD stump), but **retaining continuity of the CBD**
- Type B: end lesion that isolates a part of the biliary tree due to occlusion injury (clipping or ligation), most commonly an aberrant R hepatic duct
- Type C: similar to a type B injury, but caused by transection without occlusion
- Type D: partial (<50% and usually lateral) transection of the major bile ducts (common, right, or left)
- Type E: circumferential injury to the major bile ducts, separating the hepatic parenchyma from the lower biliary tract and subclassified into E1–5 based on the level of transection or stricture

Bismuth Classification

- Describes biliary strictures and bile duct injuries based on the level of stricture or injury before the era of laparoscopic cholecystectomy
- Each type is now incorporated into Strasburg classification as Type E injuries

Clinical Presentation

- Intra-operative identification
  - Less than 25% of injuries are identified in the OR
  - Persistent leakage of bile from the hepatic bed or portahepatis indicates injury
  - Discovery of an open ductal structure during completion of the cholecystectomy
- Postoperative identification
  - **More common. The timing of presentation (days to months after) and the constellation of symptoms depend on the type (Strasburg type) of injury**
  - Type A (minor duct injury): vague symptoms of abdominal pain, anorexia, or failure to thrive. Can progress to fever, sepsis, and/or biliary–cutaneous fistulas
  - Type B (occlusion): may be silent or present very late with cholangitis or cirrhosis
  - Types C/D (transection): bile peritonitis or sepsis from an ongoing bile leak
  - Type E: usually apparent in OR or presents early with jaundice, abdominal pain

Diagnosis

- Intraoperative cholangiography: allows for earlier diagnosis
  - Consider conversion to an open procedure if aberrant or unclear anatomy is noted
- RUQ US: identifies fluid collections (bilomas or abscesses) and ductal dilatation
- HIDA scan: identify presence of leak and rate of flow
- CT: identify collections, ductal dilatation, liver damage; may identify level of injury
- **ERCP: identifies level of injury, potentially therapeutic (especially type A injuries)**
- PTC: preferred when transection or occlusion injuries are suspected; drains retrograde
- MRCP: full delineation of the biliary tree and all its radicals

Treatment

- The first attempt at repair is typically the most effective

- Intraoperative diagnosis: convert to an open procedure, unless a damage-control approach is adopted
  Type A (leakage from CD stump): meticulous closure and drainage
  Type D (partial transections and CD avulsion injuries): interrupted fine absorbable suture closure over a T-tube; bring out the T-tube through a separate incision
  Type B, C, and E (see "Technique")
  Damage control: place closed suction drains laparoscopically or percutaneously and close; **refer to a specialized hepatobiliary team once the patient is stable**
  (HPB Oxford. 2015;17(9):753–762.)
- Postoperative diagnosis
  First: percutaneously drain bilomas or abscesses
  Second: identify the type and nature of the injury (ERCP/PTC)
  Type A and D (CD stump leaks and transected ducts of Luschka): ERCP sphincterotomy and stent placement
  Type B, C, and E (transection and occlusion injuries): require operation
  PTC and drain placement to externally decompress the biliary tree
  Timing: in the first week if the patient is stable; otherwise wait 6 weeks to 3 months
- Small leaks may resolve with simple drainage when output is low (<300 cc/day)
- A continued leak after a week of drainage requires referral for ERCP

Technique
- Dissect bile ducts, identify injury, and debride back to healthy duct (good blood flow)
- End-to-end anastomosis: can attempt for complete bile duct transections and close over a T-tube; carries a 50% chance of stricture and generally not recommended
- Biliary–enteric anastomosis: Roux-en-Y reconstruction with a high hepaticojejunostomy on the hilar plate; strictures are the most common complication (15% over time) (Fig. 7-4)
- Extensive cirrhosis and hepatic insufficiency: requires hepatic resection +/- transplant

Figure 7-4 Biliary-enteric anastomosis. (From Fischer JE, Bland KI. *Mastery of Surgery.* 5th ed. Philadelphia, PA: Lippincott Williams & Wilkins; 2007.)

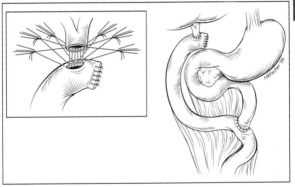

PANCREAS

MARIAM F. ESKANDER • MARK P. CALLERY

8-1: PANCREAS ANATOMY AND FUNCTION

Anatomy
Landmarks
- Head
  - Surrounded by the first and second portions of the duodenum
  - Sits to the right of the superior mesenteric vessels
- Uncinate (from the Latin for "hooked")
  - Sits inferior to the head of pancreas
  - Wraps around superior mesenteric vessels along third and fourth portions of duodenum
  - **Between superior mesenteric vein (SMV) and inferior vena cava**
- Neck: overlies superior mesenteric vessels
- Body: to the left of the superior mesenteric vessels
- Tail: most lateral (left) segment; abuts splenic hilum

Arterial Blood Supply
- Gastroduodenal artery
  - Provides superior pancreaticoduodenal artery
  - Supplies head, uncinate, and neck
- Superior mesenteric artery
  - Provides inferior pancreaticoduodenal artery
  - Supplies uncinate and head
- Dorsal pancreatic artery
  - Branch of the splenic artery (SA)
  - Releases two branches to the right—supplies neck
  - Releases one branch to the left (transverse pancreatic artery)—supplies the body
- Pancreatica magna artery
  - Branch of SA
  - Branch to the right also supplies the transverse pancreatic artery
  - Branch to the left forms caudal pancreatic artery which supplies the tail
- Caudal pancreatic artery
  - Branch from SA
  - May have more than one branch coming from SA

Venous Drainage
- Head and uncinate process: multiple veins draining into portal vein and SMV
- Body and tail: multiple veins draining into splenic vein (SV)

Ductal System
- **Main pancreatic duct (duct of Wirsung)**
  - Begins in tail and travels through the entire pancreas to the head
  - In the head, fuses with common bile duct (CBD) and **empties at ampulla of Vater**
  - Slightly more posterior throughout the pancreas
- Accessory pancreatic duct (duct of Santorini)
  - Comes off the main duct in the neck
  - Travels in a more anterior plane
  - Empties into the duodenum at the minor papilla
- Pancreas divisum (incidence 10%, most common congenital pancreatic anomaly)
  - Failure of fusion of the major and minor pancreatic ducts so that pancreas drains into minor papilla → could lead to intermittent obstruction of pancreatic duct (pancreatitis)

Pancreas Function
Endocrine
- Monitors glucose levels in portal circulation
- Hormones (insulin and glucagon) are released into the portal flow and help regulate the liver's response to meals and the processing of glucose
- Islets of Langerhans: comprise only 2% of total pancreas volume
  - Alpha cells: secrete glucagon, found on outer rim of islet, mainly in body and tail
  - Beta cells: secrete insulin, found in the islet core
  - D cells: secrete somatostatin, intermixed
  - PP cells: pancreatic polypeptide, mainly in head

Exocrine

- Produces multiple digestive enzymes that are responsible for the breakdown of food into useable nutrients
- Acinar cells: comprise 80% of pancreas volume
  - Secretin: stimulates secretion of pancreatic bicarbonate and water
  - CCK: stimulates pancreatic exocrine enzyme secretion and enhances bicarbonate
  - Somatostatin: inhibits pancreatic exocrine secretion

8-2: INFLAMMATORY CONDITIONS

Acute Pancreatitis

Etiology of Acute Pancreatitis
Alcohol (#1)
Gallstones (#2)
Iatrogenic
Pancreas divisum
Less common: medications, trauma, hypertriglyceridemia, auto-immune, hypercalcemia, ductal obstruction, malignancy, infections, familial, and idiopathic

Clinical Presentation
- Symptoms: abdominal pain, nausea, vomiting, bloating, fevers, and anorexia
- Signs: tachycardia, epigastric tenderness, distension, flank ecchymosis (Grey–Turner sign), periumbilical ecchymosis (Cullen sign), and shock

Diagnosis
- Clinical impression
- Laboratory values: elevated serum amylase and lipase levels

Imaging
- Abdominal x-ray
  - **"Sentinel loop": dilated proximal jejunum, air in duodenum,** ileus, and loss of psoas margins
- US: used to rule out gallstones, choledocholithiasis, and pseudocyst
- CT: more sensitive/specific; peripancreatic stranding, fluid collections, and necrosis

Treatment
- NPO and NGT for symptom relief
- **Aggressive IV fluid resuscitation, Foley catheter**
- Pain control
- ICU monitoring for severe cases
- Alcohol induced: withdrawal prophylaxis (Ativan or Valium)
- Stomach acid suppression may be beneficial
- Management of gallstone pancreatitis:
  - If pancreatitis severe, signs of cholangitis or persistent biliary obstruction → ERCP. (Routine use of ERCP is not advocated for patients with mild pancreatitis.)
  - Immediate surgical intervention NOT INDICATED—after resolution of pancreatitis, perform cholecystectomy to protect against further gallstone-related sequelae
  - If possibility of persistent choledocholithiasis, may also need intra-operative cholangiogram
  - Cholecystectomy should be performed prior to discharge because likelihood of recurrence is high, unless pancreatitis is severe in which case delayed cholecystectomy (after 6 weeks) is recommended
  - Elderly patients and those with multiple comorbidities who are not good surgical candidates should undergo ERCP with sphincterotomy as an alternative

Complications of Pancreatitis
• Pancreatic pseudocyst
• Endocrine and/or exocrine dysfunction
• Pancreatic necrosis
• Pancreatic duct strictures
• Hemorrhagic pancreatitis
• Chronic pancreatitis >>>
• Splenic vein thrombosis
• GI or biliary tract obstruction
• Pseudoaneurysms

Prognosis (World J Surg. 2002;26:612–619)
About 10–15% of patients will develop severe illness requiring prolonged hospitalization, extended ICU stays, and increased morbidity and mortality
- Many scoring systems and criteria: Ranson criteria, APACHE II, Imrie, and EWS
- APACHE II: can be used on admission and repeated throughout hospital stay. Points for age, previous health, temperature, heart rate, respiratory rate, mean arterial pressure, pH, Cr, K, Na, WBC, PaO_2, and GCS. A value of ≥8 means severe pancreatitis.

Ranson Criteria
On Admission (mnemonic GA LAW)
• Glucose >200 mg/dL
• AST >250 IU/L
• LDH >350 IU/L
• Age >55 yrs
• WBC >16,000
After 48 h (mnemonic CA and HOBBS)
• Calcium <8.0 mg/dL
• HCT fall >10%
• Oxygen (P_aO_2) <60 mm Hg
• BUN increase up >5 mg/dL after hydration
• Base deficit >—4 mmol/L
• Sequestration of fluid >6 L
Takes 48 h to calculate: combine criteria for both admission and 48 h
When ≥3 criteria reached → severe pancreatitis
Prognostic implications
• Score 0–2: <5% mortality
• Score 3–4: 15–20% mortality
• Score 5–6: 40% mortality
• Score 7–8: 100% mortality

(Surg Gynecol Obstet. 1974;139:69–81; Am J Gastroenterol. 1982;77:633)

Chronic Pancreatitis
Definition: chronic inflammation of the pancreas leading to scarring of the pancreatic parenchyma and/or stricturing of the pancreatic duct

Clinical Presentation
- Chronic intermittent nausea, vomiting, and abdominal pain with radiation to the back
- Weight loss
- Diabetes
- Pancreatic insufficiency with diarrhea/steatorrhea

Diagnosis
- Clinical history is the key

Imaging
- **Calcifications, gland atrophy, and dilation of pancreatic duct ("chain of lakes")**

Treatment (N Engl J Med. 1995;332:1482–1490)
- Acute setting: same as acute pancreatitis
- Remove underlying cause
- Treat underlying pancreatic enzyme insufficiency and diabetes
- Surgery: for chronic, unremitting pain
  - Generally, patients with large pancreatic duct require a decompressing procedure while those with small pancreatic duct require a resectional procedure
  - Modified Puestow procedure (lateral pancreaticojejunostomy) if large pancreatic duct
  - For focal inflammatory mass without significant dilation of the pancreatic duct, pancreatic head should be resected via either pancreaticoduodenectomy or duodenum-preserving pancreatic head resection (Beger procedure)
  - Transduodenal sphincteroplasty for ampullary stenosis or pancreas divisum
  - Celiac block (for pain control) if operative interventions fail

Pancreatic Pseudocyst
Definition: encapsulated collection of pancreatic secretions; wall of pseudocyst **does not** have epithelial lining (caused by inflammatory fibrosis that limits spread of pancreatic juice)

Etiology
- Acute pancreatitis
- Chronic ductal obstruction causing ductal blowout
- Trauma: acute ductal disruption

Clinical Presentation
- Symptoms: abdominal pain, nausea and vomiting (gastric outlet obstruction due to mass effect), fever, and weight loss
- Signs: jaundice (due to blockage of the intrapancreatic CBD), palpable mass in the epigastrium, and bleeding due to arterial injury from pancreatic juice

Differential Diagnosis of Pancreatic Cyst
• Pancreatic abscess
• Phlegmon or fluid collection
• Cystic neoplasm
• Serous cystadenoma/carcinoma: **low** viscosity, **low** CEA, **low** amylase
• Mucinous cystadenoma/carcinoma: high viscosity, high CEA, **low** amylase
• IPMN (intraductal papillary mucinous neoplasm): **high** viscosity, **high** CEA, **high** amylase
• Adenocarcinoma: high CA19–9
• Pseudocyst: low viscosity, low CEA, **high** amylase

Pseudocyst Treatment
- **Asymptomatic: can observe; 50% will resolve spontaneously in 4–6 weeks**
- **Pseudocyst >5 cm, persistent after 8–12 weeks: drainage**
- **Symptomatic:** endoscopic or surgical (laparoscopic vs. open) intestinal drainage procedure—allows pancreatic juice to mix with ingested food to maximize digestion
- About 5% of cysts are neoplastic; if any concern of malignancy, biopsy the wall at the time of drainage to exclude epithelium
- ERCP with pancreatic duct stenting
- Resection: rarely necessary, but used if malignancy cannot be ruled out

Drainage Procedures
- Cyst gastrostomy
  - Anterior gastrostomy (at least a 5-cm opening)
  - Palpate and needle aspiration to find cyst
  - Send part of wall for biopsy
  - Suture posterior wall stomach to mature cyst wall, interrupted absorbable sutures
- Cyst duodenostomy: for pseudocyst in head of pancreas or close to duodenum
  - Perform Kocher maneuver to check for adherence
  - Make a 3-cm opening into the first or third portion of the duodenum
- Cyst jejunostomy: when cyst is not adherent to stomach wall or multiple cysts
  - Use Roux loop
  - If not evident on imaging, open the gastrocolic omentum to look for plane between stomach and pseudocyst
- External drainage by percutaneous techniques
  - If patient unstable and as bridge to definitive treatment
  - If done open will need adequate drainage as symptoms slowly resolve and allow for slow healing of ductal disruption
- Distal pancreatectomy
  - For pseudocyst in tail of pancreas
  - If has eroded into surrounding structures

Pancreatic Necrosis
Etiology
- Acute pancreatitis (most common)
  - Can occur days to weeks after acute insult from thrombosis of pancreatic arteries
  - Aggressive resuscitation and avoidance of inotropes acutely can reduce risk
- Chronic pancreatitis
- Hypoperfusion due to nonpancreatic causes (cardiac surgery, myocardial infarction, and severe mesenteric ischemia)

Clinical Presentation
- Fever, abdominal pain, nausea, vomiting, and anorexia
- Sepsis, shock, and tachycardia

Diagnosis
- CT: nonenhancement of pancreatic tissue; fluid collections with air/gas raise concern for infection, can FNA

Medical Treatment (*Ann Surg.* 2000;232:619–626)
- **Continue aggressive fluid resuscitation**
- **Close monitoring for secondary signs of infection**

- **Antibiotics** *(Lancet. 1995;346:663–667)*
  - **ONLY if signs of infection, first-line agents Imipenem or Meropenem**
- Nutrition: enteral feeding if possible, if not, then TPN

Surgical Treatment
- If signs of infection, prompt pancreatic debridement is crucial
- Necrosectomy—surgical technique
  - Chevron incision
  - Open the lesser sac
  - Remove all dead tissue and debris
  - **Copiously irrigate the infected field**
  - Remove gallbladder if patient is stable, it is safe and easy
  - **Adequate drainage of the affected area**
  - Feeding jejunostomy tube and gastrostomy tube decompression

8-3: PANCREATIC NEOPLASMS

Endocrine Neoplasms
Familial
- Associated with MEN I and Von Hippel Lindau (see also Chapter 16, Endocrine)

Diagnosis and Workup of Pancreatic Endocrine Neoplasms			
	Clinical Sx	Lab Workup	Imaging

Gastrinoma	• **Zollinger–Ellison syndrome**
	 • Reflux
	 • Secretory diarrhea
	 • Abdominal pain
		• Fasting gastrin (pg/mL)
		   • >130 suspicious
		   • **>1,000 diagnostic**
		 • Decreased BAO (basal acid output)
		 • Secretin stimulation: gastrin level increases by >200 pg/mL
			• CT
			 • SRS (somatostatin receptor)
			 • +/– MRI
			 • EUS
			 • Intra-op US

Insulinoma	• **"Whipple's triad"** • Weakness and fatigue after meals • Fasting glucose <50 • Sx relieved with glucose	• **Fasting glucose level <60** • **Fasting insulin level >24** • Insulin : glucose ratio >0.3 • Elevated C-terminal peptide • Proinsulin level	• Triple-phase CT or MRI • EUS • **DO NOT BIOPSY** • Intraoperative US
VIPoma	• Watery, secretory diarrhea that persists with fasting (>3 L/day)	• Hypokalemia • Achlorhydria • Elevated serum VIP	• CT • SRS • Intraoperative US

Glucagonoma	Necrotizing migratory erythema
	 Type II DM, DVTs
	 Malnutrition
	 +/– stomatitis, glossitis, cheilosis
		• Fasting glucagon (pg/mL)
		   >1,000 diagnostic
		   >150 suggestive
		 • Hyperglycemia
		 • Hypoaminoacidemia
			• CT
			 • SRS
			 • Intraoperative US

Somatostatinoma	• Gallstones • Diabetes • Steatorrhea • Hypochlorhyidria	• Somatostatin >100 pg/mL • Positive stain for somatostatin on histopathology	• CT • MRI • EUS • SRS

Gastrinoma
- About 70% malignant
- Must rule out other causes of elevated gastrin levels (proton pump inhibitor [PPI] or H₂ blocker, retained antrum, gastric outlet obstruction, and short-gut syndrome)
- Most common pancreatic location is head
- Can occur elsewhere in duodenum and pancreas or rarely liver

"Gastrinoma Triangle"
• **Sweep of the third portion of duodenum**
• **Neck of pancreas**
• **Junction of cystic duct and CBD**

Gastrinoma Treatment
- Symptoms: PPI with good control
- Systemic therapy for metastases: PPI, octreotide, streptozotocin, and 5-FU
- Surgery: depends on location
  - Head of pancreas: enucleation
  - Duodenum: full thickness excision
  - Peripancreatic lymph node: dissection
  - Pancreatic body or tail: distal pancreatectomy
  - Unidentified: open duodenum and perform local full thickness resection

Insulinoma
- Most common pancreatic endocrine neoplasm
- About 5–10% malignant; increased risk if >3 cm
- 100% in pancreas, equally distributed between head and tail

Treatment
- Symptoms: diazoxide (ameliorates hypoglycemia from metastases)
- Surgery
  - Octreotide and antibiotics pre-op
  - Fully examine pancreas
  - **Intraoperative p EUS +/– rapid venous levels**
  - **Resection vs. enucleation depends on location and size of tumor**
  - Enucleation is preferred
  - Anatomic resection may be necessary if tumor >2 cm or close to main pancreatic duct
  - Malignant: debulk (beneficial if resect 90% of tumor) +/– resection liver mets
  - **If cannot find tumor using preoperative studies or intra-operative ultrasound, biopsies of pancreatic tail should be performed and distal pancreatectomy can be considered**
  - No need for lymph node dissection
  - Can give secretin intraoperative to check for leak with enucleation
  - Postoperative
- Strict blood glucose monitoring: mild hyperglycemia for 2–3 days
- Metastases: octreotide, diazoxide, and streptozocin

VIPoma
- Most are malignant
- Almost always in pancreas, most often in tail

Treatment
- Medical: octreotide, potassium, and +/– glucocorticoid with good response
- Surgery: complete resection with regional lymph node dissection and metastases

Glucagonoma (alpha cells)
- >80% malignant
- 100% in pancreas, tail > head

Glucagonoma Treatment
- Medical: octreotide with good control
- Pre-op: octreotide, anticoagulation, inferior vena cava filter, and antibiotics
- Surgery: resection including primary disease, lymph nodes, and metastases

Somatostatinoma (D cells)
- Least common of the functional pancreatic endocrine tumors
- 75% malignant, 75% have metastasized
- 55% in the pancreas (most often in the head or uncinate)

Treatment
- Surgery: resection (often via pancreaticoduodenectomy) and debulking of hepatic metastasis, if necessary
- If not surgical candidate, hepatic arterial embolization or chemotherapy

Pancreatic Ductal Carcinoma (Exocrine Neoplasms)
Epidemiology
- Most common primary pancreatic malignancy (95%)
- Includes **adenocarcinoma,** medullary, and adenosquamous
- Risk factors: smoking, alcohol, high-fat diet, occupational exposure to radiation, aluminum or acrylamide, chronic pancreatitis, and genetics/family history
- Metastases: lymph nodes, breast, lung, colorectal, melanoma, gastric, and renal

- **Vague abdominal pain, weight loss, jaundice, diabetes, diarrhea, and steatosis**
- Courvoisier sign: palpable nontender gall bladder in the setting of jaundice
- Sister Mary Joseph node: palpable periumbilical node
- Virchow node: palpable left supraclavicular node

Diagnosis
- CA19–9: **good sensitivity;** differential—pancreatitis and hepatic dysfunction
- CTA (triple phase)/MRCP: identifies lesion, vascular involvement, and arterial anatomy
- EGD/ERCP/EUS: identify lesion, biopsy, and +/– stent biliary tree if severe jaundice
  (N Engl J Med. 2010;362:129–137)
- Staging laparoscopy: can be done at the time of surgery to rule out metastasis prior to resection

Criteria for Unresectable Pancreatic Cancer
• Metastasis
• Solid tumor contact with the SMA or celiac axis of >180 degrees
• Unreconstructable SMV/PV involvement

Treatment (N Engl J Med. 2004;350:1200–1210)
- Pancreatic resection if workup suggests resectable disease
- Postoperative adjuvant therapy is necessary: chemotherapy +/– radiation → decreases local recurrence and improves survival
- Neoadjuvant chemotherapy +/– radiation if borderline resectable (controversial for resectable disease)
- If unresectable, palliative chemotherapy +/– radiation

Pancreatic Cystic Neoplasm
Serous Cystadenoma
- Location: head of pancreas
- CT: central "sunburst" calcifications, multiple small homogenous cysts
- **FNA: low CEA, variable CA-125, low amylase and lipase, + glycogen**

Mucinous Cystadenoma
- Higher malignant potential
- Ovarian stroma
- Location: body and tail
- CT: peripheral calcifications, small number of large cysts
- **FNA: high CEA, high viscosity, and + mucin**

Intraductal–Papillary Mucinous Neoplasm
- 25–40% malignant, higher rate for main duct IPMNs
- 5-year survival 40% if invasive, 77% if noninvasive
- 8% overall recurrence rate (17% if positive margins, 2% if negative margins)
- Location: head > body and tail; branch duct > main duct
- Symptoms: asymptomatic, recurrent pancreatitis, and diarrhea from malabsorption
- Diagnosis: ERCP shows mucin coming from ampulla, KRAS +
- Treatment: Resect if main or mixed duct. Resect if branch duct and has worrisome features (including size ≥3 cm), in addition to mural nodules, main duct features suspicious for involvement, or malignant cells on cytology (Sendai criteria) (Pancreatology. 2012;183–197)

Serous or Mucinous Cystadenocarcinoma
- Diagnosis: high CA-125 and positive cytology
- Treatment: resection

8-4: PANCREAS OPERATIONS

Pancreaticoduodenectomy—"Whipple" Operation (Ann Surg. 1935;102:763–779)
- History: first described by Dr. Whipple in 1935 (was a two-step procedure back then)
- Usage: tumors of the head and uncinate process, some periampullary tumors

Resection (Fig. 8-1).

Figure 8-1 Whipple specimen. (From Fischer JE, Bland KI. *Mastery of Surgery*, 5th ed. Philadelphia, PA: Lippincott Williams & Wilkins, 2007.)

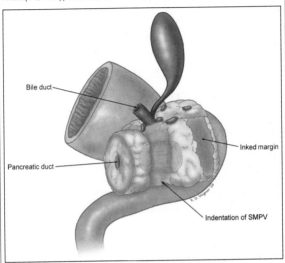

- Incision: extended right or bilateral subcostal incision
- Extensive Kocherization: mobilize the right colon to expose the duodenum
- Develop a plane under the pancreatic neck; dissect portal vein and SMV
- Cholecystectomy and transect common hepatic duct just above takeoff cystic duct
- Complete portal lymphadenectomy
- Identify and divide the gastroduodenal artery. *Be wary of aberrant arterial supply to the liver, i.e., replaced right or left hepatic arteries*
- Divide
   1. Proximal intestinal margin
      - **"Classical": divide the stomach at the level of the antrum**
      - **"Pylorus-preserving": divide just beyond pylorus (improves gastric emptying and decreases reflux)**
   2. Jejunum and mesentery
   3. Neck of the pancreas
   4. Portal vein tributaries entering the pancreas
   5. Uncinate

Anastomoses
- Pancreaticojejunostomy in two layers (+/– pediatric feeding tube duct <4 mm)
- Hepaticojejunostomy in a single layer
- Gastrojejunostomy in two layers
- Can leave a single drain near the pancreatic anastomosis if high risk for leak
- Feeding jejunostomy in select patients (malnourished, age >70)

Distal Pancreatectomy
- Usage: tumors of the body and tail

Total Pancreatectomy
- Usage: rare. Occasionally for premalignant conditions (extensive IPMN, chronic pancreatitis, and multi-focal neuroendocrine malignancy)
- **All patients will develop diabetes and pancreatic insufficiency postoperatively**

- Don't forget vaccines if performing a splenectomy—*Haemophilus influenzae, Meningococcus, Pneumococcus*

Lateral Pancreaticojejunostomy—"Puestow" Procedure
- Usage: chronic pancreatitis or obstructed pancreatic ducts (*Am J Surg*. 1987;153:207–213)

Frey Procedure (*Pancreas*. 1987;2:701–705)
- Definition: "coring out" the head of the pancreas
- Usage: if significant calcium deposition in the head of the pancreas

Transduodenal Sphincteroplasty
- Definition: sutures the mucosa of the CBD to the duodenum
- Usage: patients with ampullary stenosis or proximal pancreatic duct stricture

Ampullary Resection
- Usage: large (>2 cm) tubular or tubulovillous adenomas of papilla, villous adenomas with severe dysplasia, or pT1 N0 M0 G1/2 cancer

---

Perioperative Management of Pancreas Surgery
- **Clinical pathway: many large volume centers are utilizing preset steps of daily progress to minimize variability and maximize efficiency in postoperative management**
- Fluids: use judiciously to reduce swelling of the anastomosis and risk of leakage
- Hypotension: avoid even relative hypotension to improve pancreatic perfusion
- NGT decompression for 2–3 days
- If drains: many surgeons will remove only after drain amylase is checked with patient tolerating a diet
- Nutrition
  - Enteral feeding can be started on POD2 if feeding tube placed intraoperatively
  - TPN should be initiated and oral intake limited if significant pancreatic leak
- Octreotide (100 mg SC q8h) if soft pancreas, small pancreatic duct, or pancreatic leak suspected (*J Am Coll Surg*. 2007;205(4):546–557)

Complications of Pancreatic Surgery
Pancreatic Leak/Fistula
- Clinical presentation: fevers, elevated WBC, nausea, delayed gastric emptying, increased drain output
- Incidence of clinically relevant cases: 10–15%
- Severity (*Surgery*. 2005;138(1):8–13)
  - Grade A: biochemical only, no clinical sequelae
  - Grade B: fistula with persistent drainage (>3 weeks) usually requiring treatment
  - Grade C: severe clinical sequelae generally requiring reoperation
- Fistula risk score—based on gland texture (highest risk on soft glands), pathology, size of pancreatic duct (highest risk with small ducts), intraoperative blood loss (*JACS*. 2013; 216(1):1–14)
- Treatment: initially octreotide, NPO; +/– ERCP or IR procedures, and surgery

Wound infection

Incisional hernia

ACKNOWLEDGMENT

The authors would like to thank Saju Joseph, MD, for his contributions to the 1st edition of this chapter, which were invaluable to the writing of the 2nd edition.

9-1: HEPATIC ANATOMY

Morphologic Divisions (Figs. 9-1 and 9-2)

Figure 9-1 Functional divisions of the liver. (From Fischer JE, Bland KI. *Mastery of Surgery*, 5th ed. Philadelphia, PA: Lippincott Williams & Wilkins, 2007.)

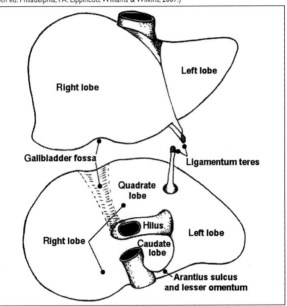

Figure 9-2 Couinaud segments. (Modified from Moore KL, Dalley AF, Agur AMR. *Clinically Oriented Anatomy*, 7e. Baltimore: Wolters Kluwer, 2014.)

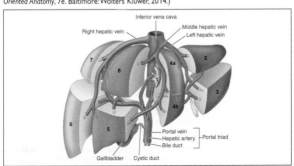

Functional Divisions
- Couinaud segments: based on branches of the portal triad (portal vein, hepatic artery, and bile duct)
- Sectors separated by three major hepatic veins
  - Caudate lobe: segment I (autonomous vasculature)
  - Left lobe: segments II, III, and IVa and IVb
  - Right lobe: segments V, VI, VII, and VIII
- Right anterior sector: segments V and VIII
- Right posterior sector: segments VI and VII
- Left medial sector: segments IVa and IVb
- Left lateral sector: segments II and III

Blood Supply
- Arterial: runs with portal vein branches and bile ducts; covered by Glisson capsule
  - Celiac → proper hepatic → common hepatic → right and left branches
  - Common variations:
    - Replaced right hepatic artery: from SMA (20%)
    - Replaced left hepatic: from left gastric (15%)
- Hepatic veins: drain segments; no capsular covering
- Portal veins: divides liver into functional segments

Bile Ducts
- **Confluence in hilum anterior to right portal vein;** many anatomic variations

---

9-2: PORTAL HYPERTENSION

Types of Obstruction Leading to Portal Hypertension

- Presinusoidal
  - Portal vein thrombosis
  - Schistosomiasis (lodge in portal vein tributaries where they incite chronic inflammation and subsequent marked fibrosis)
- Sinusoidal
  - Cirrhosis
  - Infiltrative disease (Wilson disease or hemochromatosis)
- Postsinusoidal
  - Budd–Chiari syndrome (hepatic vein occlusion)
  - Congestive heart failure

LIVER 9-2

Child–Pugh Classification

Measure of Prognosis in Chronic Liver Disease

	1 point	2 points	3 points
Bilirubin	<2	2–3	>3
Albumin	>3.5	3–3.5	<3
Ascites	None	Mild	Severe
INR	<1.7	1.7–2.2	>2.2
Encephalopathy	Absent	Grade I–II	Grade III–IV

Child class A: 5–6 points
Child class B: 7–9 points
Child class C: 10–15 points
Consider evaluating (+/– listing) for liver transplant when Child class B and MELD ≥10 (see Transplant, Chapter 18, Section 3)

Complications of Portal Hypertension
Encephalopathy
- 50–70% of cirrhotic patients will experience altered mental status
- Likely related to impaired metabolism of ammonia and other compounds
- Most common precipitating factors: infection (including SBP), variceal bleed, hyponatremia, hypokalemia, renal failure, medications (benzodiazepines, narcotics diuretics), noncompliance with lactulose, and portal vein thrombosis
- **Treatment: reduce protein intake, correct metabolic derangement, lactulose; consider oral nonabsorbable antibiotics (neomycin) or rifaximin** (antibiotics decrease gut bacterial flora that decreases nitrogen burden)

Refractory Ascites
- Effectively managed in 95% of patients with **sodium restriction and diuretics** (spironolactone and/or furosemide)
- Other options: paracentesis, transjugular intrahepatic portosystemic shunt (TIPS) placement, surgical shunt, or transplant

Bleeding and Varices
- Etiology
  - **Gastroesophageal varices: portal pressure >10 mm Hg**
  - **Bleeding: portal pressure >12 mm Hg**
  - Rebleeding varices: portal pressure >20 mm Hg
- Incidence of bleeding: 25% of patients with varices
- Risk of rebleeding within 6 weeks from first bleed: 30–40%
- Prevention: nonselective β-blocker (propranolol or nadolol), nitrates, and endoscopic variceal ligation (EVL)

Management of Acute Variceal Bleed
• Medical: volume support and transfusion (keep Hgb >8 mg/dL), antibiotic prophylaxis, somatostatin, or an analogue such as octreotide
• Endoscopic: banding (most effective), injection therapy, and sclerotherapy
• Esophageal balloon: may use as temporizing measure in patients with uncontrolled esophageal variceal bleeding until TIPS or surgical shunt
• Surgical: surgical shunt or transplant (see "Surgical Options" below)
• Prevention after bleed
• Nonselective β-blocker, + banding (best) or nitrates
• If Child class A or B: consider TIPS or surgical shunt if recurrent hemorrhage, transplant for appropriate candidates

Surgical Options
Transjugular Intrahepatic Portosystemic Shunt (TIPS)
- Indications (N Eng J Med. 2000;342:1701–1707; N Engl J Med. 2010;362:2370–2379)
  - Child class A or B
  - Hepatic vein pressure gradient >20 mm Hg
  - High-risk surgical patient
  - Bridge to transplant in patients with variceal hemorrhage
  - Refractory ascites
- **Contraindications: portal vein thrombosis, severe hepatic encephalopathy, or severe liver dysfunction (Child class C, high MELD score) right heart dysfunction or failure, intrahepatic malignancy, and +/- poor access to regular medical or surgical follow-up**
- Complications: **encephalopathy** (~25% of patients), stenosis or thrombosis of shunt requiring multiple procedures, and right heart failure

Surgical Shunts
- Indications
  - Limited indication for surgical shunts in the current era
  - Portal hypertension in absence of cirrhosis
  - Child A cirrhotic with gastric varices
  - Poor access to regular medical or surgical follow-up
- Nonselective shunts
  - End-to-side portacaval shunt
  - Central splenorenal shunt
  - Side-to-side portacaval shunt: high incidence of encephalopathy
    - Ideally for patients who are not transplant candidates
    - Acceptable in acute bleed because of rapidity of portal dissection
- Selective shunts
  - Lower incidence of encephalopathy
  - Distal splenorenal (Warren) shunt: decompresses gastrosplenic system
    - No porta hepatis dissection (good if potential transplant candidate)
    - Contraindicated if severe ascites (lymphatic dissection worsens ascites)
- Mesocaval shunt
- H-graft (Sarfeh shunt): small diameter (8–10 mm), preserves prograde portal flow

Distal Splenorenal Shunt
Open gastrocolic ligament and ligate R gastroepiploic vein
Mobilize splenic flexure
ID and dissect free splenic vein posterior to distal pancreas, divide tributaries
Dissect free L renal vein
Divide adequate length of splenic vein and anastomose to L renal vein
Ligate coronary vein at junction w/portal system

9-3: BENIGN LIVER LESIONS

Amoebic Abscess
Epidemiology
- Endemic areas: tropics and developing countries, 2% of adult population
- Amoebiasis: the third most common cause of parasitic death worldwide
- Patients: younger, healthier than pyogenic; recent travel to/from endemic area

Pathogenesis
- Causative organism: *Entamoeba histolytica*
- Transmitted via fecal to oral route, usually by contaminated food or water
- More commonly affects the **right lobe**

Clinical Presentation
- Symptoms: fever and RUQ abdominal pain
- Labs: leukocytosis without eosinophilia and elevated liver enzymes
  - Agglutination/compliment fixation test
  - **ELISA test for antibodies of *E. histolytica*:** highly sensitive and quick

Imaging
- Ultrasound: hypoechoic lesion with internal echoes, 90% accuracy
- CT: well-defined, complex, fluid-filled mass; wall enhancement and peripheral edema
- MRI: low-level intensity on T_1 images, high-signal intensity on T_2-weighted images with peripheral edema

Treatment
- **Metronidazole (Flagyl): usually shows clinical improvement in 48–72 hours**
- Tinidazole is an alternative to metronidazole
- Diloxanide furoate or another luminal amebicides must also be given afterward
Complications: rupture into the peritoneum, pleura, or pericardium which generally requires operative exploration and drainage.

Pyogenic Liver Abscess
Epidemiology
- Median age 50–60 years
- Risk factors: HIV, IV drug use, travel, and recent abdominal infections

Clinical Presentation

Source of Pyogenic Liver Abscesses
• Portal: diverticulitis, appendicitis, and inflammatory bowel disease
• Biliary: cholecystitis, cholangitis, or malignancy
• Trauma: penetrating or chemoembolization
• Bloodborne: endocarditis, dental infection, or other source of bacteremia
Causative organisms: *Escherichia coli, Klebsiella, Bacteroides,* and *Enterococcus*

- Symptoms: fever, abdominal pain, weight loss or failure to thrive, and sepsis
- Labs: leukocytosis and elevated liver function tests

Imaging
- Ultrasound: hyperechoic in early disease; hypoechoic as pus formation occurs
- CT: 95% sensitivity
- MRCP: can reveal biliary connection

Treatment
- **Broad-spectrum antibiotics until culture data final (then tailor) + percutaneous drainage for abscesses >2 cm**
- Operative drainage via laparotomy or laparoscopy if failure of percutaneous drainage, multiple abscesses, and/or contraindication to percutaneous drainage
- Treat underlying etiology, i.e., drain diverticular abscess and decompress biliary tract

Surgical Technique: Pyogenic Liver Abscess
Posterior approach through bed of 12th rib or transperitoneal via subcostal incision
Needle aspiration to identify abscess cavity
Hepatotomy with opening of abscess cavity
Biopsy of abscess wall
Suction and large volume irrigation
Place large bore drains

Hydatid Cyst

Pathogenesis
- Endemic to sheep-grazing areas (Mediterranean, Middle East, and East Africa)
- Causative organism: *Echinococcus* **species**
- Oral–fecal route of spread

Clinical Presentation
- Symptoms: abdominal pain and jaundice
- Sequelae: cholangitis; rupture into biliary tract, pleural space, or peritoneum
- **Labs: ELISA for antibodies, 90% sensitive**

Imaging
- Ultrasound may reveal daughter cysts but limited by operator dependence
- CT: thick-walled calcified cysts, often with daughter cysts
- ERCP: determine whether connection exists between cyst and biliary system

Treatment
- Medical: albendazole 10 mg/kg/day; success <30% when used alone
- **PAIR procedure (puncture, aspiration, injection, reaspiration): excellent results in uncomplicated cyst disease**
  - **Patients should be pretreated with antibiotics for at least 10 days**
  - The cyst is alternately percutaneously aspirated, then filled with saline multiple times
- Surgical treatment (gold standard)
  - **Pretreat with albendazole (minimizes risk of anaphylaxis if spillage of cyst contents into the abdomen)**
  - Conservative: remove cyst contents
  - Radical: total excision of cyst via pericystectomy or resection and pack with omentum. May consider hepatic resection if unable to perform pericystectomy or unroofing with aspiration
- Surgical technique
  - Pack field with hypertonic saline-soaked gauzes in case of spillage
  - Partially open cyst and suction contents
  - Completely unroof cyst and irrigate with scolicidal agent (NOT if: bile staining or evidence of connection to biliary tree)
  - If a biliary connection is identified, oversew and pack cyst cavity with omentum or perform cyst excision

Simple Cysts

Epidemiology
- Congenital or sporadic, more common in females
- Variable sizes, single or multiple (polycystic liver disease)
- Microscopically lined by cuboidal or columnar epithelium

Clinical Presentation
- Most asymptomatic
- Symptoms: abdominal pain, nausea, early satiety from gastric compression; jaundice from large cysts compressing bile duct

Imaging: Ultrasound
- Ultrasound: anechoic well-defined lesion
- If ultrasound, CT or MRI reveals internal septations, evidence of hemorrhage, or enhancement of the capsule, suspect cystadenomas or cystadenocarcinoma

Treatment
- Reassurance in the asymptomatic patient
- Symptomatic patients
  - Chemical sclerosis with ethanol or minocycline: contraindicated if cyst aspiration reveals bile; large cysts generally do not respond. Is painful, so requires general anesthesia.
  - Laparoscopic cystectomy or marsupialization.
  - If biliary communication: ligate connection and marsupialize or resect the cyst

- If cystadenoma or malignancy suspected: formal liver resection
- Liver transplantation in the presence of liver failure and polycystic liver disease

Cavernous Hemangioma
Epidemiology
- Congenital or sporadic
  - **No malignant potential**
- Females, third to fourth decade
- Dilated vascular spaces lined by endothelium and separated by fibrous septa

Clinical Presentation
- Symptoms: usually none unless >5 cm
- Symptoms: RUQ abdominal pain (stretching of Glisson capsule), right scapula pain (referred); N/V, fever, or early satiety from left lobe lesions; infants or children may have high output CHF
- **Kasabach–Merritt syndrome**
  - **Consumptive coagulopathy related to hemangiomas**
  - **Present with thrombocytopenia and hypofibrinogenemia**
- Physical examination may reveal a mass or bruit
- Labs: normal liver function tests

Imaging
- Often discovered incidentally
- Ultrasound: echogenic mass of uniform density, distinct margins, and acoustic enhancement
- CT with IV contrast: peripheral to central enhancement
- MRI: peripheral nodular enhancement on dynamic enhanced T_1; very bright on T_2

Treatment
- Reassurance for asymptomatic lesions of definite diagnosis
- Most large hemangiomas that are asymptomatic can be safely followed.
- **Needle biopsy is contraindicated secondary to the risk of bleeding**
- Resection ONLY if symptomatic, Kasabach–Merritt syndrome, CHF, and uncertain diagnosis
- Surgical technique
  - Occlude inflow by Pringle maneuver and/or ligation of individual feeding arteries
  - Patient may require segmental or lobar resection for giant hemangioma
- Transarterial embolization may be considered when high surgical risk or as an adjunct to surgical therapy.

Hepatic Adenoma
Epidemiology
- **Most often in females between third and fifth decades of life**
- **Associated with oral contraceptive use; risk increases with estrogen dose and duration of use**
- **May undergo rupture, hemorrhage (25% incidence), or malignant transformation (<10% incidence)**
- Pathology reveals benign-appearing hepatocytes without ducts or portal triads

Clinical Presentation
- Symptoms: usually none; may present with abdominal pain, rupture, and hemorrhage
- Liver function tests usually normal

Imaging
- Often discovered incidentally
- Ultrasound: well-circumscribed heterogeneous lesion
- CT without contrast: hypodense mass
- Triple phase contrast CT: heterogeneous, **hypervascular lesion on arterial phase,** hypodense or isodense mass on portal phase
- Standard MRI: isointense on T_1, hyperintense on T_2 (similar to focal nodular hyperplasia [FNH])
- **MRI with gadobenate dimeglumine: delayed images show hypointense adenoma (vs. hyperintense with FNH)—gold standard**
- **Radionuclide imaging with sulfur colloid or gallium-67: decreased uptake due to lack of Kupffer cells**

Treatment
- Discontinue OCPs
- Small asymptomatic lesions can be observed closely with serial imaging
- Resection if symptomatic or >5 cm or uncertain diagnosis

- **In acute life-threatening bleed: arterial embolization followed by resection**

Focal Nodular Hyperplasia
Epidemiology
- Females between the second and third decades
- **No malignant potential**
- Pathology: central scar with regenerating nodules and connective tissue (gross), normal hepatic cells and bile ducts divided by fibrous septa (microscopic)

Clinical Presentation
- Symptoms: usually none, may rarely include pain and/or hemorrhage
- Liver function tests often normal

Imaging
- Ultrasound: hypoechoic or isoechoic lesion
- CT without contrast: hypodense central scar
- **Contrast CT: hyperintense lesion that becomes iso- or hypodense in portal phase**
- Standard MRI: hypointense on T_1, isointense or slightly hyperintense lesion on T_2
- **MRI with gadobenate demeglamine: delayed images show FNH to be hyperintense or isointense** (vs. adenoma which is hypointense)
- **Radionuclide scans with sulfur colloid and gallium-67: increased uptake due to the presence of Kupffer cells**

Treatment
- Resect if symptomatic, increased tumor growth, or diagnosis in question
- If surgery indicated, attempt enucleation
- **Tumors usually have large feeding vessels that should be ligated initially**

9-4: MALIGNANT LIVER LESIONS

Metastatic Colorectal Cancer
Most common secondary hepatic neoplasm

Clinical Presentation
- Symptoms: usually none, may present with malaise, weight loss, and abdominal pain
- Signs of advanced disease include hepatomegaly, jaundice, and ascites
- Labs: elevated CEA or abnormal LFTs may be present

Imaging
- Ultrasound: sensitive for lesions >2 cm
- CT: hypodense masses; can delineate lesions <1 cm
- MRI: hypodense lesions on T1 and hyperintense T2 images

Treatment
- **Biopsy rarely indicated; risk of bleeding and dissemination of cancer along needle track**
- Surgical resection: best hope for long-term survival. 30–50% 5-year survival after successful resection.
- Portal vein embolization: induces hypertrophy of planned liver remnant to better avoid postoperative liver failure. This is done if predicted liver remnant is <30%.
- Neoadjuvant chemotherapy (FOLFOX) may help downstage disease in liver prior to resection.
- No survival benefit with adjuvant chemotherapy.
- Alternative treatment options include radiofrequency ablation (RFA), microwave ablation, transarterial chemoembolization (TACE), Ytrium-90 embolization, and conventional or stereotactic radiation therapy either for downstaging prior to surgery or as an alternative to surgery (high risk patients, unresectable disease).

Prognosis
- Five-year survival following surgical resection: 30–50%
- **Predictors of poor outcome**
  - Lymph node involvement
  - >3 lesions, bilobar
  - Size >5 cm
  - Preoperative CEA >200
  - Disease-free interval <12 months
- Overall survival rates for resection of recurrent metastases similar to initial procedure

Indications for Resection for Noncolorectal Liver Metastases

- Renal cell carcinoma
- Breast cancer
- Sarcoma
- Gastrointestinal neuroendocrine tumors (if primary disease resectable and at least 90% of hepatic tumor burden resectable or ablatable)
- Melanoma
- Ovarian and endometrial tumors

Hepatocellular Carcinoma

Epidemiology

- About 90% of all primary liver tumors, more common in males
- Highest incidence in Asia, sub-Saharan, and western coastal Africa
- **Associated with chronic liver disease, particularly HBV and HCC cirrhosis**
  (N Eng J Med. 2002;347:168–174)

Clinical Presentation

- Symptoms: malaise, weight loss, and abdominal pain; spontaneous rupture 5–15%
- Labs: elevated LFTs and elevated AFP (**higher levels with more aggressive tumor**)

Imaging

- Ultrasound: hypoechoic, may find 80–90% of lesions
- CT: early uptake of contrast with a mosaic pattern to the tumor
- MRI: mosaic pattern with **hypointensity on T_1 and hyperintensity on T_2**

Treatment

- **Biopsy rarely indicated** (risk of dissemination)
- Noncirrhotic: resection—consider preoperative portal vein embolization of lobe to be resected (may reduce postoperative complications by 50%)
- Cirrhotic: transplant (if candidate) → Milan criteria. May consider resection in well-compensated cirrhotic (Child A, platelets >100,000, <2 segments being resected)
- Cirrhotics who are not transplant candidates may be treated with RFA, TACE, or radiation therapy.

Milan Criteria

- A single Tumor ≤5 cm or up to three tumors, none >3cm
- No extrahepatic manifestations
- No vascular invasion

- TACE or RFA as bridge to transplant

Prognosis

- About 50% 5-year survival rates in noncirrhotic patients undergoing resection
- TACE and RFA improves survival in unresectable disease or patients unfit for surgery

Other Primary Liver Malignancies

Fibrolamellar Variant of HCC

- Younger patients, Western hemisphere
- AFP elevated in <15% of patients
- Better prognosis than HCC

Intrahepatic Cholangiocarcinoma

- Often occurs in the absence of chronic liver disease; therefore presents late
- Risk factors: parasitic infection, thorotrast exposure, and Caroli disease
- Labs: CEA, CA19–9, and CA125
- Imaging: CT shows fibrotic lesion which enhances late after IV administration
- Surgical resection, best chance for long-term cure
- Five-year survival rates of 25–50% following resection

9-5: Major Hepatic Resection

Indications (Ann Surg. 2002;236:397–407)

- Large tumor, >5 cm
- Tumor involving most of the right or left liver lobe
- Small tumor close to hilum or near portal pedicle

Preoperative Assessment

- CT volumetry
  - Healthy liver with >30% remnant
  - Chronic liver disease needs >40% remnant

- Indocyanine green clearance (ICG): retention >14% at 15 minutes = increased mortality

Intraoperative Considerations
- Intraoperative ultrasound: identify occult lesions and define vascular/biliary anatomy
- Staging laparoscopy: relative indication if high likelihood of unresectable disease
- Parenchymal dissection options: harmonic scalpel, bipolar device, water jet dissection, CUSA, finger fracture, or Kelley clamp crushing techniques
- Maintenance of low CVP (<5 mm Hg) decreases blood loss
- Methods to control excessive bleeding
  - Pringle maneuver: clamping of gastrohepatic ligament
  - Total vascular exclusion: combines the Pringle maneuver with clamping of suprahepatic and infrahepatic vena cava

Complications
- Liver failure: most common cause of postoperative death
- Other: hemorrhage, cardiopulmonary collapse, renal failure, biliary leak, and abscess

---

Technique: Major Hepatic Resection

Right Hepatectomy (Fig. 9-3)
Right subcostal incision with midline xiphoid extension (+ left subcostal if needed)
Mobilize right lobe by incising right triangular and coronary ligaments
Perform cholecystectomy
Divide hepatoduodenal ligament
Identify and ligate right hepatic artery to the right of common bile duct
Isolate and divide right portal vein with vascular stapler or suture ligation
Isolate and divide right hepatic duct after taking down hilar plate
Divide caudate portal vein branches
Isolate and transect right hepatic vein, preferably with vascular stapler; vascular demarcation between right and left liver should become apparent
Mark transection plane with electrocautery, which should lie to the right of the middle hepatic vein, and in line from the IVC to the gallbladder fossa
Transect liver along line of demarcation; divide terminal branch of middle HV
Ensure hemostasis: manual pressure, argon beam, electrocautery, and sutures
If diaphragmatic resection necessary, close with nonabsorbable suture

If Adding Caudate Lobectomy
Dissect caudate hepatic vein and divide
Separate the caudate lobe from hilar plate
Remove caudate by dividing the left IVC ligament and ligamentum venosum

Right Lobectomy (Right Trisegmentectomy)
Expose feedback vessels to segment IV from left pedicle by opening bridge of tissue at the base of the umbilical fissure which connects segments III and IV
Identify and ligate all vessels entering segment IV from the umbilical fissure
Divide liver to right of falciform; dissect back to point of transection of right HV
Transect middle hepatic vein found in the upper part of the dissection

Left Hepatectomy
Perform cholecystectomy and cannulate cystic duct for cholangiogram (optional)
Divide lesser omentum and enter liver hilum to left of hepatoduodenal ligament
Expose and ligate left HA after confirming patency of right HA via palpation and/or Doppler
Ligate left portal vein and divide branches to caudate (if it is to be preserved)
Isolate and divide left hepatic duct and left hepatic vein
Divide parenchyma down to left hilum
Remove specimen and complete remainder of operation as described above

Left Hepatic Lobectomy (Left Trisegmentectomy)
Dissect and expose right hepatic duct and inflow structures deep into right liver hilum until the right anterior duct, artery, and portal vein are identified
Confirm with cholangiography, occlusion, palpation, and/or Doppler
Divide right anterior structures
Line of demarcation created between segments V and VIII, VI, and VII
Divide right triangular ligament
Divide along line of demarcation caudally to right posterior portal structures while preserving these structures
Divide left and middle hepatic veins along with ligamentum venosum
Remove specimen and complete operation as described above

Figure 9-3 Standard hepatic resections. (Modified from Moore KL, Dalley AF, Agur AMR: Clinically Oriented Anatomy, 7e. Baltimore: Wolters Kluwer, 2014.)

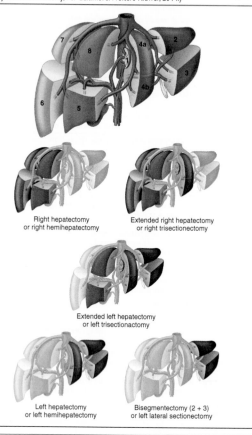

Right hepatectomy or right hemihepatectomy

Extended right hepatectomy or right trisectionectomy

Extended left hepatectomy or left trisectionactomy

Left hepatectomy or left hemihepatectomy

Bisegmentectomy (2 + 3) or left lateral sectionectomy

SPLEEN

SAILA T. PILLAI • STEVEN D. SCHWAITZBERG
• MARK A. KASHTAN • MORGAN A. BRESNICK

10-1: SPLEEN—GENERAL INFORMATION

Anatomy
Suspensory Ligaments: Splenocolic, Splenorenal, Gastrosplenic, and Phrenosplenic
- **Gastrosplenic: contains short gastric and gastroepiploic arteries**
- **Splenorenal: contains splenic vessels and the tail of the pancreas**

Vasculature
- Arteries
  - Splenic artery: directly from the celiac trunk
  - Short gastric arteries: most often from the left gastroepiploic artery
- Veins
  - Follow corresponding arteries and generally posterior
  - Splenic vein joins the inferior mesenteric vein then the superior mesenteric vein (behind the neck of the pancreas) to form the hepatic portal vein
- Geographic distribution of vessels: important for operative planning
  - **Distributed** (70%): short splenic trunk and 6–12 long branches
    - Branches enter the spleen over ~75% of the medial surface
  - **Magistral** (30%): long main splenic artery dividing near the hilum
    - Branches enter the splenic hilum over ~30% of the medial surface
- Splenic vasculature is highly variable

Accessory Spleens
- Incidence: 10–30%, higher among patients with hematologic disorders
- Seeded along path of organ migration during embryonic development

---

Location of Accessory Spleens (Fig. 10-1)

Figure 10-1 Dark dots indicate possible location of accessory spleens. (From Fischer JE, Bland KI. *Mastery of Surgery*, 5th ed. Philadelphia, PA: Lippincott Williams & Wilkins, 2007.)

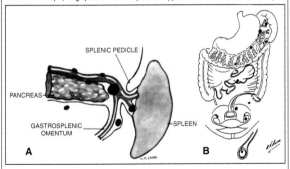

- Splenic hilum (40–60%) and lower pole
- Tail of the pancreas
- Suspensory ligaments
- Greater omentum
- Rare: presacral region, adjacent to left ovary, and in scrotum next to left testicle

---

"Hypersplenism" vs. "Splenomegaly"
- Splenomegaly: large spleen
- Hypersplenism: accelerated splenic function causing decrease in ≥1 formed blood elements

SPLEEN 10-1

Cystic Masses
- Congenital: epidermal (true) cyst
  - Usually solitary, unilocular, and asymptomatic unless enlarged
  - May have elevated CA19-9, CEA
- Posttraumatic: hematoma and posttraumatic pseudocyst (most common)
- Inflammatory: pyogenic abscess, echinococcal cysts, and fungal abscess
- Vascular: infarction and peliosis (widespread blood-filled cystic spaces)
- Neoplastic: hemangioma (most common primary neoplasm of the spleen. If consumptive coagulopathy, splenectomy is indicated), and lymphangioma
- **Nonparasitic cysts may be treated with aspiration (high recurrence rate), cyst fenestration, partial or total splenectomy**

Solid Masses
- Congenital: solid splenic lobulation
- Nonneoplastic: hamartoma and inflammatory pseudotumor
- Benign neoplasm: hemangioma, fibroma, lipoma, and angiomyolipoma
- Malignant neoplasms: may appear cystic due to hemorrhagic or necrotic foci
  - Lymphoma: most common malignant neoplasm of the spleen
  - Angiosarcoma
- Metastases: uncommon, usually only with disseminated disease
  - Most common primary cancers: breast, lung, colorectal, ovarian, melanoma, and gastric

---

10-3: DISORDERS REQUIRING SPLENECTOMY

Indications for Splenectomy
Trauma (possibly)
Hematologic: hereditary spherocytosis/elliptocytosis, autoimmune hemolytic anemia, idiopathic thrombocytopenic purpura (ITP), Felty syndrome, refractory thrombocytopenia–associated with SLE/HIV/AIDS, and persistent and refractory hypersplenism
Splenic Masses
Other: refractory TTP, pyruvate kinase deficiency, sickle cell anemia, thalassemias, lymphoma, leukemias, hypersplenism w/Chediak–Higashi, Wiskott–Aldrich, and Gaucher's

Trauma
Nonoperative Management
- Criteria
  - Hemodynamic stability
  - Negative abdominal examination
  - Low-grade injury (I–III)
  - Absence of contrast extravasation on CT scan (consider angio embolization, see below)
  - Absence of other clear indications for exploratory laparotomy
  - Absence of comorbidities that carry an increased risk of bleeding (e.g., portal hypertension) or concurrent injuries that carry inability to tolerate hypotension in event of re-bleed (e.g., brain injury)
- Failure rate of nonoperative management: 2–28%, depending on injury grade, injury severity score, presence of hemoperitoneum, and patient age
  - Angiographic embolization: potential option for splenic salvage or in poor operative candidates. Increased risk of failure in higher-grade injuries.

American Association for the Surgery of Trauma—Spleen Injury Scale	
Grade	**Description**
I	Nonexpanding subcapsular hematoma <10% of surface area. Nonbleeding capsular laceration with parenchymal involvement <1 cm deep
II	Nonexpanding subcapsular hematoma 10–50% of surface area Nonexpanding intraparenchymal hematoma <5 cm in diameter Bleeding capsular tear or parenchymal laceration 1–3 cm deep without trabecular vessel
III	Expanding subcapsular or intraparenchymal hematoma Bleeding subcapsular hematoma or subcapsular hematoma >50% of surface area Intraparenchymal hematoma >5 cm in diameter Parenchymal laceration >3 cm deep or involving trabecular vessels

IV	Ruptured intraparenchymal hematoma with active bleeding
	Laceration involving segmental or hilar vessels producing major devascularization (>25% splenic volume)
V	Completely shattered or avulsed spleen
	Hilar laceration that devascularizes entire spleen

Hematologic and Other Indications

Hematologic

- Hereditary **spherocytosis**/elliptocytosis: 90% response rate
- ITP: thrombocytopenia, no splenomegaly
  - Most common hematologic disorder requiring splenectomy
  - Spleen is both a site of autoantibody production and platelet destruction
  - Surgery is indicated if bleeding or thrombocytopenia <20–30,000/μL persists despite treatment with glucocorticoids
  - Splenectomy can result in complete (66%) or partial (22%) response with young age being the most significant predictor of success
- Autoimmune hemolytic anemia: warm antibody type
  - Splenectomy indicated after the failure of management with glucocorticoids
  - Of the 66–75% that respond, 50% will require lower steroid dosages, 30% will relapse and 20% will achieve cure
- Felty syndrome: rheumatoid arthritis associated with neutropenia and splenomegaly
  - Splenectomy indicated if severe or recurrent neutropenia and infections despite DMARDs
  - 80% response rate, although 25% experience some level of recurrence
- Refractory thrombocytopenia associated with SLE or HIV/AIDS
- Persistent and refractory secondary hypersplenism with pancytopenia, thrombocytopenia, leukopenia, or anemia

Other Indications

- Thrombotic thrombocytopenia purpura (refractory or recurrent)
- Pyruvate kinase deficiency
- Sickle cell anemia and thalassemias
  - Indications: hypersplenism, sequestration crises, splenic abscesses, and massive splenic infarction
  - Postsplenectomy patients are particularly vulnerable to infection (see "Complications" in Section 10-4)
- Hodgkin lymphoma: historically used for staging purposes
- Non-Hodgkin lymphoma
  - Indications: symptomatic relief from splenomegaly or severe hypersplenism, occasionally for diagnosis
  - Associated with high morbidity and mortality
- Chronic myelogenous leukemia
  - For massive splenomegaly; high rate of thromboembolic complications
- Chronic lymphocytic leukemia
  - Splenectomy is associated with a survival advantage
- Hairy cell leukemia
  - Splenectomy used to be treatment of choice, now interferon-α and purine analogs
- Hypersplenism with Chediak–Higashi syndrome, Wiskott–Aldrich syndrome, and Gaucher disease
- Splenic vein thrombosis and resultant gastric varices

Splenectomy Not Indicated in the Treatment of

- G6PD deficiency
- splenomegaly as a consequence of portal hypertension

10-4: OPERATIVE TECHNIQUES

Preoperative Planning

- Vaccines: Pneumococcus (both), Meningococcus, and Haemophilus influenzae vaccines
  - Optimally at least 2 weeks prior to planned surgery
  - May give after postoperative day 14 if emergent surgery
- Perioperative antibiotics
- Type and cross-match blood
- SQ heparin/antiplatelet agents for patients prone to splenic vein thrombosis: spleen weight >200 g, cirrhotics, and malignant tumors
- Platelets should be available for patients with thrombocytopenia (<50,000)
  - Administer after splenic artery ligation to prevent splenic consumption

- Preoperative splenic artery embolization (*Am J Surg.* 2007;193(6):713–718)
  - Consider for elective patients with massive spleens; perform same day or in OR

Splenorrhaphy
- Used mostly for low-grade (I–III) injuries, now often managed nonoperatively or with angiographic embolization
- Small lacerations: compression and application of hemostatic agents
- Raw surfaces: electrocautery and argon beam coagulation
- Discrete, localized lacerations: horizontal mattress sutures with or without pledgets through the entire parenchymal surface
- May use omental pocket or buttressing, particularly with friable tissue
- May fashion pocket of absorbable mesh to approximate tissue and effect tamponade
- Possible drain placement

Partial Splenectomy
- Isolate vessels to the segment to be removed and ligate in continuity within the hilum
- Transect the parenchyma, argon beam coagulation of raw surface
- Splenopexy for small splenic remnants likely to rotate
- Omental buttress
- Optional drain placement
- Carries high risk of recurrent hemorrhage because of residual raw surface

Laparoscopic Splenectomy
- Ideal for ITP patients and staging laparotomy
- **Gold standard for total splenectomy in children**
- Order of steps similar to open technique
  - Bipolar or ultrasonic scalpel for transecting ligaments and short gastric vessels
  - May use endostapler for splenic artery and vein
  - Extraction of the spleen by morcellation of the spleen in a bag
  - May enlarge a port site to facilitate removal

Complications of Splenic Surgery
- **More common in patients with malignancy**
- Hemorrhage (1–5%): most common source is from short gastrics—can be fatal
- Thrombosis (1–5%): particularly of the portal, mesenteric, and splenic veins
  - Risk factors: myeloproliferative disorders, large spleens, and laparoscopy
- Pancreatic fistula (1.5%): suspect if left lower lobe infiltrate, slow recovery
- Subphrenic fluid collection/abscess (3–13%)
- Peripheral smear postsplenectomy
  - Heinz bodies: denatured Hb
  - Howell Jolly bodies: nuclear remnants
  - Pappenheimer bodies: iron
  - Target cells and spur cells

Overwhelming Postsplenectomy Infection (*World J Gastroenter.* 2008 14;14(2):176–179)
- Incidence: 1 per 400–500 patient years (adults); **60% of cases caused by *S. pneumonia***
- Mortality rate: 50–70%
- Risk stratification
  - Age at splenectomy: increased in children, highest under 2 years old.
  - **Highest risk in setting of malignancy, lowest in trauma**
  - Majority of cases (50–80%) occur within 3 years of splenectomy
  - Overall immune status

Symptoms
- Early (nonspecific): fever, respiratory symptoms, malaise, rigors, skin changes, abdominal pain, nausea, vomiting, diarrhea, constipation, and headache
- May progress to hypotension, pneumonia, meningitis, Waterhouse–Friderichsen syndrome, multiorgan failure, and disseminated intravascular coagulopathy. **Coma and death may occur within 24–48 hours**

Prevention
- Vaccination: most effective prior to splenectomy
- Partial splenectomy or splenorrhaphy rather than total splenectomy
- Patient education
- Medical alert card or bracelet indicating asplenia
- Reserve supply of antibiotics
- **Revaccination for *S. pneumoniae* 5 years after initial vaccination** or 2–6 years after splenectomy

HERNIAS

ALEXANDER V. CHALPHIN • CHRISTOPHER BOYD

11-1: General Background

Definitions
- "Hernia": abnormal protrusion of organ or tissue through defect in the surrounding walls
- Strangulated: blood supply to hernia contents is compromised
- Reducible: contents can be manually replaced to normal anatomic position
- Incarcerated: cannot be reduced

Types of Hernias
• Inguinal hernia: involves the inguinal canal
• Direct: "Hesselbach triangle" = medial to epigastric vessels
• Indirect: lateral to epigastric vessels
• Femoral hernia: groin hernia medial to femoral vessels
• Ventral hernia: through anterior abdominal fascia (umbilical, epigastric, and incisional)
• Sportsman hernia: groin pain without obvious hernia
• Sliding hernia (extrasaccular): sac partially formed by the wall of a hollow organ (e.g., bladder, cecum, and sigmoid mesentery)
• Pantaloon hernia: direct and indirect hernias; straddles inferior epigastric vessels
• Richter hernia: involves one sidewall of bowel
• Spigelian hernia: herniation through the linea semilunaris
• Obturator hernia: through obturator canal
• Lumbar hernia: through posterolateral abdominal wall
• Petit: through inferior lumbar triangle
• Grynfeltt: through superior lumbar triangle
• Parastomal hernia: herniation adjacent to ostomy
• Sciatic hernia: through sciatic foramen
• Littre hernia: contains a Meckel diverticulum
• Amyand's hernia (appendicocele): inguinal hernia containing the appendix
• De Garengeot's hernia: femoral hernia containing the appendix
• Beclard hernia: through the opening for the saphenous vein

Epidemiology
- Most common general surgical operation (~700,000 repairs per year in the United States)
- **Groin hernias 25 × more common in males**
  - Females are more likely to develop femoral (10:1), umbilical (2:1), and incisional hernias (2:1). But, **the most common groin hernia in females is still indirect inguinal**
- Risk of strangulation
  - 0.0037% per year in patients with inguinal hernias (Surg Clin N Am. 2008;88:127–138)
- Risk factors for hernia (if present should be addressed prior to repair)
  - **Increased intra-abdominal pressure,** usually straining at stool or urination, BPH (needs citation (Surgery. 2007;141:262–266); says no significant association)
  - Obesity; COPD; excessive coughing; pregnancy; ascites; connective tissue diseases; heavy lifting; cigarette smoking; and arterial aneurysms

Anatomy

Inguinal Canal
Boundaries
• Superficial: external oblique aponeurosis
• Superior: internal oblique + transversus abdominis musculoaponeurosis
• Inferior: inguinal and lacunar ligaments
• Posterior (floor): transversalis fascia + transversus abdominus aponeurosis
Spermatic Cord Contents (Males)
• Cremasteric muscle fibers (from internal oblique)
• Testicular artery and veins
• Genital branch of genitofemoral nerve
• Vas deferens
• Lymphatics
• Processus vaginalis

Vessels
- Iliac: if a suture is placed through the vessel it should be immediately removed (not tied down) and pressure applied
- Inferior epigastric: can retract and bleed if inadvertently injured; can be divided if necessary
- Superficial epigastric: in subcutaneous tissue, above Scarpa's fascia

Nerves
- Genital branch of genitofemoral: innervates the anterolateral surface of the scrotum and cremaster muscle
- Ilioinguinal: innervates the anterior surface of the scrotum and medial thigh
- Iliohypogastric: innervates the lateral gluteal region (lateral branch) and the skin above the pubis (anterior branch)
- Lateral cutaneous: innervates the lateral thigh

Hesselbach Triangle
- Epigastric vessels (superiorly)
- Inguinal ligament (inferiorly)
- Lateral border of rectus sheath (medially)

Patient Assessment
Differentials

Groin Pain and Groin Mass	
Differential Diagnosis of Groin Mass	**Differential Diagnosis of Groin Pain (w/out mass)**
Inguinal hernia	Occult hernia
Femoral hernia	Ligament and muscle strains
Lipoma	Avulsion fractures
Hematoma	Nerve entrapment
Femoral artery aneurysm, pseudoaneurysm	Osteitis pubis
Sebaceous cyst	Stress fracture
Hidradenitis	Hip pathology: labral tears, articular cartilage injuries, avascular necrosis of femoral head
Lymphoma or metastatic lymph node	
Inguinal/femoral adenitis	UTI
Male	Nephrolithiasis (in addition to differential on left column)
Spermatocele	
Hydrocele	Athletic pubalgia (sports hernia)
Varicocele	
Undescended testes	
Epididymitis	
Testicular torsion	
Testicular carcinoma	
Female	
Ovary in canal of Nuck	
Endometriosis	

Physical Examination
- Examine groin and abdomen lying supine and standing, bilaterally
  - Inspect for asymmetry and masses
  - Have patient stand, cough, or Valsalva
  - Repeat with one finger invaginating the scrotum to palpate the inguinal canal
  - No need to differentiate direct from indirect in the average patient
- Examine for skin changes or erythema overlying the hernia
- Examine for ascites

Imaging
- Only necessary to assess for occult hernia or rule out other condition
- Ultrasound very operator dependent
- CT and MRI may also be performed. MRI is the most sensitive/specific modality
  (JAMA Surg. 2014;149(10):1077–1080)
- Difficult to differentiate direct vs. indirect hernias preoperatively

11-2: GROIN HERNIAS

Inguinal Hernia
Direct
- Herniation through weakened transversalis fascia (inguinal floor)
- Location: **within** Hesselbach triangle = above inguinal ligament and medial to the epigastric vessels
- Palpated anteriorly (protrudes directly through the abdominal wall)

Indirect

- Herniation through internal ring, may protrude through external ring and into scrotum
- Location: **lateral to** Hesselbach triangle, above inguinal ligament
- Palpated and reduced, with finger invaginating scrotum directed toward external ring (sac will touch fingertip)

How to Reduce Hernia
• Sedation to relax patient
• Ice pack to reduce swelling
• Place patient in Trendelenburg (head down)
• Gently apply pressure in the proper direction to reduce the hernia contents

Nonoperative Management
• Patients with ascites
• Truss: belt system to keep hernia reduced, mainly for symptom relief, does not prevent progression or complications, and for patients unfit to undergo surgery
• Watchful waiting: acceptable when symptoms are minimal, but most patients will eventually require surgery within 10 years due to progression of symptoms (usually pain) (Ann Surg. 2013;258:508–515)
• Reduction of incarcerated hernia: reasonable to attempt if no concern for strangulation or bowel necrosis (not for femoral hernias)

Operative Considerations

Principles of Open Inguinal Hernia Repair
Look for superficial epigastric vein (often encountered superficial to Scarpa's fascia)
⇩
Divide Scarpa's fascia
⇩
Open canal (external oblique fascia) through external ring
⇩
Clear cord structures off external oblique fascia
⇩
Control (circumferentially dissect) cord at the level of the pubic tubercle
⇩
Examine inguinal floor (medial to epigastric vessels)
⇩
Dissect the cord and look for indirect sac, separate and free sac from cord structures and identify any cord lipoma (high ligation [kids] vs. reduction of sac)
⇩
+/– plug through internal ring
⇩
Specific repair (see below)
⇩
Close external oblique fascia (+/– close Scarpa's fascia)

Anesthesia

- General
- Local/regional w/MAC
  - Ideal for high-risk patients
  - Allows for patient to be awakened and Valsalva to test the repair
- Have shorter recovery in PACU and may have less urinary retention. Tips for local anesthesia:
  - Use combo of short- and longlasting (e.g., lidocaine and bupivacaine)
  - Infiltrate prior to scrubbing, prepping, and draping
  - **Inject 10 cc two fingerbreadths medial to ASIS: blocks ilioinguinal nerve deep to internal oblique (can dull needle to feel it pass through each fascial layer)**
  - **Infiltrate 5 cc just deep to external oblique fascia: hydrodissects away nerve and cord structures prior to opening canal and further anesthetizes ilioinguinal nerve**
  - **Consider ultrasound-guided block**

When to Repair a Hernia?

- **Incarceration or strangulation**
- **Symptomatic**
- Prevention, progression, or complications
- Economic/employment/workers compensation issues

Anterior, Prosthetic Open Hernia Repairs
- Lichtenstein: tension-free mesh repair
  - **Considered to be the superior method to repair hernias** (Br J Surg. 2002 89:45–49)
  - Initial approach and control of the spermatic cord is the same.
  - **Place and anchor a polypropylene "keyhole" mesh to the pubic tubercle. If mesh has an asymmetric slit, the wide portion is placed medial to cover the floor.**
  - **Fix the mesh to the inguinal ligament laterally and the conjoined tendon medially.**
  - **Encircle the spermatic cord via a slit in the mesh.**
  - **Secure the two mesh edges to one another to recreate the internal ring.**
- Mesh plug and patch (Modified Lichtenstein)
- Use a preformed flower-shaped plug or rolled flat mesh
- Indirect: place in internal ring; direct: place through the fascial defect in the floor
- Place a mesh patch on top, similar to Lichtenstein
- Consider ramifications of non-absorbable plugs, including erosions and challenges in future operations

Complications
- Injury to
  - Femoral vessels when suturing laterally (inguinal ligament or iliopubic tract)
  - Bladder or bowel (especially w/sliding hernias)
  - Deep inferior epigastric vessels (can cause retroperitoneal bleeding)
  - Vas deferens
- Injury ± entrapment of nerves
  - **Affected nerves: ilioinguinal, genital branch of genitofemoral, and Iliohypogastric**
  - Roughly 10% experience chronic postherniorrhaphy pain lasting at least 3 months, 2–4% have severe pain interfering with lifestyle (Hernia. 2009;13:343–403)
  - Onset is usually immediate
  - Transient neuralgias usually resolve within a few weeks
  - Persistent neuralgias cause pain and hyperesthesia; palpation over the point of entrapment, usually reproduces pain, and hyperextension of the hip
  - If pain continues and appears to be nerve entrapment or injury, operation is triple neurectomy (ilioinguinal, iliohypogastric, and genital branch of the genitofemoral)
- Recurrence: extremely variable depending on technique, surgeon experience and follow-up
  - Can be as low as 1–3% in experienced centers
    Data varies, but several recent meta-analyses suggest open repair superior to laparoscopic in terms of recurrence in first time inguinal hernia repair (Agency Healthcare Qual. 2012:1–1219; Ann Surg. 2012;255:846–853)
  - **Most commonly recurs medially in the floor near the pubic tubercle**
  - Most recurrences occur within the first two years, direct hernias
  - **Repairing a recurrence: choose a different approach than the initial operation; can open posterior or laparoscopic; and mesh is usually needed**
- Failure to identify and reduce an indirect hernia sac (common cause of "recurrence")
- Wound infection
  - Occurs in 3–4% of open repairs (Cochrane Database Syst Rev. 2012;(2):CD003769) and 1% of laparoscopic repairs (Surg Endosc. 2013;27:3505–3519). Mesh does not increase the risk of infection.
  - Decrease risk by clipping hair (not shaving), antibiotics if mesh used
- Ischemic orchitis: thrombosis of pampiniform plexus veins
  - Incidence of 0.7%, regardless of open or laparoscopic technique (Hernia. 2009;13:343–403)
  - Testis becomes swollen and tender 2–5 days postoperatively
  - Lasts for 6–12 weeks and usually results in testicular atrophy
  - **Minimize unnecessary dissection in the spermatic cord**

Laparoscopic Inguinal Hernia Repair
Transabdominal Preperitoneal (TAPP)
- Make a small periumbilical incision in peritoneum at medial umbilical ligament; extend laterally over the direct and indirect spaces
- Fold and place a piece of mesh through a 10-cm port into abdomen
  - Mesh should cover myopectineal orifice (Cooper ligament medially, the internal ring laterally, and above the defect superiorly)
  - May fix the mesh with tacks, suture or fibrin glue) to Cooper ligament medially, the rectus muscle superiorly, and the lateral abdominal wall
  - The tacks need to be above the iliopubic tract to avoid nerve injury
  - Fibrin glue avoids neurovascular injury
  - All mesh repairs of direct inguinal hernias should have mesh fixated
- Bilateral repairs should be done with individual pieces of mesh

Laparoscopic Repair—Considerations
- Advantages: decreased postoperative pain and earlier return to activity
- Risks: major complication rate may be higher in laparoscopic vs. open repair; visceral injury; and vascular injuries
- Absolute contraindications: intra-abdominal infection and coagulopathy
- Relative contraindications: intra-abdominal adhesions, ascites,, and inability for general anesthesia
- **Current indications: recurrent hernia, bilateral hernias, or patient choice**

(Cochrane Database Syst Rev. 2003;1:CD001785; N Engl J Med. 2004;350:1819–1827; Agency Healthcare Res Qual. 2012:1–1219; Ann Surg. 2012;255:846–853)

Totally Extraperitoneal Repair (TEP) (Fig. 11-1)
- Does not violate the peritoneal cavity
- Uses a large preperitoneal mesh to cover hernias (12×15 cm^2)
- Surgical technique
  - Incision just lateral to the umbilicus, dissect down to medial border of rectus sheath, open the anterior fascia, and retract the muscle laterally
  - Bluntly dissect with a dissecting balloon
  - Place a 10-mm camera port and two 5-mm working ports between umbilicus and pubis. Place mesh and secure to Cooper ligament

Figure 11-1 Anatomy of the inguinal space. Essential landmarks of the inguinal anatomy when performing laparoscopic repair include epigastric vessels, Cooper's ligament, internal ring, and major vessels. (From Fischer JE, Bland KI. *Mastery of Surgery*, 5th ed. Philadelphia, PA: Lippincott Williams & Wilkins, 2007.)

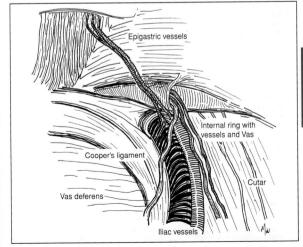

Complications (Fig. 11-2)

Figure 11-2 Anatomic detail of inguinal region. Note the Triangle of Doom and Triangle of Pain location. Both potential pitfalls of laparoscopic inguinal hernia surgery. (Illustrations reprinted with permission from Jones et al., *Atlas of Minimally Invasive Surgery*, Cine-Med, 2006. Copyright of the book and illustrations are retained by Cine-Med.)

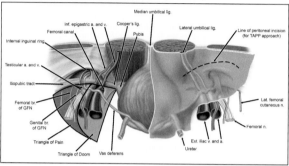

- **Triangle of Doom**
  - Zone bordered laterally by spermatic vessels and medially by the ductus deferens
  - Apex is at the deep inguinal ring
  - External iliac vessels are contained in this space
- **Triangle of Pain**
  - Zone bordered medially by spermatic vessels and superolaterally by iliopubic tract
  - Contains the genitofemoral nerve and the lateral femoral cutaneous nerve

Femoral Hernia
Definition
- Inferior to inguinal ligament, medial to femoral vessels
- **High incidence of incarceration and strangulation**
- Cooper hernia: through femoral canal travels into scrotum or labia majoris

Surgical Technique—Always Repair!!!!
- McVay (tension repair)
  - Used with femoral hernias since it narrows the femoral canal
  - Similar to the Bassini, except pectineal (Cooper) ligament is lateral attachment
  - **Need to perform a relaxing incision**
    - Bluntly dissect external oblique aponeurosis away from internal oblique
    - Make a 7–8-cm cephalad incision 1.5 cm above the pubic tubercle
    - Make a 7–8-cm incision in the anterior rectus sheath
- La Roque counter incision
  - Allows access to peritoneal cavity without performing a laparotomy when approaching an incarcerated hernia from a standard groin incision to inspect bowel and resect if necessary
  - Clear the subcutaneous tissue off the abdominal fascia cranially and make a separate incision into the peritoneum
  - Inspect bowel for necrosis or perforation prior to returning it to the peritoneum
  - Divide the inguinal ligament if necessary to reduce swollen hernia contents

Pediatric Hernias
Epidemiology
- Most common: indirect, due to patent processus vaginalis, R > L
- Higher incarceration rates than in adults
- Risk factors
  - Age (most important): **preterm—13% of babies <32 weeks** (*Surg Clin N Am.* 2012;92:487–504)
  - Undescended testis, hypospadias/epispadias, cystic fibrosis, other abdominal wall abnormality, and connective tissue disease

Diagnosis
- Clinical only
- On palpation, may feel "silk glove" sign: thickened cord of hernia sac within the spermatic cord feels like two silky gloved fingers rubbing together
- Passing fingers over pubic tubercle may reveal patent processus vaginalis

Treatment
- Surgical repair is indicated for all inguinal hernias
- 70–80% can be reduced, thus initial management is often conservative
  - Sedate child and attempt to reduce
  - Go to OR if not reduced after 6 hours; any signs of peritonitis
- Repair is often just high ligation of sac or Marcy repair (high ligation with suture narrowing of deep inguinal ring) if the internal ring is large
- Laparoscopic repair has similar operative time, length of hospital stay, recurrence and complication rates in the hands of experienced operators, and is superior to open repair for bilateral inguinal hernias in pediatric cases (*J Ped Surg.* 2011;46:1824–1834)

11-3: ABDOMINAL HERNIAS

Ventral Hernias
Umbilical: Herniation Through the Umbilical Ring
- More common in females; mostly acquired in adults
- Risk factors: obesity, chronic cough, and ascites

Epigastric: Herniation Through the Linea Alba Above the Umbilicus
Incisional: Herniation Through an Incision Site
- Risk factors: **wound infection** (#1 cause), re-incision, advanced age, male sex, smoking, steroid use, diabetes, and obesity
- Occurs in 11% of noninfected, 23% of infected wounds after abdominal surgery
- 80% develop within the first 3 years after surgery
- Traditional primary repair had recurrence rate ~50%; **use of mesh in hernias 0.2 cm decreases recurrence rate to 0–10%** (*Ann Surg.* 2004;240:578–583)
- Open and laparoscopic approaches of fairly equal efficacy

Open Repair
- Primary: for hernias <2 cm, closed transversely or vertically
- Mesh
  - Dissect the hernia sac free and reduce its contents
  - Clear a 1-cm fascial edge above and below
  - Place polypropylene mesh in the preperitoneal space and suture the edges
  - Close the fascia over the mesh
- Component separation: may be done with or without mesh
  - Clear the rectus fascia of overlying tissue out to 5 cm lateral to lateral border
  - Open medial border of oblique fascia
  - Transverse abdominis release (make sure this step is in the appropriate location)
  - Separate the anterior portion of the muscle and advance medially
  - Divide the external oblique aponeurosis cranially and caudally, allowing the external oblique to be advanced medially
  - Close the rectus fascia in the midline

Laparoscopic
- Allows for examination of the entire abdominal wall
- Good for obese patients, large and recurrent hernias >2.5 cm or so
- Surgical technique
  - Initial scope placement can be lateral with 2–3 additional lateral working ports
  - Reduce contents using blunt graspers and take down thin filmy attachments
  - Roll and insert a mesh of choice (enough for 4 cm of mesh coverage on all sides) through a 10- or 12-mm port
  - Secure mesh with either tacks or transabdominal U stitches via suture passer
- Seroma formation is common and should be managed expectantly
- Abdominal binder

Parastomal Hernias
Epidemiology
- Occurs in 3–39% of colostomies and 6% of ileostomies (*Br J Surg.* 2003;90:784–793)
- High recurrence rate since you must leave a fascial opening
- Placement of mesh in either preperitoneal or sublay positions at time of stoma creation has been shown to decrease rates of parastomal hernias and rates of parastomal hernias requiring surgical repair without any added morbidity (*J Am Coll Surg.*

2010;211:637–645). Consider repair if skin breakdown, difficulty applying appliance, and incarceration/strangulation

Surgical Options (Arch Surg. 1994;129(4):413–418; Ann Surg. 2012;255:685–695)
- Re-site stoma (33% recurrence)
- Primary suture (tightening of fascial defect): high recurrence (76%)
- Keyhole mesh repair (33% recurrence)
  - Open intra-abdominal, open interfascial, or laparoscopic approaches
  - Slit in mesh can act as a weak point for recurrence
- Sugarbaker method: mesh repair without a slit
  - Mesh is sutured to the peritoneum on all sides of the fascial defect
  - Bowel is brought out on one side of the mesh

11-4: BIOPROSTHESES/MESH

Nonabsorbable Mesh
- Polypropylene
  - Monofilament: Marlex, Proline
  - Polyfilament: Surgipro
- Mersilene
- e-PTFE
- Polyester
- Infection may necessitate removal of synthetic mesh; chronic pain may require removal
- Synthetic mesh: relative contraindication in infected field and when there is necrotic/perforated bowel; consider mesh selection carefully

Absorbable Mesh: Polyglactin (Vicryl)
Biologic Mesh
- Decellularized extracellular matrix
- Cross-linked vs. noncross-linked
- Properties: thought to maintain growth factors to allow ingrowth of new tissue; potentially useful in infected field; more expensive
- Types
  - Porcine: dermis or intestinal submucosa
  - Human: dermis
  - Bovine pericardium

DRE M. IRIZARRY • DEBORAH NAGLE

12-1: BASICS OF COLON SURGERY

Anatomy
- Cecum: largest diameter of colon (up to 9 cm normal)
- Ascending and descending colon: retroperitoneal, fixed along paracolic gutters by areolar lateral peritoneal reflections, "white lines of Toldt"
- Transverse colon: intraperitoneal, has greater omentum on antimesenteric border
- Sigmoid colon: smallest caliber of colonic segments, fixed distally to rectum
- Taenia coli: three bands of longitudinal muscles along colon that coalesce proximally at the origin of the appendix and splay out at rectosigmoid junction
- Haustra: bulges in the colonic wall seen between taenia
- Histology
  - Mucosa: glandular epithelium with crypts and goblet cells, underlying lamina propria
  - Submucosa: strength layer
  - Muscular layer: circumferential and longitudinal fibers, strength layer
  - Serosa: overlying peritoneal surface
- Function: slows transit of enteric contents, resorbing water as contents move through

Arterial Supply
- Follows embryologic development of midgut and hindgut (*Fig. 12-1*)

Figure 12-1 Colonic arterial supply. (From Fischer JE, Bland KI. *Mastery of Surgery*, 5th ed. Philadelphia, PA: Lippincott Williams & Wilkins, 2007.)

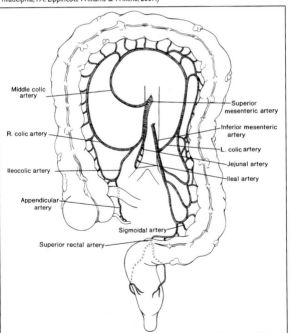

- SMA: midgut—majority of small bowel, ascending, and transverse colons
  - Branches: jejunal, ileal, ileocolic, right colic (diminutive), and middle colic

- IMA: hindgut—distal colon (descending, sigmoid, and upper rectum)
- Marginal artery of Drummond: runs parallel to colonic wall; provides collateral circulation in areas of decreased flow
- Splenic flexure: "watershed area" of SMA/IMA; at risk for ischemia in hypotension

Nerves and Lymphatics: Follow Arterial Supply
- Sympathetic innervation from thoracic splanchnic nerves/superior mesenteric and inferior mesenteric ganglion: inhibits peristalsis and stimulates internal anal sphincter
- Parasympathetic innervation from vagus and pelvic splanchnic nerves: stimulate motility and relax internal anal sphincter
- External sphincter: somatic innervations from pudendal nerve

Minimally Invasive Surgery
- Advantages of laparoscopic vs. open: faster return of bowel function, less postoperative pain, fewer pulmonary complications, shorter hospital stays, and lower incidence of postoperative infection, small bowel obstruction, and hernias
- Laparoscopic vs. robotic: postoperative outcomes equivalent aside from increase in operative time and shorter length of stay in robotic group (*J Am Coll Surg.* 2016;7515(16): 30073–30074. Doi10.1016/jamcollsurg.2016.03.041)
- Lateral to medial approach: similar to open
  - Take down line of Toldt to mobilize colon to points of resection
  - Divide corresponding mesentery last
- Medial to lateral approach
  - Takes advantage of the lateral tension provided by the peritoneal folds
  - Divide the target mesenteric vessels first, then mobilize and divide the colon

Stomas
- Artificial diversion of enteric contents through the anterior abdominal wall
- Indications
  - Inability to safely reconnect the colon at surgery because of sepsis, hypotension, and extensive soiling of the abdomen or technical issues
  - Divert stool away from a worrisome anastomosis or site of sepsis
  - Incontinence or disease in the anorectum (IBD, cancer)
- Patients should be seen and marked preoperatively by a stoma therapist
- Location
  - Traditionally placed within the rectus sheath on a flat portion of abdomen
  - End colostomies: usually left-sided
  - Ileostomies: usually on right side
- Output
  - Right-sided colostomies: higher volume and frequent output
  - Left-sided colostomies: intermittent, solid outputs, with an associated odor
- Surgical technique: permanent end colostomy
  - Mobilize proximal colon to reach anterior abdominal wall without tension
  - Create stoma tunnel through abdominal wall and rectus sheath
  - After closing wound, mature colostomy with full-thickness suture

---

12-2: DIVERTICULITIS

Colonic Diverticula
- Incidence: 30% by age 60 and 60% by age 80
- Risk factor: thought to be diets low in fiber and higher in red meat
- Etiology
  - Sigmoid: acquired diverticula, most common site of diverticulosis
  - Cecal: congenital diverticula; young Asian males
- Pathophysiology: increased intraluminal pressure leads to mucosal outpouchings between the taenia where the vasa recta enter the colonic wall

Clinical Presentation of Diverticulitis
- Symptoms: fever + constant LLQ pain (RLQ if cecal or "floppy" sigmoid colon)
- Complications: abscess, free perforation, stricture, large bowel obstruction, fistulization to vagina, uterus, or bladder

Imaging: CT Scan

Hinchey Classification
Defines the degree of perforation in complicated diverticulitis • I: localized pericolonic abscess or inflammation • II: confined pelvic abscess • III: purulent peritonitis from abscess perforation • IV: fecal peritonitis from colonic perforation

Treatment
Conservative
- Antibiotics covering colonic flora
- +/– Admission for IV hydration and bowel rest
- Percutaneous drainage if abscess present and technically feasible. Abscesses 3 cm and under generally do not require drainage.
- Repeat imaging in 3–4 days if no improvement in symptoms
- Colonoscopy at 6 weeks to rule out an occult cancer or another etiology for the patient's symptoms after the first episode IF not scoped within the last 3 years.

Surgical Indications
- Acute
  - Free air (controversial)
  - Peritonitis
  - Failure of medical therapy
  - Immunocompromised (lower threshold for surgery)
  - Giant diverticulum
- Chronic/recurrent
  - Less of a role for aggressive use of antibiotics or surgery for chronic or recurrent diverticulitis than historically thought necessary. (JAMA. 2014;311(3):287–297). Surgery should be considered after four recurrent episodes of diverticulitis.

Surgical Options
- Laparoscopic lavage is controversial but it may be safe and feasible in short-term management for select patients (Ann Surg. 2016;263:117–122)
- Single stage with primary anastomosis (Br J Surg. 2001;88:693–697)
- Mikulicz operation (two stage): end colostomy with mucous fistula or with a primary anastomosis and diverting ileostomy
- Hartmann procedure (two stage): end colostomy and blind rectal pouch
  - Resect diseased segment by dividing at rectosigmoid junction (splaying out taenia) and working proximal to remove diseased segment of bowel
  - Mark or tag rectal stump
  - Close wound and fashion end colostomy in LLQ abdomen

12-3: COLITIS (NON-IBD)

Ischemic Colitis
Basics
- Epidemiology: more common in older age group
- Location: typically localized to splenic flexure due to watershed area (arc of Riolan)

Clinical Presentation
- Symptoms: vague or localized abdominal pain
- Signs: can have guaiac-positive or frankly bloody stools

Imaging
- CT scan with IV contrast: identifies vascular patency of the major vessels; wall thickening in the affected area
- Colonoscopy (but usually not in the acute setting)

Treatment
- Conservative: IV hydration, antibiotics, and bowel rest; systemic anticoagulation in setting of embolic or venous source of ischemia if no active bleeding
- Operative indications
  - Full-thickness ischemia with peritonitis
  - Persistent or worsening pain despite adequate hydration
  - Clinical deterioration

Antibiotic-Associated *Clostridium difficile* Colitis
Basics
- *Clostridium difficile*
  - Spores are not susceptible to alcohol-based hand sanitizers; wash hands with soap and water before and after examining patients with *C. difficile*
  - Increasing prevalence as well as virulence of *C. difficile* infections
  - Difficult to culture *in vitro*
- Risk factors (worst antibiotic offenders): clindamycin, fluoroquinolones, broad-spectrum penicillins, and cephalosporins
- Pathophysiology
  - Antibiotics disrupt normal colonic flora, enhancing the growth of *C. difficile*

- Antibiotics elaborate toxins that cause mucosal injury and inflammation, interrupts intercellular junctions, enhances neutrophil chemotaxis, and results in pseudomembrane formation

Clinical Presentation
- Antecedent antibiotic use or fecal–oral exposure
- Signs: watery, foul-smelling diarrhea

Imaging
- CT scan: diffuse distribution of colonic inflammation
- Endoscopy (usually limited to flexible sigmoidoscopy for diagnosis): mucosal inflammation and pseudomembrane formation

Treatment
Medical: IV hydration, PO/IV metronidazole, or oral vancomycin. Duration depends on the number of episodes.
- Surgical indications
  - Failure to respond to medical therapy
  - Fulminant sepsis
  - Toxic megacolon
  - Colonic perforation
- Surgery: subtotal colectomy with end ileostomy

12-4: INFLAMMATORY BOWEL DISEASE (IBD)

Basics
- Chronic inflammatory disorder of the GI tract
- Etiology unknown
- Risk factor: family history
- Bimodal age of onset

Crohn's Disease		Ulcerative Colitis
• Anywhere from mouth to anus • Terminal ileum: most common • Perianal disease common	Characteristics	• Begins in rectum and proceeds into colon • Continuous, uninterrupted disease • Bloody diarrhea
• Transmural inflammation w/ multiple lymphoid aggregates • Segmental disease (skip lesions) • Cobblestoning • Mucosal ulceration (aphthous) • Creeping fat • Fistulas	Pathological Features	• Only mucosa and submucosa involved • Friable mucosa
• Arthritis/arthralgias • Pyoderma gangrenosum • Erythema nodosum • Ocular diseases • Growth failure • Megaloblastic anemia from folate and B12 malabsorption	Extraintestinal Manifestations	• Peripheral arteritis • Ankylosing spondylitis • Primary sclerosing cholangitis (does not resolve with colectomy)

Treatment
- Crohn's: no definitive cure
- UC: can cure with surgery; need lifetime surveillance of any residual rectal area
- Medical therapy: to slow disease progression and decrease symptoms

Surgical Indications	
Medically refractory disease	Obstruction
Abscess (Crohn's)	Toxic megacolon
Hemorrhage	Enterocutaneous fistula (Crohn's)
Perforation	Acute fulminant ulcerative colitis (UC)
Dysplasia or cancer	Systemic complications (UC)

- Surgical principles: Crohn's
  - Resect ONLY grossly diseased bowel (e.g., ileocecectomy)

- Stricturoplasty may benefit some patients for very short-strictured segments (see Chapter 6, Section 3, for operative technique)
- Take down most fistulas, resect involved bowel, and close other organs
- Drain any intra-abdominal abscess
- Surgical principles: ulcerative colitis
  - Type of surgery depends on emergent vs. elective, extent of rectal disease
  - Elective surgery: ileoanal pouch
  - Emergent surgery and severe rectal disease: total proctocolectomy with end ileostomy

Ulcerative Colitis—Ileoanal Pouch
Perform an abdominal colectomy and proctectomy
⇩
Transect the ileum at the ileocecal valve and complete a rectal excision down to the level of the levator complex from the above. Create an ileal J pouch by folding and stapling the ileum to recreate a rectal reservoir.
⇩
+/- diverting loop ileostomy
⇩
Different pouch configurations: J-pouch construction
⇩
Close off the terminal ileum with a linear stapler
⇩
Find the longest reach of the ileal mesentery to the levators and double the ileum back on itself at that point
⇩
Strive for a length of 14–15 cm on the pouch
⇩
Make an apical enterotomy
⇩
Sequentially fire a GIA to construct the pouch
⇩
Place anvil of circular stapler in apical enterotomy and secure with purse string suture
⇩
Pass the circular stapler transanally to fashion the anastomosis

12-5: Lower Gastrointestinal Bleeding

Etiology
- Diverticulosis
- Vascular ectasia
- Colon cancer
- Ischemic colitis
- Inflammatory bowel disease
- Other: trauma, hereditary hemorrhagic telangiectasia, intussusception, volvulus, anticoagulation, rectal cancer, Meckel diverticulum, stercoral ulcer, irradiation injury, infarcted bowel, and aortoenteric fistula

Management of Lower GI Bleeding
Initial
• Access: two large bore IVs
• Type and cross-match RBC units
• Check coags
• NGT lavage to rule out upper GI source
• Anoscopy to rule out rectal source
Imaging
• Colonoscopy
• Angiography: bleeding rate must be 0.5–1 cc/min, diagnostic and therapeutic *(Tech Vasc Intern Radiol. 2009;12(2):80–91)*
• CTA: (only diagnostic) 0.3–0.5 cc/min *(Radiology. 2003;228(3):743–752)*
• Tagged red blood cell scan: bleeding rate must be 0.1–0.5 cc/min, requires active bleeding, localizes to general area *(Am J Gastroenterol. 1994;89(3):345)*
• Angiogram: bleeding rate must be >0.5 cc/min
• Capsule endoscopy
Surgical Indications in Lower GI Bleeding
• Intervention depends on etiology/location of the bleed

Etiology
- #1 adhesive disease
- #2 tumors
- #3 hernias

Imaging
- Flat and upright abdominal x-ray (KUB)
- CT scan
- Gastrografin enema
- Management
- NPO, IV fluids
- NG tube
- Serial exams
- To OR if peritoneal on exam or if fails conservative management

Perforation
- Colon perforation with obstruction: most likely to occur in cecum

$$\text{Law of Laplace: tension = pressure} \times \text{diameter}$$

- Competent ileocecal valve can lead to closed-loop obstruction in large bowel

Sigmoid Volvulus
- Risk factors: debilitated, nursing home resident, psychiatric patients, neurologic dysfunction, colonic dysmotility, and chronic constipation
- Do not attempt decompression with gangrenous bowel or peritoneal signs
- Treatment
  Decompress with colonoscopy: 77% successful reduction (Tech Coloproctol. 2013;17(5):561–569)

Cecal Volvulus
- Do not attempt decompression with colonoscopy
  - Unlikely to succeed
- Treatment: right hemicolectomy

Functional Obstructions
- Types: Ileus, Ogilvie (pseudo-obstruction), and chronic dysmotility
- Treatment
  - Check electrolytes (Na^+, K^+, and Mg^{++})
  - Discontinue drugs that slow the gut
  - Ogilvie
  Serial exams
- If fail conservative management and >12 cm: Neostigmine vs. colonoscopic decompression vs. surgical intervention. Colonoscopic decompression and neostigmine can both be repeated until pseudo-obstruction resolves.

Colon Cancer
Epidemiology
- Incidence: the third most common cancer in men and women
- Risk factor: gene mutation
  - APC: chromosome 5q21
  - k-ras: chromosome 12
  - p53: chromosome 17
  - DCC: chromosome 18q
- Metastases: no. 1 to liver and no. 2 to lungs. These two sites account for the vast majority of colorectal metastases.

Colorectal Cancer Screening (American Cancer Society Guidelines on Screening and Surveillance)
- Average risk (all following, if positive, should be followed up with colonoscopy)
  - Annual fecal occult blood test
  - Annual fecal immunochemical test (FIT)
  - Stool DNA every 3 years
  - Flexible sigmoidoscopy every 5 years
  - Double contrast barium enema every 5 years
  - CT colonography every 5 years
  - Colonoscopy every 10 years (gold standard)

- Increased risk
  - 1–2 adenomas, low-grade dysplasia, <1 cm: same interval as average risk
  - Single adenoma >1 cm, 3–10 small adenomas, villous features, or high-grade dysplasia: colonoscopy in 3 years
  - History of colorectal cancer or polyps in first-degree relative <60 years of age, or two or more first-degree relatives of any age: screen at 40 or 10 years before the youngest relative diagnosed, colonoscopy every 5 years
  - Guidelines for screening are frequently adapted based on endoscopist's perception of patient preparation and completeness of exam.
- High risk
  - FAP: yearly flexible sigmoidoscopy beginning at age 10–12; consider colectomy
  - Lynch syndrome: colonoscopy every 1–2 years starting at age 20–25 or 10 years before youngest immediate family member diagnosed
  - IBD: colonoscopy every 1–2 years with biopsies

Polyps
- Hyperplastic polyps: if small no cancer risk, some thought that larger may be precursor to sessile serrated polyps
- Adenomatous polyps: benign lesions with malignant potential, need removal
  - Tubular adenoma: most common
  - Villous adenoma: least common
  - Tubulovillous:
- Carcinoma in situ in resected specimen
  - No further surgery if margins negative
  - Close follow-up with colonoscopies
- Cancer invading the muscularis mucosa
  - Polypoid with a stalk, stalk free of tumor, and no vascular/lymphatic invasion:
    - Close follow-up with colonoscopy
- If residual sessile polyp cannot be completely resected with repeat colonoscopy, consider surgical resection

AJCC Staging
- T1 invades submucosa
- T2 invades muscularis propria
- T3 invades into subserosa or non-peritoneal colonic tissues
- T4 invades other organs and/or perforates visceral peritoneum

Treatment
Preoperative Workup
- Colonoscopy to rule out synchronous colonic lesions (5% or less chance)
- Imaging: CT chest/abdomen/pelvis
- Labs: CEA and CBC

Surgery
- Goals: en bloc resection, 5-cm margins, and regional lymphadenectomy
- Metastases: improved survival if liver or lung metastases resected
- Recurrence: operate if metastases not diffuse

Operative Management
Laparoscopic Right Hemicolectomy
Trendelenburg position with the right side up
⇩
Generally three or four ports: umbilicus, upper midline, and left mid-abdomen or lower midline
⇩
High ligation of ileocolic vascular pedicle
⇩
Divide the TI at the level of the ileal fat pad (about 5 cm from the IVC)
⇩
Mobilize the colon along the white line of Toldt around the hepatic flexure
⇩
Divide the transverse colon proximal to the middle colic vessels

⇩

Perform a side-to-side anastomoses

⇩

(In either open or minimally invasive technique, colon can be mobilized first, then bowel/mesentery are divided)

Laparoscopic Sigmoid Colectomy

Generally three or four ports: umbilicus, RLQ, LLQ, and other

Incise the peritoneal reflection of the mesocolon

⇩

Identify the left ureter

⇩

Identify and divide the IMA vessels near their origins

⇩

Mobilize and divide the rectosigmoid or distal sigmoid

⇩

Anastomosis: end-to-end with EEA stapler

Chemotherapy Options
- Capecitabine
- FOLFOX: oxaliplatin + lecovorin + 5-FU—this is the gold standard for stage III disease
- CapeOx: oxaliplatin + oral capecitabine
- Add bevacizumab (Avastin) for stage IV disease

Surveillance
- Every 3 months for 2 years: office visits with CEA level
- One-year postoperative: colonoscopy and CT chest/abdomen

Rectal Cancer
Anatomic Considerations (Compared With Colon Cancer)
- Constrained, narrow, funnel-shaped, bony pelvis. Much higher local recurrence rate. Surgery is more technically challenging
- Anal sphincters: essential for continence. Perform an abdominoperineal resection (APR) if (a) tumor invades sphincters, (b) poor preoperative continence, or (c) inability to obtain adequate distal margins without incorporating sphincters

Preoperative Workup
- CT scan: metastases
- MRI : for local T (depth) and N (nodal) staging
- Transanal EUS: T and N staging

Preoperative Chemoradiation
(4500 cGy + infusional 5-FU or oral capecitabine) for T3, T4, or Node-Positive Tumors
(N Engl J Med. 2004;351:1731–1740; Lancet. 2009;373:811–820)
- Shrink tumor: downstage
- Facilitate negative resection margins
- Allow for low anterior resection (LAR) vs. APR

Surgery
- Timing: 6–12 weeks after neoadjuvant therapy
- Diverting loop ileostomy at the time of the primary resection may be used to protect anastomosis
- Transanal excision and transanal endoscopic microsurgery
  - Benign lesions
  - Early stage (T0 and T1) low rectal tumors
  - Elderly or those who could not tolerate a major surgery
- LAR (Figure 12-2)
  - If anastomosis <6 cm from the anorectal junction, consider colonic J pouch
  - LAR syndrome
    - Decreased rectal reservoir capacity after partial or complete proctectomy
    - Symptoms: frequency, urgency, and clustering of bowel movements
    - Treatment: medical management with fiber and antiperistaltic agents

Posterior Plane of LAR Dissection

Lithotomy Position (Fig. 12-2)

Figure 12-2 Sequential mobilization of the rectum by sharp dissection of the posterior plane between the visceral layer and parietal layers of the pelvic fascia. **A:** Plane of the posterior dissection between the visceral and parietal layers of the pelvic fasciae. **B:** Sharp division of the rectosacral fascia. **C:** Division of the Waldeyer fascia, completing the posterior dissection to the anal hiatus. **D:** Complete mobilization of the rectum down to the levators. **E:** A typical level of distal level of transaction. (From Fischer JE, Bland KI. *Mastery of Surgery*, 5th ed. Philadelphia, PA: Lippincott Williams & Wilkins, 2007.)

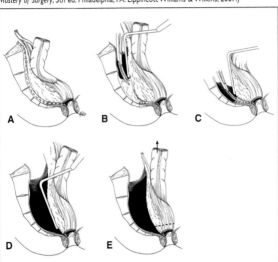

Make a V-shaped incision at the base of sigmoid mesentery on right, extending it distally to right side of the rectum and superiorly to expose the IMA at its origin

⇩

Identify the left ureter as it crosses the pelvic brim over the left common iliac artery

⇩

Divide the IMA just distal to origin of left colic artery, the IMV just distal to its takeoff from the splenic vein or the ligament of Treitz, and the mesenteric vessels

⇩

Isolate and divide the superior hemorrhoidal vessels and the lateral stalks containing the middle hemorrhoidal vessels

⇩

Divide the peritoneum on each side of rectum just medial to ureters; extend anterior until able to gain access to seminal vesicles in males or rectovaginal septum in females

⇩

Incise Denonvilliers fascia anteriorly, separating the anterior rectal wall from the seminal vesicles and posterior capsule of prostate

⇩

Divide the loose areolar tissue between the mesorectum and the presacral fascia so that the entire mesorectum can be removed intact

⇩

Divide the proximal colon with a GIA-60 stapler and the rectum with a reticulating stapler, ideally leaving 5-cm margins in the nonradiated patient

⇩

Place a purse-string 3-0 monofilament nonabsorbable suture around the opening of the proximal colon, insert the EEA anvil, and tie down

⇩

Insert an end-to-end stapler, usually 28 or 31 Fr, through the anal canal. Advance the spike just anterior to the distal staple line and engage the anvil

⇩

Check the integrity of the anastomosis by inspecting the two tissue doughnuts and performing an air leak test

Rectal Cancer—APR

Lithotomy Position

Close the anus with a heavy purse-string suture in the perianal skin before starting

⇩

Divide the distal sigmoid colon or proceed directly to dissection

⇩

Elevate the inferior mesenteric vessels

Open the peritoneum at the base of the mesentery, extending the incision from perirectal sulci to the anterior reflection

⇩

Enter the presacral space and identify ureters at the pelvic brim

⇩

Divide the superior hemorrhoidal vessels

⇩

Dissect in avascular plane circumferentially around the rectum always working from posterior to lateral to anterior. Do not enter the mesorectum

⇩

Continue the dissection laterally and then anteriorly through Denonvillier fascia
Identify the hypogastric plexus

⇩

Circumferentially mobilize the rectum down to the levator muscles

⇩

Divide the sigmoid to allow a tension-free exteriorization of the stoma

Perineal Resection

Make an elliptical incision around the anus using electrocautery

⇩

Circumferentially divide the subcutaneous tissue to the perianal/gluteal in a plane of dissection outside the sphincters

⇩

Continue in the posterior midline plane to identify the tip of the coccyx

⇩

Divide anococcygeal ligament and enter pelvis on anterior surface of the coccyx

⇩

Working from posterior to anterior, circumferentially free the anal canal from levator and transverse perineal attachments

⇩

Deliver the specimen through the perineum if performing laparoscopic resection
Approximate the divided levator muscles

⇩

Close the subcutaneous tissues and skin with absorbable, interrupted suture

⇩

Mature the colostomy by suturing full-thickness wall of colon to the skin

ANORECTAL

JOHN TILLOU • THOMAS CATALDO

First edition authored by Vitaliy Poylin, Deborah Nagle

13-1: BASICS OF ANORECTAL SURGERY

Anatomy

Anal Canal (*Semin Colon Rectal Surg.* 2013;24(2):68–71)

- Anatomic canal: anal verge to dentate line, 2 cm long
  - Anal verge: junction of anoderm and perianal epithelium (keratinized epithelium, sweat glands, hair follicles), where a finger or proctoscope contacts skin on anal examination
- Surgical canal: anal verge to anorectal ring (levator ani): 2.5–4 cm long
- Internal anal sphincter: thickened continuation of involuntary circular smooth muscle; controlled by **autonomic nervous system**
- External anal sphincter: elliptical cylinder of voluntary striated muscle, around and distal to internal anal sphincter
- **Mucosal lining**
  - Rectum: columnar epithelium
    - Columns of Morgagni (longitudinal folds above dentate line) to dentate line: transitional epithelium
      - Internal hemorrhoidal plexus lies deep to this
  - Below dentate line: squamous epithelium
- Anal crypts: 3–12 in number, attached to anal glands
- Anal columns (Morgagni): 8–14 longitudinal folds

Rectum

- Surgical margins: confluence of teniae coli proximally to anorectal ring distally, 12–15 cm
- Continuous longitudinal muscle layer
- Valves of Houston (2–3 in number)
  - Upper and lower: convex to the right
  - Middle: convex to the left

Pelvic Floor

- Components: anal sphincter complex, pelvic floor muscles, and muscles that line the sidewalls of the osseous pelvis
- Levator ani: major component of pelvic floor
  - Three striated muscles: ileococcygeus, pubococcygeus, and puborectalis
- Puborectalis: U-shaped loop of striated muscle, slings around anorectal junction from posterior aspect of the pubis. By affecting anorectal angle, it is a major component of gross fecal continence. Relaxation causes straightening of rectum during defecation

Arterial Blood Supply

- Superior hemorrhoidal artery: from inferior mesenteric artery
- Middle hemorrhoidal artery: variably from internal iliac or pudendal artery
- Inferior hemorrhoidal artery: branch of pudendal artery

Venous Drainage

- External hemorrhoidal plexus: subcutaneous, below dentate line
  - Drains via superior hemorrhoidal veins to the IMV
- Internal hemorrhoidal plexus: submucosal, superior to dentate line
  - Drains via inferior and middle hemorrhoidal veins to internal iliac and IVC

Lymphatic Drainage

- Above third valve of Houston to inferior mesenteric and internal iliac nodes
- Below third valve of Houston: along inferior rectal lymphatics to superficial inguinal nodes

Evaluation of Anorectum

Physical Examination

- Inspection and palpation
- Anoscopy +/− rigid sigmoidoscopy
- Examine in left lateral decubitus (Sims) or jackknife (Kraske) position
- Examine under anesthesia

Imaging

- Endolumenal US: Evaluate sphincter complex/defects, fistulous tracts, and abscess. Evaluate depth of invasion, nodal status in anal and rectal cancer.

- CT scan: Evaluation of perirectal abscesses.
- MRI scan: Evaluation of perirectal abscess or fistula and staging of anal and rectal cancer.

13-2: HEMORRHOIDS

(Clin Colon Rectal Surg. 2016;29(1):22–29)

Epidemiology
- 100% of individuals have hemorrhoids—contributes to normal fecal continence
- Symptomatic hemorrhoids
  - Prevalence: 4.4% in the United States, peaks between ages 45 and 65
  - Etiology: constipation, prolonged straining, increased intra-abdominal pressure, pregnancy, irregular bowel habits/incontinence, diarrhea, heredity, and age

External Hemorrhoids
- Anatomy: **distal to dentate line, covered by anoderm–somatic sensory innervation**
- Symptomatic acute thrombosed external hemorrhoid
  - **painful, palpable, blue/purple and tender lump**
  - may bleed due to pressure necrosis of covering mucosa
- Diagnosis: physical examination
- Treatment
  - Conservative: **sitz baths and topical analgesics (i.e., lidocaine-low efficacy)**
  - Surgical
    - Anesthetize with local anesthetic containing epinephrine
    - Small, radial elliptical incision over hemorrhoid (not simple incision and drainage)
    - Excise thrombus and associated vessels
    - Remove excess skin
    - Surgical treatment is most effective within the first 72 hours and is preferred to medical management

Internal Hemorrhoids

Classification of Internal Hemorrhoids
• First degree: no prolapse and **painless rectal bleeding**
• Second degree: prolapse during defecation and reduces spontaneously
• Third degree: requires manual reduction
• Fourth degree: irreducible

- Three major groups: right anterior, right posterior, and left lateral
- Symptoms: pain (if thrombosed), occasional bleeding, mucosal protrusion, sensation of incomplete evacuation, mucus discharge, and pruritus ani
- Diagnosis: digital examination and anoscopy, assess degree, and extent of the disease

Treatment	
Conservative	**Hemorrhoidectomy**

• Diet: increase water intake
• Change defecation habits
• Fiber supplementation (20–30 g/day)
• Sitz baths
• Topical anesthetics (i.e., Anusol HC)
 	
Office-Based Procedures
• Sclerotherapy—rarely used
• Infrared photocoagulation—for bleeding internal hemorrhoids
• Rubber banding
• For first- to third-degree internal hemorrhoids
• Do not perform if patient is on plavix or warfarin (may if patient is on baby aspirin)
• Can band multiple groups at the same time
	• **Caution if IBD, cirrhosis, or pregnant**
	• **For stage III or IV hemorrhoids**
	  Place patient in jackknife position; inject local anesthetic with epinephrine (perineum, submucosa, and pudendal nerves)
	  ⇩
	Grasp + retract external hemorrhoid, skin
	  ⇩
	Suture ligate proximally to internal hemorrhoid
	  ⇩
	Excise skin, external + internal hemorrhoids up to suture (minimal anoderm)
	  ⇩
	Close wound with running absorbable suture
	
	• Harmonic scalpel and Ligasure possible decrease in postoperative pain

Place patient in left lateral decubitus or jackknife position	• Complications
⇩	Urinary retention (common)
	Bleeding
Using an anoscope, check for correct placement with the "pinch test"	Pain (common)
	Incontinence
⇩	Anal stenosis (uncommon)
Place band 1–2 cm above dentate line	• Whitehead procedure (rarely used)—360° hemorrhoidectomy proximal to dentate
• Banded tissue sloughs off within 7 days	• Complications
• Complications	Whitehead deformity—mucosal ectropion
Pain	Stenosis
Bleeding	
Urinary hesitancy	
Transmural mucosal necrosis	

13-3: ANAL FISSURE

Location
- **Distal to dentate line and above anal verge**
- **Posterior midline (90%)** > anterior midline (5–10%, more common in women)
- Lateral: concerning for Crohn's disease, malignancy, HIV, tuberculosis, sexual abuse

Etiology
- Constipation/straining due to hard stools or diarrhea
- Increased resting pressure in the anal canal
- Associated decrease in the perfusion of anoderm (poorest perfusion posteriorly)

Clinical Presentation
- Symptoms: **pain during and after defecation, usually short lasting (tearing sensation)**
- Acute fissure: appears as oval ulcer resembling a longitudinal tear in anal canal
  - Majority resolve without surgical intervention
- Chronic fissure (8–12 weeks): one or all of the three cardinal features
  - Rolled edges with exposed sphincter at the base
  - Sentinel tag (external)
  - Hypertrophied papilla at the proximal margin (internal)

Treatment (Clin Colon Rectal Surg. 2016;29(1):30–7)

Conservative	Surgical
• Change bowel habits, stool bulking agents, sitz baths, topical anesthetics, and steroidal ointments	*"Tailored" Lateral Internal Sphincterotomy (Gold Standard)*
• Chronic fissure—50% healing rate	Locate intersphincteric groove
• Topical nitrates (0.2% nitroglycerine)	⇩
• 50% rate of healing	Insert knife blade lateral to the internal sphincter
• 50% recurrence rate	⇩
• May cause severe headaches	Lateral to medial division of up to one-third of distal internal sphincter vs. division equivalent to the length of the fissure
• Topical calcium channel blockers	• **98% success: best long-term results**
• 60–90% healing rate	• Complications: **incontinence of feces (10–15%) or flatus (5–7%)** and urgency
• 40% recurrence rate	*Botox and Fissurectomy*
Botulinum Toxin	• 85% successful
• Inject 30 U on both sides of internal anal sphincter or just one position in the lateral internal sphincter	• No permanent division of sphincter
• Adjust dose based on body size	• Removing chronic granulation tissue around fissure may improve healing rate
• Healing rate 60–80%	
• 40% recurrence	
• Effects last 3 mo—need to address underlying cause of fissure	

13-4: ANAL FISTULA/ABSCESS

Basics
- Different stages of the same process, from abscess (acute) to fistula (chronic)
- Etiology: 90% from cryptoglandular infections
- Other risk factors: constipation, anal fissures, Crohn's disease, hematoma, and HIV
- Fistulas present for >60 days are unlikely to heal without an operation

Clinical Presentation of Abscesses
- Symptoms
  - **Pain (rectal or gluteal) with defecation only (fissure) or constant pain (abscess)**
  - **Discharge**
  - **Fever**
  - **Urinary retention**
- Physical examination: erythema, swelling, flatulence, and tenderness
  - Intersphincteric and supralevator abscess may have minimal external signs but will have severe tenderness and fullness on rectal examination

---

Goodsall's Rule for Fistula-in-Ano

- Correlates internal and external opening of the fistula
- External fistula opening posterior to a transverse line drawn through anal opening has a tract that curves and opens at posterior midline internally
- External fistula anterior to the transverse line will extend directly to the anal canal anteriorly (more common in females)

Treatment of Abscess
- Drain as soon as possible
- Antibiotics not required unless immunosuppressed
- Packing/wicks are generally not useful
- Sequelae—up to 50% of patients will have associated fistula

Perianal Abscess (most common)
- Location: under skin of anal canal **adjacent to anal verge**
- Does not traverse external sphincter
- Treatment: incision and drainage
  - Cruciate or elliptical incision
  - Sitz baths and showers
- Association: **intersphincteric fistula**
  - Tract passes within intersphincteric space
  - Need to identify blind tract ending at rectal wall

Ischiorectal Abscess
- Location: through the sphincters, below levator ani, **fills ischioanal fossa**
- "Horseshoe" abscess: bilateral ischiorectal abscesses with midline connection within the deep postanal space
- Imaging: CT scan or MRI can be useful to delineate extent of abscess
- Treatment: incision and drainage under anesthesia in the operating room
  - Incise and drain as close to anus as possible to minimize subsequent fistula
  - Horseshoe abscess: incise anococcygeal ligament in posterior midline between coccyx and anus with counter incisions in each ischioanal fossa to drain anterior extensions
- Association: **transsphincteric fistula**
  - Tract passes from internal opening through internal and external sphincters to the ischiorectal fossa

Intersphincteric Abscess
- Location: **between internal and external sphincters,** most commonly located posteriorly
- Treatment: anesthesia in the operating room
- Transanal division of the internal sphincter over the area of the abscess
- Marsupialize to allow adequate drainage into anal canal

Supralevator Abscess (uncommon)
- Location: **above levator ani muscle**
  - Downward extension of pelvic abscess (i.e., diverticulitis, appendicitis, etc)
  - Upward extension of intersphincteric, ischiorectal abscess
- Treatment
  - If from an upward extension of intersphincteric abscess: drain though the rectum
  - If from an upward extension of ischiorectal abscess: drain through perianal skin
  - If extension of pelvic abscess: percutaneous drainage
- Association: **suprasphincteric fistula**
  - Tract arises from intersphincteric groove, passes above puborectalis, curves downward lateral to the external sphincter into the ischioanal space

Clinical Presentation of Fistula
- Symptoms: cyclic history of abscess, pain, bleeding, and drainage
- Digital examination: indurated internal opening, discharge at external opening
  May use hydrogen peroxide or methylene blue to find internal opening
- Imaging: CT scan, MRI (most useful), and endoanal US

Anal Fistula—Treatment

Preoperative: know baseline continence, rule out IBD and HIV

Lay-open technique: if limited low external sphincter fiber involvement can open most of the internal sphincter muscle. Caution with anterior fistula in a female, IBD.

Pass a probe through the fistula
⇩
Incise tissue over the probe
⇩
Curettage the granulation tissue
⇩
Marsupialize the wound edges if needed

Draining Seton: consider if fistula crosses the sphincter above the midway point, IBD patient, multiple or complex fistulas—allows for resolution of inflammation, establishes well fibrosed tract which improves success rate of other techniques. **Return to OR in 6 wk to 3 mo for definitive repair. Minimizes postoperative incontinence.**

Identify tract using above techniques
⇩
Divide lower portion of internal sphincter to reach external opening
⇩
Place non-absorbable material (i.e., silk suture, Penrose, vessel loop) through tract and tie ends

Cutting Seton: tightened at regular intervals to cut through sphincter converting high tract to a low one. **Return to OR in 6 wk to 3 mo for definitive repair.** Incontinence in up to 12%.

Endoanal advancement flap: often reserved for patients with IBD, multiple complex fistulas, or a previous fistula operation; failure in up to 40% of cases

Identify fistula's tract and enlarge external opening to allow drainage
⇩
Create full thickness flap of mucosa, submucosa, and parts of internal sphincter
⇩
Advance flap below internal opening
⇩
Close defect with absorbable sutures

Bioprosthetic plug (porcine or bovine collagen): failure in up to 85% of cases

Identify fistula tract and place rehydrated plug through the tract
⇩
Excise excess plug externally and fix internal portion with absorbable suture

LIFT procedure (ligation of intersphincteric fistula tract): primary healing rate of up to 80%, failure rate of 15–20%.
Identify the fistulous tract with probe. Incise skin/mucosa over intersphincteric groove. Dissect down and identify fistulous tract. Excise 0.5–1 cm of the tract. Suture ligate proximal and distal ends within the groove. Close mucosa over internal opening

---

Crohn's-Related Anal Fistula
- Often complex, multiple tracts
- Treatment: Avoid division of sphincter muscle, open superficial tracts, and drain abscesses. **Primary treatment is medical.** Metronidazole, Infliximab—up to 50% fistula closure rate

13-5: PILONIDAL DISEASE

Etiology
- **Foreign body reaction from burrowed hair and debris** leads to subcutaneous infection in the upper portion of gluteal cleft
- Continuum from abscess (acute) to sinuses and crypts (chronic)
- Epidemiology: males > females
- Risk factors: obesity, heredity, and sedentary lifestyle

Pilonidal Abscess

- Symptoms: fever, pain, and drainage
- Physical examination: tender and erythematous mass
- Treatment: incision and drainage
  - May curettage wound to enhance healing
  - VAC dressing may significantly simplify care and speed up recovery
- Recurrence: up to 40% will develop chronic pilonidal disease

Chronic Pilonidal Disease (Cochrane Database Syst Rev. 2010; 20(1):CD006213)

- Symptoms: pain and intermittent drainage
- Physical examination: sinuses may extend down to presacral fascia
  - Treatment: **local excision of all diseased areas.** Wound curettage to remove granulation tissue
  - Primary closure—earlier healing, earlier return to work
  - May include V-Y, Rhomboid, Karydakis, or Bascum flap techniques
  - Secondary intention or VAC-assisted—**lower likelihood of recurrence (5%)**

13-6: RECTAL PROLAPSE

Clinical Presentation

- Symptoms: **mass protruding from anus** (often with defecation), constipation, straining, fecal incontinence, and erratic bowel habits
- Physical examination
  Type I: mucosal prolapse only, radially oriented grooves
  Type II: full-thickness prolapse, concentric rings, and grooves
  Type III: if also a sliding perineal hernia
- Chronic prolapse: mucosal ulcerations, irritation, or maceration of surrounding skin; sphincter tone usually decreased

Diagnosis

- Have patient strain while on commode to reproduce prolapse—concentric mucosal rings think rectal prolapse versus "grapes" think prolapsed hemorrhoids
- Colonoscopy or flexible sigmoidoscopy with barium enema: identifies associated mucosal abnormalities, anterior ulceration
- Cinedefecography: if diagnosis is in doubt

Rectal Prolapse—Treatment (Dis Colon Rectum. 2015;58(8):799–807; World J Gastroenterol. 2015;21(16):5049–55; Gastroenterol Clin North Am. 2013;42(4):837–61)

Abdominal Procedures—dozens of named procedures—suture vs. mesh, anterior vs. posterior rectopexy, with vs. without sigmoid resection, open vs. laparoscopic vs. robotic

Laparoscopic/robotic ventral rectopexy with mesh: **recurrence rate <5% at 5 y,** mesh erosion in 2%, improved continence/constipation, preserved sexual function

Peritoneum over anterior lateral rectum is incised from sacral promontory to pouch of Douglas. Denonvillier's fascia incised

⇩

Mesh secured to ventral aspect of the rectum in the rectovaginal/rectovesical septum

⇩

Elevate rectum out of the pelvis and fixate mesh to presacral fascia below sacral promontory. Close peritoneum over the mesh.

Ripstein procedure (rectopexy with anterior mesh sling): **rarely preformed**
  Complications: mesh erodes into rectum, obstruction

Perineal procedures: elderly patients or those with significant comorbidities, young men to avoid possible sexual dysfunction after low rectal dissection—
low morbidity, high recurrence rates

Altemeier procedure (perineal rectosigmoidectomy)

High recurrence rate: up to 35%, high rates of fecal incontinence and urgency

Place the patient in prone or high lithotomy position

⇩

Make circumferential incision in rectal wall 2 cm above dentate, then full thickness

⇩

Pull down cut edge, ligate, and divide the mesorectum, progressively taking the incision cephalad until all redundant rectum is mobilized

⇩

Divide the rectum and hand sew a coloanal anastomosis

Levatorplasty, both anterior and posterior, is frequently performed as well to help recreate a more normal anorectal angle and hopefully improve continence

Delorme Procedure (perineal mucosal proctectomy)—circumferential stripping of prolapsed mucosa with plication of the seromuscular layer, rarely performed in US

13-7: ANAL CANCER

Epidemiology
- Risk factor: longstanding co-infection of HIV and HPV
- Spreads by direct extension and lymphatics
  - **Tumors distal to third valve of Houston: to superficial inguinal nodes**
  - **Tumors proximal to third valve of Houston: to internal iliac and inferior mesenteric nodes**

Anal Canal Cancer
Squamous Cell Carcinoma
- Most common

Clinical Presentation
- Symptoms: bleeding, anal pain, pruritis, fecal incontinence, and change in bowel habits
- Physical examination: digital rectal, proctoscopy, and lymph nodes
  - **Assess tumor size, mobility, and distance from the anal verge**
  - **All atypical anal masses/polyps/fissures should be biopsied**

Imaging
- **Endoanal/endorectal US:** assess extent of the local disease, perirectal nodal disease—suspicious nodes should be biopsied
- **Pelvic MRI**
- PET-CT to rule out metastatic disease

Staging
Risk of nodal spread correlates with size and depth of wall invasion
- At presentation: 45% have positive nodes (15–20% inguinal) and 10% distant metastasis
- Stage I: T1 < 2 cm
- Stage II: T2, T3 > 2 cm without adjacent organ invasion
- Stage IIIA/B: Nodal disease or T4 (adjacent organ invasion)
- Stage IV: M1 disease

Treatment (Clin Colon Rectal Surg. 2011;24(1): 54–63; Clin Colon Rectal Surg. 2011;24(3): 177–192)
- Radiation: external beam, brachytherapy, or combination
  - Best results seen at levels of 54 Gy or above
  - Local control: up to 70%; less than 50% if tumor >5 cm or positive lymph nodes
  - Balance benefit of higher radiation doses with increased morbidity
- **Chemoradiation—first-line therapy**
  - **Originally based on the Nigro protocol: mitomycin—C + 5-FU + XRT**
  - Combination offers best chance for cure—5-year survival up to 75%
  - Primary treatment of squamous cell cancer of the anal canal
- Surgery: second-line therapy for recurrent or persistent disease localized to the pelvis
  - Salvage APR after re-staging, may require myocutaneous flap if large tissue defect
  - 5-year survival 30–64%

Adenocarcinoma
- Uncommon
- **Wide local excision** if <2 cm and well differentiated, otherwise APR with neoadjuvant chemoradiation

Anal Margin Tumors
Clinical Presentation
- Symptoms: anal pain, bleeding, pruritis, and incontinence
- Physical examination: assess size of the mass and lymph node involvement

Squamous Cell Carcinoma
- Most common anal margin tumor
- More common in men, prior HPV exposure, HIV

Staging
- Size of tumor and lymph node involvement correlates with prognosis
- Lymph node involvement: 0.1% in tumors <2 cm and 67% in tumors >5 cm

Treatment

- **Wide local excision** (WLE) of T1/T2 tumors when >1 cm margin and intact sphincter can be achieved; consider APR for patients with persistent and recurrent disease
  - For bulky, poorly differentiated tumors APR does not provide survival benefit over WLE
  - WLE with adjuvant radiotherapy—5-year survival rate up to 86%
- Chemoradiation: consider for patients with large tumors, nodal involvement, or sphincter involvement

Paget Disease—Intraepithelial Adenocarcinoma

- 50% of patients have a synchronous colorectal neoplasm
  - Full colonoscopy required
- Surgery: **wide local excision,** may require APR if synchronous neoplasm or extensive lesion
- Chemoradiation: consider topical 5-FU

Melanoma

Epidemiology

- Most common site for primary gastrointestinal melanoma
- More common in women
- Up to 35% of patients present with metastatic disease

Clinical Presentation

- Symptoms: bleeding, pain, discharge, change in bowel habits, and weight loss
- Physical examination: most lesions are lightly pigmented
  - Early lesions may appear polypoid
  - Larger lesions may have ulcerations, raised edges

Treatment

- **Wide local excision, APR reserved for cases of sphincter involvement with incontinence**
- APR conveys no survival benefit over wide local excision
- Do not operate if evidence of metastatic or loco-regional disease; patients with tumors >1 cm are not cured by any treatment

VASCULAR SURGERY

PATRIC LIANG • ALLEN HAMDAN

Based on prior chapter by Gautum V. Shrikande, Thomas S. Monahan,
Frank B. Pomposelli

14-1: CAROTID DISEASE

Surgical Indications
Symptomatic Patients
- Symptoms: ipsilateral transient ischemia attacks (TIAs), previous nondisabling stroke <6 months, amaurosis fugax (transient monocular vision loss), and crescendo TIAs
- Carotid stenosis is unlikely to cause vertigo or syncope
- North American Symptomatic Carotid Endarterectomy Trial (*N Engl J Med.* 1991;325:445–453)
  - 659 patients w/stroke or TIA in last 120 days. Patients randomized to carotid endarterectomy (CEA) vs. medical treatment with internal carotid artery (ICA) stenosis >70%
  - Trial was terminated early because of evidence that CEA was beneficial
  - Patients undergoing CEA had lower 2-year stroke rates (9% vs. 26%)
  - Subanalysis of patients undergoing CEA for 50–69% ICA stenosis showed moderate benefit in terms of 5-year stroke rates (16 vs. 22%)
- European Carotid Surgery Trial (*Lancet.* 1998;351:1379–1387)
  - 3,024 patients w/stroke or TIA in last 6 months. Patients randomized to CEA vs. medical treatment regardless of their degree of stenosis.
  - For patients with >80% stenosis, CEA had significantly lower 3-year stroke rate (2.8 vs. 16.8).
- **Many surgeons extend indications for CEA to symptomatic patients with >50% stenosis**

Asymptomatic Patients
- Asymptomatic Carotid Atherosclerosis Study (*JAMA.* 1995;273:1421–1428)
  - 1,662 patients with >60% ICA stenosis randomized to CEA vs. medical treatment
  - Patients undergoing CEA had lower 5-year risk of stroke or stroke/death rate (5.1 vs. 11%)
- Asymptomatic Carotid Surgery Trial (*Lancet.* 2004;363:1491–1502)
  - 3,120 patients with >60% ICA stenosis randomized to CEA vs. medical treatment
  - Patients undergoing surgical treatment had a lower 5-year risk of stroke or stroke/death (6.4 vs. 11.8%)
- **As a general rule, CEA in asymptomatic patients should be reserved for good- to moderate-risk patients with stenoses >70% and a life expectancy of greater than 2 years**

Diagnosis
Imaging
- Noninvasive carotid duplex scans
  - Quantifies the degree of stenosis and extent of lesion. Provides information regarding the contralateral side and direction of flow in the vertebral arteries
  - Duplex findings suggestive of >70% stenosis: peak systolic velocity (PSV) >230 cm/sec, end diastolyic velocity (EDV) >100 cm/sec, ICA/CCA PSV ratio >4
  - Carotid occlusion: no color flow, no diastolic flow, and systolic velocity <40 cm/sec; no surgical intervention indicated for asymptomatic carotid occlusions
  - CCA velocities <50 cm/sec is suggestive of more proximal stenosis; ostial carotid stenosis
  - Contralateral severe stenosis can falsely elevate PSV of the ipsilateral artery
- CTA and MRA: can assist in surgical planning including evaluation of aortic arch for carotid stenting (CAS)

Carotid Stenting
SAPPHIRE Trial (N Engl J Med. 2004;351:1493)
- Demonstrated equivalency of CAS with carotid endarterectomy for patients with a high operative risk for the combined primary endpoint of stroke, perioperative death, or myocardial infarction at 1 year
- Many patients in this study were not randomized
- High risk criteria: severe cardiac disease, severe pulmonary disease, age >80, prior ipsilateral endarterectomy, prior neck surgery or radiation, contralateral carotid occlusion, or contralateral laryngeal nerve palsy

CREST Trial (N Engl J Med. 2010;363(1):11)
- 2,502 symptomatic and asymptomatic patients randomly assigned to CEA or CAS
- Similar outcomes in composite outcome of stroke, myocardial infarction, or death
- Stenting had higher rates of stroke or death (4.4 vs. 2.3%)
- CEA had high rates of myocardial infarction (2.3 vs. 1.1%)

CREST-2 Trial (Active Enrollment)
- Medical treatment has improved for treatment of hypertension, hyperlipidemia, diabetes, smoking cessation
- Two parallel, randomized control trials comparing carotid revascularization + intensive medical management vs. medical management alone in patients with asymptomatic high-grade carotid stenosis
- Carotid revascularization groups: CEA vs. no CEA, CAS with embolic protection device vs. no stenting

Carotid Disease—Surgical Technique

Standard Endarterectomy

Make an oblique incision along anterior border of sternocleidomastoid muscle
⇩
Transect facial vein and laterally retract the jugular vein
⇩
Dissect out external carotid artery (ECA), ICA to the level of the hypoglossal nerve, and common carotid artery (CCA) along its medial border (Fig. 14-1)
⇩
Avoid injury to vagus (most common), hypoglossal, glossopharyngeal nerves
⇩
Place vessel loops around CCA, ICA, ECA, superior thyroid artery
⇩
Heparinize (80–100 units/kg of body weight)
⇩
Sequentially clamp ICA, CCA, ECA
⇩
Begin arteriotomy on proximal CCA, extend onto ICA beyond level of plaque
⇩
If shunt is to be used, insert into the distal ICA beyond the level of the vessel loop and proximally into the CCA
⇩
Perform endarterectomy
⇩
Place tacking sutures if needed at the distal end point
⇩
Close with prosthetic or vein patch (remove shunt prior to completing patch)
⇩
Flush all vessels before closure
⇩
Restore flow initially to the ECA and then to ICA
(prevents residual debris from traveling to the brain)

Eversion Endarterectomy
- ICA is elongated or kinked and reduction in length is desired
  Identical to above until the arteriotomy is made, then transect origin of the ICA
⇩
Atheroma is intussuscepted from the ICA by peeling back the deep media and adventitia of the distal vessel
⇩
Place tacking sutures
⇩
Begin single circular suture line in middle of posterior wall, carry around bulb

Cerebral Monitoring
- No single best method, based on surgeon preference
- Techniques:
  - Awake operation, monitor motor function deficits and speech impairment
  - EEG—monitor for delta waves
  - Stump pressure measurement (systolic <40 mm Hg should be shunted)
  - TCD and cerebral oximetry

Complications
- Cranial nerve injuries
  - Vagus nerve is the most commonly injured nerve; manifests as dysphagia or hoarseness (recurrent laryngeal nerve)
  - Hypoglossal nerve injury results in tongue deviation toward side of injury
  - Mandibular branch of the facial nerve injury results in ipsilateral facial droop, drooling
- Expanding neck hematoma—can lead to dysphagia, difficulty breathing, stridor
  - Treatment: emergent re-exploration
- Cerebral hyperperfusion syndrome—ipsilateral headache, focal seizures, focal neurologic deficit, ipsilateral intracerebral hemorrhage, and edema after CEA
  - Prevention: postoperative blood pressure control
- Recurrent stenosis: 1–20%
  - Within the first 2 years: myointimal hyperplasia; treat when >80% stenosis
  - After 2 years: atherosclerosis; treat with the same original indications
- Stroke
- Infection

Figure 14-1 Carotid artery anatomy. The first branch off the external carotid artery is the superior thyroid artery. The hypoglossal nerve crosses the carotid artery at or near the carotid bifurcation. The vagus nerve typically travels in the posterior carotid sheath behind the carotid artery. (From Fisher JE, Bland KI. *Mastery of Surgery*, 5th ed. Philadelphia, PA: Lippincott Williams & Wilkins, 2007.)

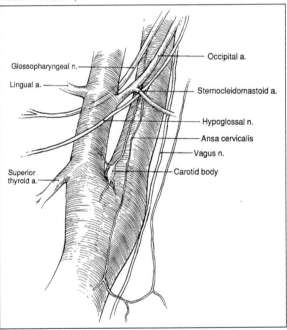

Labels:
- Glossopharyngeal n.
- Lingual a.
- Superior thyroid a.
- Occipital a.
- Sternocleidomastoid a.
- Hypoglossal n.
- Ansa cervicalis
- Vagus n.
- Carotid body

14-2: ABDOMINAL AORTIC ANEURYSMS

General Considerations
Etiology
- Inflammatory and degenerative processes
- **Risk factors: smoking, family history, peripheral vascular disease, and coronary disease**

- Associated findings: popliteal or femoral aneurysms
- Majority of AAAs occur infrarenally (90%)

Diagnosis
- Ultrasound: can be used for screening and routine follow-up
- CTA and MRA for operative planning
- Arteriography: may underestimate the size when aneurysm contains significant mural thrombus

Screening
- USPSTF recommends one-time ultrasound screening for AAA in men ages 65–75 who have ever smoked

Rupture
- ***Natural history of abdominal aortic aneurysms (AAA)***
- **Untreated AAA rupture is associated with 50–90% mortality**
- Risk factors: smoking, hypertension, COPD, expansion >1 cm/y, female, familial
- Clinical presentation: **hypotension, back pain, and pulsatile epigastric mass**
- Incidence of AAA rupture per year by aneurysm size
  - 4 cm: 0.5–5%
  - 5 cm: 3–15%
  - 6 cm: 10–20%
  - 7 cm: 20–40%
  - 8 cm: 30–50%

Current Recommendations (UK Small Aneurysm Trial, ADAM trial)
- Repair all aneurysms >5.5 cm or showing rapid growth (>0.5 cm over 6 months)
- For aneurysms <5 cm, follow with interval imaging

Postoperative Complications
Ischemic Colitis
- Clinical presentation: **bloody diarrhea**, acidosis, elevated WBC, increased fluid requirements
- Diagnosis: if stable, immediate **flexible sigmoidoscopy**
- Management
  - Full thickness necrosis: OR for sigmoid colectomy/Hartman procedure
  - Ischemia limited to mucosa: fluid resuscitation and antibiotics

Aortic Graft Infections
- **Early graft infections: *Staphylococcus aureus***
- **Later graft infections: *Staphylococcus epidermidis***
- Management
  - First: antibiotics
  - Second: extra-anatomic bypass (usually axillary–bifemoral)
  - Third: graft excision

Aortoenteric Fistulas
- Clinical presentation: **"herald bleed"**
- Diagnosis: EGD (can sometimes confirm if graft is seen); CT angiography
- Management: **emergent laparotomy,** obtain vascular control, repair of the GI fistula, remove the graft after extra-anatomic bypass
  Other Complications: bleeding, MI, ARF, and false aneurysm formation

Endovascular Repair of Aneurysms (EVAR) (*NEJM.* 2004;351:1607–1618; *NEJM.* 2008;358(5):464–474; *NEJM.* 2015; 373(4):328–338)
- Patients undergoing EVAR have lower perioperative morality rates compared to open AAA repair (1.2 vs. 4.8, $P < 0.001$)
- EVAR is associated with higher rates of late rupture (5.4 vs. 1.4%) and reinterventions

Anatomic Requirements and Considerations for EVAR
- Aneurysm neck: 10–15 mm
  - Area between renal arteries and start of aneurysmal dilatation
- Aortic angulation: <60 degrees
- Femoral and iliac artery diameter and tortuosity

Endoleaks
- Type I: inability of the proximal or distal end of the device to completely seal
  - Risk factors: initial aortic neck >25 mm, >10% dilation of aortic neck
- Type II: back bleeding into the aneurysm sac from the lumbars or IMA
- Type III: occurs when component pieces of the endograft break apart
- Type IV: leaks from graft porosity
- **In general, type I and type III endoleaks need to be repaired urgently**

Open AAA Repair—Surgical Technique

Transabdominal Aortic Tube Graft

Relative indications: rupture, coexistent intra-abdominal pathology, bilateral large iliac aneurysms, need for access to both renal arteries, uncertain diagnosis

Midline incision

⇩

Reflect transverse mesocolon cephalad and incise ligament of Treitz

⇩

Pack small bowel to right, make longitudinal incision in posterior peritoneum

⇩

Identify left renal vein as well as renal arteries; heparinize systemically

⇩

Place proximal clamp on aorta in infrarenal position if there is room

⇩

Place distal clamps on bilateral iliac arteries

⇩

Sew in graft in an end-to-end fashion

⇩

Close residual aneurysm over graft and close retroperitoneum

⇩

Check distal pulses when finished

Consider re-implanting the IMA if history of visceral angina, post-AAA repair pressure <40 torr, loss of Doppler signal at anti-mesenteric border

If AAA ruptured:
Emergent OR, prep chin to knees, **cross 10 units pRBCs, + FFP, platelets**

⇩

Divide hepatogastric ligament, pull stomach to left
Retract left hepatic lobe superiorly

⇩

Can compress aorta against the spine until an aortic clamp is placed (alternatively a percutaneous aortic occlusion balloon can be placed prior to abdominal incision)

⇩

Distally clamp the iliac arteries

⇩

Enter the retroperitoneal hematoma (watch for ureters near iliac bifurcation)

⇩

Identify aneurysm neck and place proximal clamp in infrarenal position

⇩

Open the aneurysm, evacuate the thrombus, suture ligate any lumbars, sew in tube graft end-to-end

⇩

Check distal pulses when finished

14-3: AORTOILIAC OCCLUSIVE DISEASE AND AORTIC DISSECTION

Aortoiliac Disease

Clinical Presentation: LeRiche Syndrome
- **Thigh and buttock claudication**
- **Impotence**
- **Diminished or absent femoral pulse**

Surgical Management: Aortobifemoral Bypass
- 85% 5-year patency
- Increased patency with patent profunda
- Patency risk factors: small aortas, women, and patients <50 years old

Aortic Dissections
Classified based on the location of the origin of the dissection

Debakey Classification
- Type I: involves the ascending and descending aorta
- Type II: isolated to the ascending aorta
- Type III: exclusively involves descending aorta

Stanford Classification
- Type A: involves ascending aorta (with or without the descending aorta)
- Type B: involves only the descending aorta

Clinical Presentation
- Chest and back pain
- Mediastinal widening, asymmetric pulse examination

Treatment
- Location of the origin of dissection determines the treatment strategy

Dissections of the Descending Aorta (DeBakey III, Stanford B)
- If no acute ischemic complications, manage with blood pressure control
- Delayed repair if retroperitoneal hematoma, contaminated wound, burns, blunt cardiac injury, and old age

Dissections Involving the Ascending Aorta
- **Needs emergent surgical intervention**
- Complications: aortic rupture, CVA from carotid involvement, occlusion of coronary vessels leading to myocardial infarction, and pericardial tamponade

14-4: VISCERAL AND PERIPHERAL ANEURYSMS

Visceral Artery Aneurysms
Splenic Artery
- Epidemiology: **60% of all splanchnic aneurysms,** 20% multiple, 2% rupture
- Pathophysiology: male, atherosclerosis; female, medial wall dysplasia
- Risk factors: women with multiple pregnancies, portal hypertension, trauma, and inflammatory disease (e.g., pancreatitis)
- Diagnosis: angiography or CTA; eggshell calcifications on XR
- **Surgical repair indicated: pregnancy, women of childbearing age; symptomatic or asymptomatic if >2 cm**
- Surgical options
  - Aneurysmectomy
  - Exclusion with splenic artery ligation without arterial reconstruction
  - Endovascular stent placement

Hepatic Artery
- Epidemiology: 20% of splanchnic artery aneurysms; can be life threatening
  - Excluding trauma, most in patients >50 years of age
  - 80% extrahepatic, 20% intrahepatic
- Clinical presentation: most diagnosed incidentally
- Surgical repair: **all should be surgically treated**
  - Aneurysm exclusion without reconstruction
  - If blood flow to the liver appears compromised, reconstruct the artery

Superior Mesenteric Artery
- Epidemiology: third most common, 5.5%
  - Mycotic aneurysms: secondary to bacterial endocarditis
- Clinical presentation: majority are symptomatic
- Surgical repair: **most should be repaired surgically**
  - May be a role for endovascular stent placement
  - Exclusion and intestinal revascularization by an aortomesenteric graft

Celiac Artery (4%)
- Clinical presentation: asymptomatic, incidental finding, and vague abdominal pain
  - Rupture can be seen and carries a high mortality.
- Surgical repair: **repair all**
  - Aneurysmectomy with repair or stenting
    - Gastric and gastroepiploic artery: **repair all with excision or ligation;** high risk of rupture
    - Jejunal, ileal, and colic arteries: **all need to be ligated or excised;** most are symptomatic

Peripheral Aneurysms
Iliac Artery Aneurysms
- Epidemiology: majority associated with abdominal aortic aneurysms, most in common iliac artery, 10–20% involve the internal iliac artery, one-third bilateral
- Clinical presentation: incidental, lower abdominal pain, flank pain
- Surgical repair
  - Elective if >3 cm in good-risk patients or symptomatic with pain
  - Excision and interposition graft vs. endovascular repair using covered stents

Femoral Artery Aneurysms
- Clinical presentation: can cause pain and acute thrombosis; do not commonly rupture
- Surgical repair: **asymptomatic >3.5 cm, all symptomatic,** during planned aortic repair
  - Excision and an interposition graft

Femoral Artery Pseudoaneurysm
- Can occur after percutaneous common femoral artery access procedures
- Treatment
  - Ultrasound-guided compression
  - Ultrasound-guided thrombin injection into pseduoaneurysm sac
  - Open surgical repair

Popliteal Aneurysms
- Definition: external diameter >2.0 cm or 1.5 times the size of normal proximal artery
- Epidemiology
  - AAAs are present in one-third of patients with popliteal aneurysms
  - Popliteal aneurysms occur in approximately 10% of patients with AAA
  - 50–60% are bilateral
- Clinical presentation:
  - Thrombosis or distal embolization—claudication, rest pain, or acute limb ischemia
  - Venous compression—leg swelling
  - Aneurysm rupture is rare
- **Requires surveillance of contralateral popliteal artery and abdominal aorta**
- **#1 complication is distal embolization**
- Surgical repair: **asymptomatic >2 cm, all symptomatic**
- Open surgical technique: proximal and distal ligation of the aneurysm + femoral to below-knee popliteal bypass with saphenous vein either via medial or posterior approach
- Endovascular repair: covered stent

14-5: MESENTERIC ISCHEMIA

Acute Mesenteric Ischemia
Etiology
- Arterial (70%)
  - Embolic (45%): typically spares the proximal jejunum
  - Thrombotic (25%): involves small bowel from ligament of Treitz distally
- Venous (10%)
- Nonocclusive (20%)

Clinical Presentation
- Sudden abdominal pain, gut emptying (diarrhea)
  - Peritonitis is a late finding suggesting transmural ischemia
- Labs: elevated white blood count, serum lactate, and serum amylase

Imaging
- CTA findings (if high clinical suspicion)
  - Portal venous air (sensitivity 12%, specificity 100%)
  - Pneumatosis intestinalis (sensitivity 42%, specificity 100%)
  - Superior mesenteric artery (SMA) filling defect (12%, specificity 100%)

Surgical Treatment
- Exploratory laparotomy to assess bowel viability
  - Resect obviously necrotic bowel and attempt to preserve small bowel length
  - **Plan for "second look" laparotomy at 48 hours to reassess remaining bowel**

Revascularize Ischemic Bowel
- Embolectomy
  - Reflect transverse mesocolon cranially, identify middle colic, and trace to SMA
  - Obtain proximal and distal control of SMA, make a transverse arteriotomy
  - Systemically heparinize
  - Pass a Fogarty catheter proximally and distally to remove clot
- Catheter-directed thrombolysis: limited to case reports; up to 48 hours needed
- Open surgical reconstruction
- Endovascular revascularization

Open Surgical Reconstruction
- Conduit: patency rates similar for prosthetic and vein graft; vein should be used in contaminated field
- Inflow
  - Supraceliac aorta
    - Divide the gastrohepatic ligament to access aorta as it passes through the diaphragmatic hiatus
    - Divide the ligament of Treitz and open the retroperitoneum between the superior mesenteric vein and duodenum
    - Graft can be tunneled behind the pancreas
    - Drawbacks: need for supraceliac clamp, less familiar exposure
  - Infrarenal aorta
    - Distract the transverse colon superiorly and move viscera to right
    - Drawbacks: high incidence of atherosclerosis of the infrarenal aorta
  - Common iliac artery
- Outflow
  - Expose SMA as described above
  - Make a longitudinal arteriotomy for endarterectomy or patch angioplasty
  - Anastomosis is typically end-to-side

Chronic Mesenteric Ischemia
Etiology: arterial or venous thrombosis, women > men

Clinical Presentation
- History of weight loss, intestinal angina (postprandial pain), and "food fear"
- Risk factors for atherosclerosis

Imaging
- Mesenteric duplex
  - Measure celiac and SMA peak systolic and end diastolic velocities
  - Celiac artery PSV >200 cm/sec and SMA PSV >275 cm/sec suggestive of >70% stenosis
  - Limited examination in obese and nonfasting patients
- CTA

Endovascular Revascularization
- Number of vessels to be treated is controversial; classically revascularize two vessels
- Technical considerations
  - Brachial artery vs. common femoral access
  - Catheter tip should be positioned at the T12 level
  - Lesions are treated with angioplasty and stenting

14-6: ACUTE AND CHRONIC LIMB ISCHEMIA

Acute Limb Ischemia
Etiology
- **Embolism (>90%); #1 source is cardiac** (recent MI with mural thrombus, a fib) (Fig. 14-2). Typically lodge at an **arterial bifurcation**, often distal SFA or popliteal artery
- Thrombosis of aneurysm
- Thrombosis of atherosclerotic lesion
- Inflammatory arteriopathies (giant cell arteritis)
- Bypass graft thrombosis: most common cause of nonembolic acute limb ischemia

Clinical Presentation
- History: acute onset, known embolic source, no prior history of claudication
- **Physical examination (the "6 p's"): paresthesia, pain, pallor, pulselessness, paralysis, poikilothermia (cool extremity);** normal pulses in contralateral limb

Classification: Rutherford Criteria
- Class I: limb is viable and remains so without therapeutic intervention
- Class II: limb is threatened and requires revascularization for salvage
- Class IIa: limb is not immediately threatened
- Class IIb: limb is threatened and urgent revascularization is necessary
- Class III: limb is irreversibly ischemic and salvage is not possible

Treatment
- All patients are started on a heparin drip
- Thrombolytic therapy: local, catheter-directed infusion with plasminogen activators (urokinase, alteplase, and reteplase); consider if significant medical comorbidities and cannot tolerate open procedure

- Embolectomy
- Mechanical thrombectomy: rapid restoration of blood flow, decrease in duration of systemic anticoagulation
- Monitor for lower extremity compartment syndrome
  - Ischemia causes buildup of toxic free radicals, leakage of protein and fluid from capillary bed, causes increased extravascular pressure, and impedes venous outflow

Figure 14-2 A: Common sources of emboli include the heart and large vessels especially the aorta. Thrombus from AAA can also embolize. **B:** The extremities are the most common end point of emboli although cerebral and mesenteric emboli also occur in the percentages listed. (From Fisher JE, Bland KI. *Mastery of Surgery*, 5th ed. Philadelphia, PA: Lippincott Williams & Wilkins, 2007.)

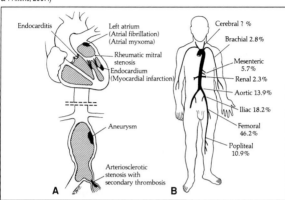

Open Surgical Revascularization

- **Bilateral femoral pulses absent**
  - Prep abdomen and infraclavicular area
  - Explore bilateral groins
  - Consider thrombectomy/embolectomy with iliac stent if needed
  - Rarely require aortobifemoral bypass (or axillary–bifemoral bypass)
  - Longitudinal arteriotomy for femoral artery thrombosis
  - Transverse arteritomy for embolization
- **Unilateral femoral pulse absent**
  - Iliac embolism or thrombosis of stenotic iliac artery
  - May require fem–fem bypass
- **Unilateral popliteal pulse absent with good femoral pulse**
  - Transverse arteriotomy in common femoral artery
  - May require fem–pop bypass
- **Pedal pulses absent**
  - Perform thromboembolectomy for all three tibial arteries
- **Always perform completion angiogram in the OR and check foot pulses**
- **Consider fasciotomy**
  - Single incision: begin one fingerbreadth anterior to head of fibula and extend to the lateral malleolus or two incisions (medial and lateral)
  - Lateral: start 2 cm lateral to anterior tibial border
  - Medial: 1–2 cm posterior to medial tibial border
- Longitudinal incision of the entire fascia investing each of the compartments
  - Anterior (tibialis anterior)
  - Lateral (peroneal)
  - Superficial posterior (gastrocnemius)
  - Deep posterior (soleus)
  - **Most common nerve injury: peroneal nerve causing foot drop and loss of sensation over the first web space**

Chronic Limb Ischemia

Indications for Intervention
- Rest pain: occurs in forefoot, awakens patient from sleep, and relieved by dependency
- Tissue loss: nonhealing, ischemic wounds; foot salvage requires restoration of pulsatile flow to the foot
- Gangrene
- Disabling claudication (claudication alone is not an indication for revascularization)

Distribution of Disease
- Aortoiliac disease: patients with atherosclerotic disease or a history of tobacco abuse
- Distal tibial vessel disease: diabetics

Preoperative Evaluation
- **Ankle brachial index (ABI) interpretation**
  - **Normal >0.9–1.3, claudication 0.4–0.9, rest pain 0.2–0.4, tissue loss or gangrene <0.2**
  - Disadvantages: does not indicate level of disease; may be falsely elevated (>1.3) in patients with heavily calcified vessels (**medial calcinosis**)
  - Cuff size must be at least 1.5× diameter of limb for accurate measurement
- **Toe brachial index (TBI)**
  - Normal TBI >0.7
  - Toe pressures <30 mm Hg is not compatible with healing toe ulcers or toe amputation
- Noninvasive vascular studies: pulse–volume recordings
  - Advantages: provides information about the level of disease
  - Disadvantages: does not provide anatomic detail
- Angiogram
  - Diagnostic and therapeutic if atherosclerotic lesion is amenable to endovascular angioplasty and/or stenting
- Assessment of bypass conduit
  - Venous duplex and mapping to assess vein size and abnormalities (>3 mm preferred)
  - Mark path of saphenous vein and significant collaterals on leg preoperatively

Operative Technique
Adequate inflow, patent distal target vessel (outflow), and adequate conduit

Proximal Exposure
- Common femoral artery: vertical skin incision over CFA, dissect out SFA and profunda; can divide inguinal ligament if necessary to get nondiseased artery (Fig. 14-3)

Distal Exposure
- Above-knee popliteal artery: medial thigh incision
  - Reflect the sartorius muscle posteromedially, adductor magnus anteriorly
- Below-knee popliteal artery, tibial peroneal trunk
  - Incision on upper third of lower leg, 1 cm posterior to tibia
  - Retract medial head of the gastrocnemius posteromedially
- Posterior tibial, peroneal artery
  - Incision on distal third of lower leg, posterior to the medial border tibia
  - Reflect the soleus muscle posteromedially, flexor digitorum longus anterolaterally, exposing the posterior tibial neurovascular bundle
  - Retract the PT neurovascular bundle posteromedially to expose the peroneal neurovascular bundle medial to the fibula
- Dorsalis pedis artery
  - Longitudinal incision over artery, carry dissection through extensor retinaculum
  - Locate the DP artery just distal to ends of malleoli and 1 cm lateral to extensor hallucis longus tendon
  - Want inner diameter >1 mm

Conduit Considerations
- **Graft of choice: long saphenous vein > short saphenous vein > arm veins > PTFE**
- Reversed vein graft: theoretically less traumatic to endothelium; no valve lysis
- In situ graft: vein left in native position; valves lysed with valvulotome +/− angioscopy
  - Less size discrepancy
- Prosthetic grafts: Dacron (woven polyester) or ePTFE (Gore-tex®)
  - For patients with inadequate autogenous conduit
  - Advantages: shorter operative times and less morbid procedure
  - Disadvantages: significantly diminished patency rates for infrainguinal bypasses, cannot be used in a contaminated field, and greater risk for graft infection

Figure 14-3 The anatomic relationship of the structures in the right groin. The femoral artery lies medial to the femoral nerve and lateral to the femoral vein. The common femoral artery branches into the superficial and deep (profunda) femoral arteries. (From Fisher JE, Bland KI. *Mastery of Surgery*, 5th ed. Philadelphia, PA: Lippincott Williams & Wilkins, 2007.)

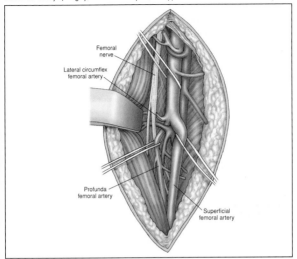

Postoperative Considerations
- Anticoagulation: aspirin for all patients; no consensus on routine anticoagulation
  - Warfarin is reserved for patients with grafts at high risk for failure
- Graft surveillance: 6 months to yearly duplex surveillance
  - Most lesions found 1–2 years after bypass are due to the formation of intimal hyperplasia

Outcomes
- Vein graft 5-year patency: 80% both popliteal and infrapopliteal, 60% dorsalis pedis
- ePTFE grafts have similar patency rates for suprapopliteal bypasses, but have much poorer patency rates for infrapopliteal bypasses

Lower Extremity Ulcers
Clinical Presentation
- **Venous: painless, large, superficial; red granulation base over medial malleolus**
- **Arterial: painful, small, deep; punched-out appearance and no granulation**
- Risk factors: chronic vascular disease, diabetic neuropathy, DVT

Treatment
- Venous
  - Unna boot with compression, elevation, and various topical remedies
  - May consider surgical intervention to improve venous flow
- Arterial: consider surgical intervention to improve blood flow

14-7: MAJOR LOWER EXTREMITY AMPUTATIONS
Indications
- Myonecrosis as a complication of acute arterial insufficiency
- Nonhealing wounds and one or more failed attempts at revascularization as a final course for chronic critical limb ischemia (most common reason for amputation)
- To control life-threatening sepsis

Goals of Amputation
- Eliminate nonviable tissue
- **Provide a stump that has the best chance to heal**
  - Palpable pulse at a level immediately proximal to a proposed amputation has a high rate of healing
  - Other parameters: skin temperature, hair growth, tissue bleeding, muscle viability.
  - Dependent rubor: indicates tissue ischemia, avoid amputation through this level.

Above-Knee and Below-Knee Amputations
- General principles: vessels should be suture ligated; divide bones with saw to avoid spiral fractures; may need to debride muscle to avoid bulbous stump
- Above-knee amputation (AKA)
  - Easier to heal than below-knee amputation (BKA)
  - Less potential at rehabilitation and prosthetic use
  - Flaps: equal anterior and posterior flaps
  - Preferred if: cannot heal BKA, unlikely to mobilize after amputation, and presence of significant knee contracture
- BKA
  - Higher rehabilitation potential than AKA
  - Flaps: long posterior myocutaneous flap or equal anterior and posterior flaps (Fig. 14-4)
- Guillotine amputations: removes the septic focus quickly, leaves wound open to drain
  - Return to OR for complete amputation once fever, edema, and leukocytosis resolve

Figure 14-4 Below-knee amputation with long posterior myocutaneous flap. (From Fisher JE, Bland KI. *Mastery of Surgery*, 5th ed. Philadelphia, PA: Lippincott Williams & Wilkins, 2007.)

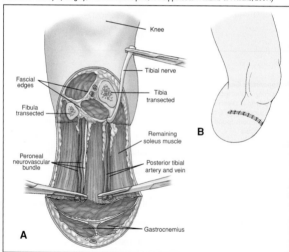

Amputation-Associated Mortality (Arch Surg. 2004;139:395–399)
- 30-day mortality: 16% for AKA, 6% for BKA
- **Worse survival in patients with diabetes and end-stage renal disease**

14-8: DEEP VENOUS THROMBOSIS
Clinical Presentation
- Calf pain, edema, venous distension, and pain on dorsiflexion of the ankle (Homan sign)
- Only one-third of patients present with physical examination findings
- Phlegmasia alba dolen—painful white edema

- Phlegmasia cerulean dolens—painful blue edema; extensive thrombotic occlusion that can lead to limb gangrene

Imaging
- Requires a high clinical suspicion
- Ultrasound: often poor imaging quality of iliac veins
- CT venography with intravenous contrast if iliocaval clot burden is suspected

Risk Factors for DVT	
Condition	**Relative Risk**
Inherited conditions	
Antithrombin deficiency	25
Protein C deficiency	10
Protein S deficiency	10
Factor V Leiden mutation	
Heterozygous	5
Homozygous	50
G20210A prothrombin-gene mutation	2.5
Dysfibrinogenemia	18
Acquired conditions	
Major trauma or surgery	5–200
History of DVT	50
Cancer	5
Major medical illness	5
Age	
>50	5
>70	10
Pregnancy	7
Estrogen therapy	5
Tamoxifen therapy	5
Obesity	3

Medical Treatment
Initial Therapy (N Engl J Med. 2004;351:268–277)
- **Unfractionated heparin:** 80 units/kg bolus followed by 18 units/kg IV drip
  - Titrate to PTT 1.5–2.5 times normal (monitor every 6 hours)
  - Risks: major bleeding complications (7%), heparin-induced thrombocytopenia (3%)
- Low–molecular-weight heparin (enoxaparin, Lovenox®): 1 mg/kg every 12 hours
  - Inhibits factor Xa
  - Lower risk of heparin-induced thrombocytopenia
  - Risks: similar bleeding risk, cannot reverse effects as quickly
- Thrombolysis: reserved for patients with limb-threatening thrombosis

Long-Term Therapy
- **Warfarin therapy with a goal INR 2.0–3.0**
  - Duration of treatment: 3–6 months
  - Absolute contraindications: active bleeding, platelet count <20,000, neurosurgery or intracranial bleeding within 10 days
  - Relative contraindications: thrombocytopenia, brain metastases, recent major trauma, major abdominal surgery within 2 days, GI or GU bleeding within 14 days, endocarditis, and severe hypertension
- Inferior vena cava filters indications:
  - Contraindication to or complication from anticoagulation
  - Breakthrough pulmonary embolism despite anticoagulation

Invasive Treatment
Open Surgical Thrombectomy
- Ileofemoral venous thrombectomy with ligation of femoral vein
- Goal: restore venous outflow and decrease the risk of pulmonary embolism
- Indication: acute ileofemoral DVT in patients with contraindication to thrombolysis or patients with poor response to thrombolysis or mechanical thrombectomy

Mechanical Thrombectomy
- Devices are either rotational (fragments thrombus) or hydrodynamic (aspirates thrombus based on the Venturi effect)
- Indication: acute ileofemoral DVT
- Often used in conjunction with pharmacological thrombolysis

Invasive Therapy for Pulmonary Embolism
- Indications
  - SBP <90 or rapid decrease in SBP of >40 mm Hg
  - Systemic hypoperfusion and hypoxia; need for CPR
  - Right ventricular failure
  - Arterial oxygen alveolar gradient >50 torr
  - Contraindication to anticoagulation
- Catheter-directed thrombolysis: continuous infusion for 12–24 hours
- Percutaneous embolectomy: performed in conjunction with catheter-directed lysis
- Surgical embolectomy: most definitive and invasive treatment; high mortality
- Pulmonary artery stenting: extraordinary circumstances when all else fails

14-9: THORACIC OUTLET SYNDROME

Etiology
- Extrinsic compression of neurovascular bundle serving the arm as it passes through the thoracocervical region to the axilla
- Abnormal anatomy: cervical rib, rudimentary first rib, laxity of costoclavicular joint, enlarged C7 transverse process, fibrosed posterior aspect of anterior scalene, and fibrous bands in scalene triangle
- **85–90% neurogenic or mixed** in presentation: 5–8% venous, 1–5% arterial

Imaging
- X-rays: visualize bony abnormalities
- MRI: cervical disc disease and brachial plexus compression
- Ultrasound/angiography: if vascular disease suspected

Clinical Presentation and Treatment
- Neurogenic presentation (95%)
  - Most commonly in **females aged 20–40**
  - Symptoms: **pain, numbness, weakness, and thenar muscle wasting**
  - Treatment: physical therapy and NSAIDs initially
  - Surgical repair: **first rib resection** (if present) + **anterior/middle scalenectomy**
- Arterial presentation
  - 90% have a bony abnormality, most commonly a complete cervical rib
  - Signs: focal aneurysm and secondary embolization; can see poststenotic dilatation of subclavian artery
  - Symptoms: cold intolerance, forearm exertional pain, gangrene; rarely stroke, aneurysm rupture
  - Surgical repair: resection of affected arterial segment with an interposition graft + correction of any bony abnormality
  - Consider anticoagulation if patient is not surgical candidate or with mild symptoms

14-10: SUBCLAVIAN AXILLARY VEIN THROMBOSIS (PAGET–SCHROETTER SYNDROME)

Etiology
- Associated with thoracic outlet syndrome, malignancy, trauma, and indwelling lines
- Compression of the subclavian vein at costoclavicular space
- Can have narrowing at costoclavicular joint (most common), abnormal anterior scalene, subclavian muscle, pectoralis, or scalene minimus muscles
- Most common in **young males who have repetitive strenuous activity**
  Clinical Presentation: **upper extremity swelling without neurogenic symptoms**

Treatment
- If thoracic outlet syndrome, can try catheter-directed thrombolysis for clots detected within 10–14 days
- If this fails can try operative thrombectomy
- Always need to **correct any underlying anatomic abnormality** (e.g., first rib resection)
- Place **all patients on anticoagulation**

15-1: CORONARY ARTERY DISEASE

Coronary Anatomy

Left System

- **Left main coronary artery:** emerges from left coronary ostium, runs between pulmonary artery and left atrial appendage, and bifurcates early into **left anterior descending coronary artery (LAD)** and **left circumflex coronary artery (LCX)**. In some patients the left main coronary artery trifurcates into the ramus intermedius, LAD and LCX.
  - LAD: gives off ~2–6 *diagonal and septal branches* and ~3–5 *septal perforator branhes*; anastomoses with **posterior descending coronary artery (PDA)**
  - LCX: gives off *obtuse marginal branches*
- Left system supplies the anterior and lateral left ventricle and the interventricular septum

Right System

- **Right coronary artery (RCA):** emerges from right coronary ostium, runs in the right AV groove, and terminates in the **PDA;** gives off *acute marginal branches*
- Usually supplies AV node *and* SA node, as well as the right ventricle and interventricular septum

Dominance of Circulation

- **Right dominant:** 85–90% of patients: PDA arises from the RCA
- **Left dominant:** 10–15% of patients: PDA arises from the LCA, which also supplies the AV node
- **Codominant:** The PDA may also be supplied by *both* the left and right systems

Venous Drainage

- Primarily via the **coronary sinus** (85%) and empties into right atrium (and right ventricular veins)
- **Thebesian veins** drain directly into the cardiac chambers

Coronary Artery Disease (CAD)

Etiology

- Endothelial injury, inflammation, and lipid deposition → coronary arterial **atherosclerosis;** plaque formation that eventually obstructs the arterial lumen
- **Myocardial ischemia:** decreased perfusion of heart muscle due to arterial narrowing, plaque rupture, or thrombosis
- **Myocardial infarction:** cell death and necrosis associated with more than 20 minutes of ischemia

Clinical Presentation

- **Angina pectoris:** chest pain, heaviness, or tightness that may radiate to shoulder, back, or arm with exercise, eating, or emotional stress, usually subsides with rest (compromised coronary blood flow)
- **Unstable angina:** pain at rest or with minimal exertion; may last more than 20 minutes; associated with >90% obstruction of coronary artery
- **Silent ischemia:** no chest pain (about 15%); most common in diabetics
- **Acute myocardial infarction:** crushing, sudden chest pain; may be associated with nausea, diaphoresis, dizziness, fatigue, and dyspnea

Diagnostic Studies

- **Chest x-ray:** cardiomegaly, pulmonary edema, or aortic/coronary calcifications
- **EKG:** ST elevation/depression, Q-waves, arrhythmias, or bundle branch blocks
- **Cardiac echocardiography,** with or without **dobutamine (stress echo):** new wall motion abnormalities and reduced ejection fraction
- **Exercise or pharmacologic stress test:** EKG or functional changes
- **Spiral CT:** visualizes coronary lesions or myocardial thinning
- **Cardiac catheterization:** visualize cardiac anatomy, identify location and severity of coronary disease, assess systolic and diastolic function, and intervene with angioplasty or stenting

Coronary Artery Bypass Grafting

Indications for Coronary Artery Bypass Grafting (**CABG**) *(Circulation. 1999;100:1464–1480; Circulation. 1997;96:1761–1769)*

Indications for Coronary Artery Bypass Grafting

Condition	Extent of Disease
Asymptomatic or mild angina	• Left main stenosis ≥60% • "Left main equivalent"—proximal LAD and LCX stenoses >70% • Three-vessel disease (LAD, LCX, and RCA)
Chronic stable angina	• Diabetic patients • Left main stenosis ≥60% • Left main equivalent • Three-vessel disease • Two-vessel disease with EF <50% or ischemia on non-invasive testing • One-vessel disease with proximal LAD stenosis • Disabling angina despite maximal medical therapy
Unstable angina/ NSTEMI	• Left main stenosis ≥60% • Left main equivalent • One- or two-vessel disease with proximal LAD stenosis • Ongoing ischemia unresponsive to maximal nonsurgical therapy
STEMI/acute myo-cardial infarction	• Ongoing ischemia/infarction unresponsive to maximal nonsurgical therapy

CABG: Surgical Technique

Midline sternotomy
⇩
Dissect left internal mammary artery (LIMA) under left sternum
⇩
with simultaneous harvesting of greater saphenous vein or radial artery
⇩
Systemic heparinization to activated clotting time >400
⇩
Arterial cannulation of ascending aorta; venous cannulation of right atrium
⇩
Initiation of bypass
⇩
Retrograde cardioplegia into coronary sinus, antegrade cardioplegia into aortic root
⇩
Systemic cooling to 30°–32°C, cardiac cooling with saline slush
⇩
Cross clamping of aorta, infusion of cardioplegia
⇩
Distal anastomoses of LIMA, reversed saphenous vein or radial artery
⇩
Proximal anastomoses to aorta
⇩
Systemic rewarming, wean off bypass
⇩
Reversal of anticoagulation with protamine
⇩
Removal of bypass catheters
⇩
Placement of pacing wires, pleural and mediastinal chest tubes
⇩
Sternal closure with steel wires

Cardiopulmonary Bypass
• Collects venous blood, filters, and oxygenates it; returns it to aorta to perfuse systemic circulation
• Allows for operation on the open heart in a nearly bloodless field
• Flow rate can be adjusted to maintain systemic perfusion pressure

Cardioplegia
• Cold potassium-containing solution that cools and arrests heart while preserving the myocardium
• Can be blood- or crystalloid-based

Choice of Conduit
- **LIMA** is always used if possible (mostly used for LAD), as it has the *highest patency rate* (>90% at 10 years)
- **Right internal mammary artery (RIMA)** can sometimes be used to graft the RCA
  - Bilateral internal mammary arteries should be avoided in patients at risk of sternal wound complication because blood flow to the sternum will be compromised and may prevent adequate healing.
- **Greater saphenous vein**
  - All patients should undergo preoperative vein mapping to assess adequacy of veins (at least 3.5 mm in diameter, without varicosities or strictures)
  - Dissection and harvest of vein can be open or endoscopic
  - Patency rate: 81% at 1 year, 75% at 5 years, 50% at 15 years
- **Other arterial grafts:**
  - **Radial artery** grafts may provide some survival benefit
  - **Right gastroepiploic artery** may be considered in patients with poor conduit options or as an adjunct to complete arterial revascularization

Complications
- Wound infection (especially sternal)—caution with bilateral IMA grafts
- Persistent bleeding
- Atrial fibrillation, other arrhythmias
- Stroke/neurocognitive dysfunction
- Pulmonary effusions; pneumothorax; respiratory failure
- Renal insufficiency
- Gastrointestinal dysfunction

Variations (Circ J. 2010;74(6):1031–1037)
- **Off-pump CABG:** avoids whole-body inflammatory response induced by CP bypass; special instruments stabilize the beating heart and shunt blood flow;
  - Has been shown to reduce postoperative bleeding, neurocognitive dysfunction, fluid retention, and organ dysfunction, but results are mixed
  - Debate whether graft patency is inferior with off-pump CABG
- **Minimally invasive/robotic CABG:** performed via small thoracotomies with a videoscope and laparoscopic or robotic instruments
  - Reduced incidence of atrial fibrillation, transfusion requirements, and hospital stays in some studies
  - Steep learning curve, difficult to teach, prolonged operative times limit widespread use
- **Hybrid CABG:** minimally invasive LIMA to LAD graft, in conjunction with catheter-based stenting of the RCA or LCX; avoids sternotomy while still offering complete revascularization
  - Prolonged patency and outcome data still pending

15-2: Valvular Disease

	Etiology	Patho-physiology	Symptoms	Physical Examination
Valvular Disease				
Mitral stenosis	• #1: Rheumatic fever (RF) • Congenital defects • Malignant carcinoid • Lupus	• Inflammatory infiltration of valves • Thickening/fusion of valve structures • Left atrial enlargement • Increased left atrial pressure • Pulmonary HTN	• **Dyspnea** with exertion or with a fib • Dysphagia or hoarseness • Occasional **hemoptysis**	• Low-pitched crescendo–decrescendo diastolic murmur, often with opening snap • JVD, ascites, hepatomegaly, peripheral edema, loud second heart sound (P_2)

Mitral regurgitation	• #1: RF • Trauma • Endocarditis • MI • Mitral valve prolapse (5%)	• Leaflet perforation, laxity or chordal rupture • Increased left atrial pressure • Pulmonary HTN • Increased preload • Cardiac dilatation • LV hypertrophy • Heart failure	• Shortness of breath • Dyspnea on exertion • Exercise intolerance	• **Holosystolic murmur** at apex, radiating to axilla
Aortic stenosis	• Calcification (advanced age) • RF • Congenital **bicuspid aortic valve:** develop aortic stenosis much younger	• LV hypertrophy • Decreased compliance • Increased O_2 requirement • Decreased coronary perfusion	**Classic triad** • Angina • Syncope • Heart failure	• Systolic murmur at base, radiating to carotids • *Pulsus parvus et tardus*—slow, prolonged rise in arterial pulse
Aortic Regurgitation	• **RF** • Congenital defects • Endocarditis • Aortic root dilatation: Marfans, Ehlers–Danlos, or cystic medial necrosis	• Decreased diastolic pressure • Decreased coronary perfusion pressure • LV volume overload • LV dilatation or ischemia • Myocardial fibrosis	• Dyspnea on exertion • Paroxysmal nocturnal dyspnea	• **Widened pulse pressure** → "water hammer pulse" • **Decrescendo diastolic murmur**

Diagnostic Studies
• **ECG:** RV/LV hypertrophy, left atrial enlargement, T-wave inversion, and ST depressions
• **Echocardiogram:** determine *severity* of disease (valve area, transvalvular pressure gradient)
• **Cardiac catheterization:** measure transvalvular pressure gradient, exclude coronary artery disease, and indirectly calculate valve area

Indications for Surgery

Valvular Disease, Indications for Surgery			
Mitral Stenosis	**Mitral Regurgitation**	**Aortic Stenosis**	**Aortic Regurgitation**
• Valve area ≤ 1cm • Symptomatic despite medical management • Pulmonary hypertension • Systemic emboli • Endocarditis	• Symptoms despite medical management • Severe mitral regurgitation with structure abnormality (ruptured chordae or perforated leaflet) • Pulmonary HTN • Deteriorating LV function • **EF <60%** or **end-systolic diameter >45 mm**	• Symptomatic • Asymptomatic if LV decompensation or transvalvular blood flow gradient of >4 m/sec • **Congestive heart failure: urgent treatment** • Angina, syncope: elective treatment	• Symptoms despite medical management • Systolic dysfunction • Decreasing ejection fraction
Medication: beta- or calcium-channel blockers	Medication: Diuretics, ACE inhibitors (reduce afterload, increase cardiac output)		Medication: ACE inhibitors, calcium-channel blockers (afterload reduction)

Asymptomatic patients: prophylaxis against bacterial endocarditis is sufficient antibiotic coverage

Mitral Stenosis—Surgical Options

- **Balloon valvuloplasty:** percutaneous inflation of a balloon in the valve to dilate it
  - Contraindications: mitral regurgitation, thickening and calcification of the mitral leaflets, or scarring and calcification of the papillary muscles or chordae tendineae
  - Low risk (0.5–2% mortality rate)
  - 66% of patients free of subsequent intervention at 3 years
- **Open mitral commissurotomy:** allows division of fused commissures and leaflets, mobilization of scarred chordae, and debridement of calcification, as well as removal of atrial clot
  - Requires midline sternotomy or right thoracotomy, cardiopulmonary bypass, and cardioplegia
  - Slightly higher risk than balloon valvuloplasty (2% mortality rate)
  - 75% of patients free of subsequent intervention at 5 years
- **Mitral valve replacement:** tissue or mechanical
  - Indicated when dense calcifications or mitral regurgitation make valvuloplasty impossible
  - Attachments of chordae tendineae should be preserved if possible
  - 2–10% mortality rate

Mitral Regurgitation—Surgical Options

- Mitral valve repair vs. replacement—repair is always preferred, if possible
- Better residual LV function by preserving chordae and papillary muscles
- Less risk of thromboembolism, endocarditis, and valve deterioration
- Lower mortality (0–2% in repair vs. 4–7% in replacement)

Aortic Stenosis

- Valve replacement or repair is the only effective therapy
- Mortality rate: 2–8%; increases exponentially with decreasing LV function
- Nonoperative options:
  - Historically poor operative candidates could undergo palliative **balloon valvuloplasty**—high incidence of symptom recurrence, restenosis, and death
  - Transcatheter aortic valve replacement (TAVR):
    - Recent endovascular techniques allow aortic valve replacement for patients with severe symptomatic AS who are deemed poor operative candidates based on comorbidities (based on surgical risk scores) and other considerations (including frailty, reoperative chest, irradiated chest, unfavorable anatomy)
      - Delivered via transfemoral approach versus transapical or transaortic depending on the anatomy of the iliac arteries and aorta (calcifications/tortuosity/size, etc.)
        - Transfemoral approach is becoming more feasible (>80% are now delivery transfemorally) as valves have become smaller.
      - Valve options include balloon expandable valves and self-expandable valves
    - Recent clinical trials have demonstrated efficacy of TAVR as a safe option for patients at high operative risk and even intermediate risk. Further multicenter studies investigating lower operative risk patients are in process.
      - Long term durability remains a question. However, valve-in-valve deployment is a well-described option for patients with recurrent disease

Aortic Insufficiency

- Mortality rate: 4–6%

Prosthetic Valves

Prosthetic Valves		
Mechanical Valves	**Bioprosthetic Valves**	**Pulmonary Autograft (Ross Procedure)**
• More durable • Require lifelong anticoagulation	• Porcine or bovine pericardium • Undergo structural deterioration, requiring reoperation • Do not require anticoagulation • Preferred for patients in whom anticoagulation is contraindicated or more elderly patients	• Uses patient's own pulmonary root to replace aortic root, pulmonary root replaced with allograft • Technically more challenging • Does not require anticoagulation and complications rates are low

OLIVER S. CHOW • JENNIFER L. WILSON • SIDHU P. GANGADHARAN

16-1: THORACIC ANATOMY

Thoracic Cavity

Skeletal
- Intercostal arteries: supply the posterior and lateral aspects of chest wall; **run inferior to each rib in the intercostal neurovascular bundle;** first two intercostal arteries originate from subclavian arteries, inferior 10 from the descending thoracic aorta
- Diaphragm: primary muscle involved in inspiration and expiration
- Accessory muscles
  - Inspiratory: scalenes, sternocleidomastoid, and external intercostal muscles
  - Expiratory: abdominal wall musculature and internal intercostal muscles

Pleura
- Visceral pleura
- Parietal pleura

Right Lung
- **Comprised 3 lobes and 10 segments**

Left Lung
- **Comprised two lobes and eight segments**

Fissures
- Right major or oblique: separates RLL from RUL and RML
- Right minor or horizontal: separates RUL and RML
- Left major: separates LUL from LLL

Mediastinum
Anterior: thymus, lymph nodes, and pericardial fat
Middle: heart, ascending aorta, lymph nodes, trachea/main stem bronchi, lung hila, esophagus, phrenic and vagus nerves
Posterior: descending aorta, azygous vein, sympathetic chain, nerve roots of thoracic spinal cord, and thoracic duct

16-2: LUNG CANCER

Epidemiology
- Most common cause of cancer death for men and women

Risk Factors
- Smoking (>30 pack-years significantly higher risk for malignancy)
- Older age
- Asbestos, uranium, radon exposure
- Family history (particularly first-degree relatives)
- Previous diagnosis of lung cancer

Screening
- Based on the National Lung Screening Trial (NLST), the USPSTF recommends low-dose CT chest for adults age 55–80 with a ≥30 pack-year smoking history who are current smokers or quit within past 15 years, if their health and life expectancy would allow for curative lung surgery

16-3: LUNG LESIONS

Solitary Pulmonary Nodule

Goal
- Determine whether the nodule is malignant or benign
- Decide whether to biopsy, resect, or follow with serial imaging

Fleischner Society Recommendations for Small Pulmonary Nodules		
Nodule Size (mm)	**Low-Risk Patient**	**High-Risk Patient**
≤4	No follow-up needed	Follow-up CT at 12 mo; if unchanged, no further follow-up
>4–6	Follow-up CT at 12 mo; if unchanged, no further follow-up	Follow-up CT at 6–12 mo, then at 18–24 mo if no change

| >6–8 | Follow-up CT at 6–12 mo, then at 18–24 mo if no change | Follow-up CT at 3–6 mo, then 9–12, and 24 mo if no change |
| >8 | Follow-up CT at 3, 9, and 24 mo, dynamic CT, PET, and/or biopsy | Same as low risk |

MacMohan H, et al. Fleischner Society recommendations for small pulmonary nodules. *Radiology.* 2005;237:395–400.

Fleischner Society Recommendations for Subsolid Pulmonary Nodules		
Nodule Type	Management Recommendations	Additional Remarks
Solitary Pure GGNs		
≤5 mm	No CT follow-up needed	Obtain contiguous 1-mm-thick sections to confirm as pure GGN
>5 mm	Follow-up CT at 3 mo to confirm persistence, annual surveillance for minimum 3 y	PET not recommended
Solitary part-solid nodules	Follow-up CT at 3 mo to confirm persistence, annual surveillance CT for minimum 3 y; if solid component >5 mm, biopsy or resection	Consider PET for part-solid nodules >10 mm
Multiple Subsolid Nodules		
Pure GGNs ≤5 mm	Follow-up CT at 2 and 4 y	Consider alternate causes for multiple GGNs ≤5 mm
Pure GGNs >5 mm without dominant lesion(s)	Follow-up CT at 3 mo to confirm persistence, annual surveillance for minimum 3 y	PET not recommended
Dominant nodule(s) with part-solid or solid component	Follow-up CT at 3 mo to confirm persistence. If persistent, biopsy or resection recommended, especially for >5 mm solid component	Consider lung-sparing surgery

Naidich DP, et al. Fleischner Society recommendations for subsolid pulmonary nodules. *Radiology.* 2013;266(1):304–317.

Radiographic Characteristics		
	Malignant	Benign
Size (among smokers)	8–20 mm: 18% malignant >20 mm: 50% malignant	<3 mm: 0.2% malignant 4–7 mm: 0.9% malignant
Borders	Irregular and spiculated	Smooth and discrete
Calcification	Eccentric	**"Popcorn," central, concentric, or diffuse homogeneous calcification**
Growth	Rapid growth—solid nodules Slow growth—ground glass or semi-solid nodules	No growth

- Nodules that are high risk for malignancy or PET + should undergo excisional or needle biopsy

Diagnosis and Staging
- Bronchoscopy with biopsy or endobronchial ultrasound-directed transbronchial needle aspiration (TBNA)
- Percutaneous core needle biopsy
- Cervical mediastinoscopy to access to LN stations 1, 2, 4, 7, or anterior mediastinotomy (Chamberlain procedure) to gain access to levels 5 and 6
- Video-assisted thoracic surgery (VATS) wedge biopsy

Non–Small Cell Lung Cancer
Pathology
- Adenocarcinoma (50–60%): #1, peripheral location; more common in women
  - Subcategories: invasive adenocarcinoma, minimally invasive adenocarcinoma (<5 mm invasive component), and in situ adenocarcinoma (formerly bronchoalveolar carcinoma)
- Squamous cell carcinoma (15–25%): central location; more common in men
- Large cell carcinoma (10–15%): aggressive

Clinical Presentation
- Asymptomatic
- **Symptoms often imply higher stage: cough (50–75%), hemoptysis, weight loss, chest wall pain, and/or hoarseness**
- Pancoast tumors are associated with Horner's syndrome (ptosis, miosis, anhydrosis)

Imaging and Evaluation
- Chest and upper abdomen CT (through adrenals): extent of disease + adenopathy
- Whole-body PET/CT: metastases
- Invasive staging (EBUS, EUS, mediastinoscopy, and/or anterior mediastinotomy) should be considered for all tumors >2 cm (>cT1a), central tumors, or in cases where adenopathy is discovered on imaging.
- MRI of head (clinical stage II and higher or neurological symptoms): brain metastases
- **Pulmonary function tests: all operative candidates (calculated postresection FEV_1 and DLCO >40% predicted)**
  - CPET (cardiopulmonary exercise testing) functional assessment when suitability equivocal (VO_2 max <15 mL O_2/kg/min—high risk for resection, <10 mL O_2/kg/min—prohibitive risk for resection)
- Cardiac workup based on history, cardiac risk factors, and if pneumonectomy is planned.

Surgery
- Clinical stages I, II, selected IIIA (if response to induction chemotherapy or chemo-XRT)
- Open thoracotomy or VATS with **anatomic resection and lymph node dissection for patients with NSCLC**

Staging by TNM System *(AJCC, 8th ed., 2017)*

8th Edition of the TNM Classification for Lung Cancer
T Stage
• T1: ≤3 cm, surrounded by lung, not involving any bronchus proximal to lobar bronchus
• T1a: ≤1 cm
• T1b: >1 and ≤2 cm
• T1b: >2 and ≤3 cm
• T2: >3 and ≤5 cm, or involving main bronchus ≥2 cm from carina, invades visceral pleura, associated with atelectasis, or pneumonitis extending to hilar region
• T2a: >3 and ≤4 cm
• T2b: >4 and ≤5 cm
• T3: >5 and ≤7 cm, or invasion chest wall, phrenic nerve, parietal pericardium, main bronchus within 2 cm of carina, or separate nodule in same lobe
• T4: >7 cm, or invading diaphragm, mediastinum, heart, great vessels, trachea, recurrent laryngeal nerve, esophagus, vertebrae, carina, or separate nodule in a different ipsilateral lobe
N Stage
• N1: Hilar, interlobar, peripheral nodes
• N2: Ipsilateral mediastinal or subcarinal nodes
• N3: Contralateral mediastinal, ipsilateral scalene, or supraclavicular nodes
M Stage
• M1a: separate tumor nodule(s) in a contralateral lobe, pleural or pericardial nodules, malignant pleural or pericardial effusion
• M1b: single extrathoracic metastasis in a single organ
• M1c: multiple extrathoracic metastases in one or several organs
Stage Groupings

Occult Carcinoma	Tx	N0	M0
Stage 0	Tis	N0	M0
Stage IA1	T1a	N0	M0
Stage IA2	T1b	N0	M0
Stage IA3	T1c	N0	M0
Stage IB	T2a	N0	M0
Stage IIA	T2b	N0	M0
Stage IIB	T1a–T2b	N1	M0
	T3	N0	M0
Stage IIIA	T1a–T2b	N2	M0
	T3	N1	M0
	T4	N0, N1	M0

Stage IIIB	T1a-T2b	N3	M0
	T3/T4	N2	M0
Stage IIIC	T3/T4	N3	M0
Stage IVA	Any T	Any N	M1a/M1b
Stage IVB	Any T	Any N	M1c

Five-Year Survival for NSCLC (AJCC, 7th ed., TNM Staging)

Stage	Based on Clinical Stage	Based on Pathologic Stage
IA	50%	73%
IB	43%	58%
IIA	36%	46%
IIB	25%	36%
IIIA	19%	24%
IIIB	7%	9%
IV	2%	13%

J Thorac Oncol. 2007;2:706–714.

Chemotherapy
- Induction chemotherapy or chemoradiotherapy considered for stage IIIA (T1–2N2 or T3 [separate nodules] N2) tumors that are possibly resectable (NCCN Guidelines 2016 for NSCLC)
- Adjuvant chemotherapy for tumors stage II or greater, or also high-risk stage IB (poorly differentiated, vascular invasion, close margins, wedge only with insufficient margins); most common regimen: cisplatin based
- Permetrexed—antifolate agent effective for adenoca
- Bevacizumab—anti-VEGF, used for adenoca but not used for squamous cell due to particularly high bleeding risk
- Tyrosine kinase inhibitors (e.g., erlotinib)—for tumors with EGFR mutation
- MET/ALK inhibitors (e.g., crizotinib)—for tumors with EML4/ALK translocation

Radiation
- Definitive treatment (along with chemotherapy) for stage IIIB
- IIIA: mediastinum
- 45–50 Gy if neoadjuvant, no planned pneumonectomy; 60–75 Gy for definitive treatment
- Treatment of positive surgical margins
- M1 disease: single lesion
- Role for stereotactic radiotherapy for surgically operable lung tumors still under investigation

Surveillance
- First 2 years: chest CT and H&P every 6–12 months
- Years 3 and onward: annual chest CT and H&P

Recurrence
- Locoregional and/or distant (brain, adrenals, contralateral lung)
- Role for resection, external beam radiation therapy, or other modalities should be evaluated by multidisciplinary teams

Small Cell Lung Cancer
General Information
- Develops from basal cells of bronchial epithelium
- **100% smoking related**
- **Metastasize early and widely: poor prognosis**

Treatment
- Chemotherapy
- Radiotherapy added for limited-stage disease confined to chest
- Stage I disease (node negative) occasionally may be treated with resection and chemotherapy

Carcinoid
Epidemiology
- 80% centrally located, arising in lobar or segmental bronchi
- Neuroendocrine (Kulchitsky cell) carcinomas derived from amine precursor uptake derivative cells

Clinical Presentation
- Hemoptysis and/or recurrent pneumonia
  Diagnosis: bronchoscopy and biopsy
  Treatment: complete resection (lobectomy) + hilar/mediastinal nodal sampling

Types
- Typical: 0–2 mitoses/high power field, no necrosis, and no nodal involvement
- Atypical: 2–10 mitoses/high power field, necrosis, nodal involvement more likely, generally more aggressive, present later in disease process, possible role for adjuvant chemotherapy, and mean survival of 2 years

Malignant Pleural Mesothelioma
Epidemiology
- Rare malignancy
- 85% associated with asbestos exposure
- Diagnosis made best with pleural biopsy
- Median survival with palliation or chemotherapy alone 6–12 months
- Surgical approaches include extrapleural pneumonectomy (EPP) and pleurectomy/decortication
  - Multimodality therapy appears to have the most favorable outcome

Pulmonary Metastasis
Operative Patient Selection
- Control of the primary tumor
- All of the metastatic cancer may be removed with planned resection
- Adequate pulmonary reserve to tolerate resection
- No other sites of metastasis

Operation
- Preserve as much lung tissue as possible
- Bilateral disease may be treated with sternotomy, staged bilateral thoracotomy, or bilateral VATS

Five-Year Survival for Solid Tumors That Have Metastasized to the Lungs
- Soft tissue sarcoma: 25%
- Colon/rectal cancer: 8–37%
- Renal cell cancer: 13–50%
- Breast cancer: 14–49%
- Melanoma: 25%

Benign Lung Lesions
Principles
- Most are incidentally found on CXR or CT
- Lesions that are stable for 2 years or more on imaging are likely benign
- Presence of fat or calcifications (dense, central, or "popcorn" shaped), tissue positive for fungal, mycobacterial, or bacterial growth
- **When diagnosis cannot be established by other means, resection is required.**
  - Endobronchial lesions can be excised bronchoscopically
  - Non-anatomic resection (wedge) if peripheral for diagnosis
  - Lobectomy or segmentectomy may be required for more central lesions

Classifications/Tissue Origin
- Epithelial: papilloma, adenomatous hyperplasia, and polyps
- Mesodermal: fibroma, lipoma, leiomyoma, chondroma, granular cell tumor, and sclerosing hemangioma
- Unknown: hamartoma (#1), teratoma, and clear cell tumor
- Other: amyloid, MALT, xanthoma, and myofibroblastic tumor

16-3: SURGICAL OPTIONS AND TECHNIQUES

Cervical Mediastinoscopy
- Use: diagnose N2 or N3 disease
- Level 1 (R and L): partially accessed via cervical incision, before introducing mediastinoscope; low cervical, supraclavicular, and sternal notch, from inferior aspect of cricoid to superior aspect of clavicles and manubrium
- Level 2 (R and L): paratracheal superior to innominate
- Level 4 (R and L): paratracheal inferior to innominate artery
- Level 7: subcarinal

Complications
- **Left: recurrent laryngeal nerve palsy**
- **Right: azygous vein injury**
- **Esophageal injury posterior to station 7**

Thoracoscopy/VATS (Video-Assisted Thoracoscopic Surgery)
- Diagnostic indications
  - Pleural disease
  - Lung biopsy for parenchymal disease or indeterminate nodule
  - Nodal sampling (neoadjuvant therapy, previous mediastinoscopy, and laryngectomy)
  - Alternative approach to anterior mediastinotomy (Chamberlain procedure) to sample subaortic and paraortic nodes for staging (levels 5 and 6)
- Therapeutic indications
  - Bleb and bullae resection with stapler
  - Mechanical pleurodesis
  - Apical pleurectomy
  - Decortication for empyema
  - Ligation of thoracic duct for chylothorax
  - Lobectomy for cancer
- Mediastinal disease
  - Pericardial window for malignant pericardial effusions
  - Resection of tumors including posterior, thymoma, and cysts
  - Sympathectomy
    Chest wall resection with reconstruction en bloc: stage III disease

Complications
- Bronchopleural fistula
- Atrial fibrillation
- Prolonged air leak
- Mortality: 1.5% lobectomy (*Ann Thorac Surg. 2016 Apr;101(4):1379–1386*) and 6% pneumonectomy (*Ann Thorac Surg. 2010 Sep;90(3):927–934*)

16-4: ACQUIRED THORACIC PATHOLOGY
Pneumothorax
Primary PTX
- Etiology: rupture of small subpleural blebs in otherwise normal lungs
- Risk factors: young, tall, male, Marfan syndrome, smoking history, familial history, and prior pneumothorax
- Location: most on the right, 10% bilateral
- Recurrence: after first episode, 20–30% will recur within 2 years

Secondary PTX
- Pulmonary disorders: COPD, asthma, cystic fibrosis, pulmonary fibrosis, sarcoidosis, infectious (bacterial, mycobacterial, parasitic, fungal, *Pneumocystis carinii*, AIDS), and neoplasm (bronchogenic, metastatic lymphoma, or sarcoma)
- Nonpulmonary disorders: catamenial (thoracic endometriosis), Marfan syndrome, Ehlers–Danlos syndrome, histiocytosis X, scleroderma, collagen disorders, and lymphangiomyomatosis
  Clinical presentation: chest pain, dyspnea, and crepitus

Diagnosis
- CXR: erect PA and lateral plain films fastest and easiest; expiratory films if small
- CT: can be helpful to identify blebs and predict possible future pneumothoraces

Management
- First episode
  - Clinically stable and small: supplementary oxygen + observation with serial CXRs +/- small-bore catheter evacuation (e.g., pigtail, dart)
  - Clinically stable and large: tube thoracostomy or small-caliber catheter evacuation
  - Clinically unstable: needle decompression followed by tube thoracostomy
- **Indications for surgery**
  - **First episode: persistent air leak (>4 days), failure to re-expand, bilateral, associated hemothorax, tension pneumothorax, occupational risk, and lack of medical care in isolated area**
  - **Subsequent episodes: ipsilateral or contralateral recurrence after initial pneumothorax**
- Surgical goal: resect blebs/bullae and obliterate pleural space
- Surgical options
  - Resection: VATS wedge resection of blebs and bullae

- Apical +/– superior segment wedge resection (30–40% will have normal lungs without identified blebs)
- Pleura: mechanical pleurodesis, parietal pleurectomy, or chemical pleurodesis (typically talc, doxycycline, or bleomycin)

Traumatic PTX

- Etiology: blunt or penetrating trauma
- **Will usually warrant tube thoracostomy**
- Large/persistent air leak: may require bronchoscopy to rule out central airway injury
- Associated hemothorax may require surgical evacuation

Retained Hemothorax

- Etiology: postoperative complication, blunt, or penetrating trauma
- Observation: if small (<25% of hemithorax), usually resolves without complication
- Tube thoracostomy: usually requires large tube (32 Fr or greater); most resolve
- Surgical evacuation: if large or failed tube thoracostomy drainage, typically VATS
  - Goal: prevent development of empyema or trapped lung secondary to fibrothorax
  - Ideally want to perform within 7 days of injury, before loculations form

---

Tube Thoracostomy—Technique

Tube Thoracostomy (Fig. 16-1)

Figure 16-1 A: Blunt dissection of the subcutaneous tissue and intercostal musculature. **B:** Insertion of the tube is facilitated by mounting the tube on a Kelly clamp. **C:** The tube is directed posteroapically through a 180-degree rotation of the clamp. **D:** Advancement of the tube with drainage openings well within the thorax. **E:** Final position of the chest tube. (From Fischer JE, Bland KI. *Mastery of Surgery*, 5th ed. Philadelphia, PA: Lippincott Williams & Wilkins, 2007.)

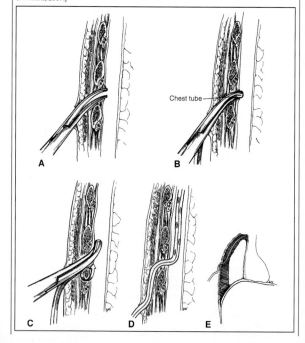

Anesthetize skin, subcutaneous tract, periosteum of rib and just outside parietal pleura (remember intercostal nerves run posterior to anterior, under rib; intercostal blocks above and below site of insertion ideal)

⇩

Make 2–3 cm incision in the 4th or 5th intercostal space between the anterior and midaxillary line

⇩

Bluntly dissect soft tissue with a Kelly clamp to create a subcutaneous tunnel

⇩

Push the Kelly clamp through the intercostal muscle and parietal pleura in the **space above the rib** to avoid neurovascular bundle injury

⇩

Place a finger through the tract to ensure absence of adhesions

⇩

Clamp chest tube at proximal end; insert through the tract into the pleural space

⇩

Direct apically for pneumothorax, inferiorly and posteriorly for effusion

⇩

Advance the tube until the proximal hole is 2 cm beyond the rib
Connect tube to water seal or suction system, close skin with suture, secure tube

- Equipment: Silastic tube (size depending on indication, 20–36 Fr), Kelly clamp, scalpel, suture, needle driver, lidocaine, and water seal or suction system (e.g., Pleurovac®)
  Position: supine with ipsilateral arm above the head in a comfortable position
  Small-bore tube thoracostomy (e.g., pigtail catheter, 8–14 Fr)
  Inserted using Seldinger catheter-over-wire techniques
  Anesthetize skin and subcutaneous tract; anterior 2nd intercostal space commonly used for pneumothorax, though lateral 4th or 5th intercostal space along anterior to midaxillary line can also be used; ultrasound guidance is especially useful when effusion is present
  Introducer needle inserted while aspirating to enter pleural cavity without advancing or probing deep into thorax
  Flexible guidewire placed into pleural cavity
  Small skin incision made to allow dilator placement
  Dilator used to expand tract over guidewire, followed by drainage catheter
  Some devices included a trocar
  Catheter connected to one-way valve and collection device (e.g., Pneumostat, Heimlich)

Empyema
Definition: localized infection of the pleural space

Clinical Presentation
- Symptoms: pleuritic chest pain, fever, cough, and dyspnea
- Etiology: pneumonia, esophageal perforation, bronchopleural fistula, recent surgery, subphrenic abscess, undrained pleural effusion, and hemothorax

Imaging
- CXR: difficult to tell whether benign effusion or empyema; decubitus films may help
- Ultrasound: identify fluid and loculations; can direct aspiration
- CT: differentiates consolidated lung from effusion, assesses for loculations, thickened pleura, and trapped lung
- Diagnostic thoracentesis: fluid aspirated should be sent for gross examination, cytology, Gram stain, culture (aerobic, anaerobic, fungal, and mycobacterial), and biochemical analysis (**pH <7, glucose <50 mg/dL, LDH 1000 IU/L suggestive of empyema**)

Stages of Empyema

- **Stage I: exudative (acute phase), first week**
  - Fluid is free flowing and thin; lung is still able to expand
- **Stage II: fibrinopurulent (transitional phase), second week**
  - Loculations start to form as fibrin deposits increase
  - Rind begins to form, causing some limitation of lung expansion
  - Fluid becomes turbid or frankly purulent, more gelatinous in texture
- **Stage III: organizing (chronic phase), third week and later**
  - Fluid becomes thick and purulent
  - **Thick rind forms over the lung, limiting expansion**
  - Chronic empyema progresses to fibrothorax with trapped lung and chest wall retraction

Treatment
- All: treat underlying cause, antibiotics
- Exudative stage (first week)
  - Tube thoracostomy, pigtail catheter drainage, or repeat aspiration
- Fibrinopurulent (second week): tube thoracostomy
  - Fibrinolytic agents (urokinase, streptokinase, or tPA, plus DNAse) to break up loculations
  - **Surgical evacuation may be needed for large or complex empyemas**
- Organizing (third week and later): decortication
  - VATS for early, simple cases; open thoracotomy if more complex or chronic
- **In cases of delayed diagnosis, inadequate antibiotic therapy, failed drainage in the more acute phases, continued reinfection from bronchopleural fistula or abscess, and in TB or fungal infections, more extensive therapy is needed**
  - Open drainage with rib resection: Eloesser flap or Clagett window
  - Collapse and sterilization of the empyema cavity
  - Eventual space-filling procedure with a muscle transposition flap

Chylothorax
Epidemiology
- Definition: accumulation of lymph in pleural space secondary to lymphatic obstruction or injury (usually iatrogenic)
- Incidence: 0.4–0.5% of thoracic surgeries
- Morbidity
  - Malnutrition: loss of proteins, lipids, and fat-soluble vitamins
  - Electrolyte imbalance and dehydration
  - Immunologic compromise: loss of lymphocytes

Anatomy of the Thoracic Duct
- Originates in abdomen at cisterna chyli
- Enters thorax at aortic hiatus and ascends extrapleurally between aorta and azygous vein posterior to esophagus, **crosses midline at T5–7**
- Terminates **at junction of left internal jugular and subclavian veins**

Injury
- **Vulnerable in esophageal (#1) and aortic surgery**
- Location: just posterior to left subclavian artery
- Prevent: prophylactic ligation in high-risk surgery

Clinical Presentation
- Nonoperative: dyspnea
- Postoperative: milky white drainage from chest tube 2–8 days after feeding

Diagnosis
- Fluid for pH, gram stain and culture, triglycerides (>110 mg/dL is diagnostic), and protein

Treatment
- Low output: low-fat diet + medium-chain triglycerides
- Best: **NPO + elemental tube feeds or TPN, chest tube drainage, +/– octreotide**
- Surgical intervention if
  - output >1,000 mL/day
  - 500–1,000 mL/day after enteral feedings have resumed
- Options: VATS > thoracotomy for thoracic duct ligation, percutaneous coil embolization of duct by interventional radiology

Surgical Treatment for Select Emphysema patients
Emphysema definition: abnormal and permanent enlargement of airspaces distal to the terminal bronchioles (hyperinflation) associated with destruction of alveolar wall and subsequent loss of lung elastic recoil
Giant bullectomy: removal of air space occupying more than one-third to half of the hemithorax and compressing otherwise normal lung parenchyma
- Types of bulla: open communication with bronchial tree vs. closed
- severe dyspnea is common if a large bulla occupies >30% of hemithorax
- Technique: thoracoscopy or thoracotomy with excision of the bulla with stapler; median sternotomy and resection for bilateral disease

Lung Volume Reduction Surgery (LVRS)
- National Emphysema Treatment Trial (NETT): enrolled 1,218 patients with emphysema, randomly assigned to best medical therapy vs. surgery

- Benefit in patients with upper lobe predominant emphysema
  - Reduced short- and long-term mortality if baseline low exercise capacity
  - Durably improved exercise capacity and quality of life
- Benefit in the following conditions
  - Disability despite maximal rehabilitation
  - Quit smoking for >6 months
  - Marked airflow obstruction but reasonable alveolar gas exchange, normal heart
- Technique: bilateral stapling through median sternotomy or bilateral thoracoscopy
  Bronchoscopic lung volume reduction (investigational): occlusion of airway using
  fibrin-based glue, or endobronchial one-way valves

Lung Transplant
Types of Transplantation
- Single lung
- Bilateral lung
- Living-related lobar
- Heart–lung

Immunosuppression
- Induction therapy: controversial; polyclonal-ATG vs. monoclonal OKT-3
- Triple maintenance therapy: calcineurin inhibitor (Cyclosporin A, Tacrolimus) +
  steroids + Immuran vs. Mycophenolate

Complications
- Primary graft dysfunction (reperfusion)
- Acute rejection
- Infection (bacterial, viral, fungal, and protozoan)
- Anastomotic (dehiscence or stricture)
- Malignancy (PTLD, skin, native lung, and donor lung)
- Chronic rejection (BOS—bronchiolitis obliterans syndrome)

16-5: DISEASES OF THE CHEST WALL

Chest Wall Neoplasms
Characteristics
- Rare tumors, typically malignant (50–60%)
- Origin: bone, cartilage, soft tissue, and 85% from ribs
- Slow growing pain is usual presenting symptom
- Diagnosis based on history, examination, imaging (CT), and excisional biopsy

Primary Neoplasms of Chest Wall
- Benign: chondroma, desmoid, fibroma, lipoma, rhabdomyoma, and schwannoma
- Malignant: malignant fibrous histiocytoma, malignant schwannoma, chondrosarcoma,
  neurofibrosarcoma, hemangiosarcoma, lymphoma, liposarcoma, and leiomyosarcoma

Metastatic Lesions to Chest Wall
- **Metastases to rib: most common malignant chest wall neoplasm**

Thoracic Outlet Syndrome
Definition: compression of the subclavian vessels and brachial plexus at the superior
aspect of the thorax (technically the thoracic inlet) from a cervical rib, anterior scalene
hypertrophy, or trauma to the structures forming the thoracic outlet

Anatomy
- Anterior and middle scalenes: insert onto first rib
- Subclavian vein: anterior to anterior scalene, over the first rib, posterior to clavicle
- Subclavian artery and brachial plexus: anterior to middle scalene, over the first rib,
  posterior to anterior scalene

Clinical Presentation
- Worsened with arm abduction
- **Neurogenic: #1, ulnar distribution most common,** lower trunk of plexus
  - Pain, paresthesias, motor weakness, and (rarely) atrophy of intrinsic muscles of hand
- Vascular
  - Arterial: coldness, weakness, unilateral Raynaud's, pain, and fatigue of arm and hand
  - Venous: edema, aches, pains, discoloration, and venous distension arm and shoulder
- Physical examination: Adson's or scalene test (loss of radial pulse with head turned
  to ipsilateral side with head extended), costoclavicular, and hyperabduction tests
- Imaging: chest and cervical spine radiographs, EMG, nerve conduction studies,
  angiography, and venography

Treatment
- Conservative therapy: if neurogenic symptoms
  - Physical therapy, postural modification, rest periods, cervical rolls for sleeping, and physical therapy
- Effort-induced venous thrombosis (Paget–Schroetter syndrome)
  - Thrombolytics, anticoagulation, and surgical decompression
  - Thrombectomy and venous bypass rarely required
- Surgical decompression
  - Indication: neurogenic symptoms that fail conservative management and those with vascular compromise
  - Technique: divide anterior scalene muscle, first rib resection, or a combination.
  - Cervical ribs should be resected if present

16-6: MEDIASTINAL TUMORS AND CYSTS

Anterior Mediastinal Masses
Classification
- **Most common mediastinal tumors**
- **4 T's (95%): thymoma, teratoma (germ cell tumors), thyroid goiter, and "Terrible" lymphoma**
- Other less common: thymic carcinoma, thymic carcinoid, and parathyroid adenoma

Thymoma
- Most common anterior mediastinal mass
- Gland normally enlarges until puberty, then degenerates and is replaced with fat
- Symptoms: vague cough and dull chest pain
- Myasthenia gravis (MG): 30–50% of patients with a thymoma have MG
- Only 15% of patients with MG have thymoma
  - Labs: positive serum anti-acetylcholine receptor antibodies
- Paraneoplastic syndromes (5–10%): red cell aplasia, systemic lupus, Cushing syndrome, hypogammaglobulinemia, and SIADH
- Imaging: CT with IV contrast
  - Early: well-circumscribed, round masses
  - Advanced: irregularly shaped or invasive
  - Must rule out teratoma or lymphoma: look for lymphadenopathy
- Operative management: resect all thymic tissues and pericardial fat en bloc
  - Median sternotomy provides best access; VATS and robotic VATS also used
  - Masaoka staging based on encapsulation (stage I), invasion of capsule (stage II) or adjacent organs (stage III) and pleural/pericardial implants or distant metastases (stage IV)
- Invasive or unresectable tumors: biopsy for tissue diagnosis, neoadjuvant therapy

Lymphoma
- **Not a surgical disease, goal is typically to provide adequate tissue for diagnosis**
- Types: Hodgkin disease >>> primary mediastinal or lymphoblastic lymphoma
- Diagnosis: parasternal core-needle biopsy under ultrasound or CT guidance is preferred, cervical or anterior mediastinotomy, and VATS

Germ Cell Tumors (10–20%)
- Principles: most common extragonadal site of germ cell tumors
- Three main types:
  - Teratomas: most common, typically benign
  - Seminomatous: more likely to be malignant
  - Nonseminomatous: malignant tumors more likely symptomatic from mass effect
- Diagnosis: CT with IV contrast, tumor markers (AFP, beta-hCG, and LDH)
  - Teratoma: none
  - Seminomatous: low-level beta-hCG elevation
  - **Nonseminomatous: 80% elevated AFP, 30–50% elevated beta-hCG, 80–90% elevated LDH,** directly related to tumor volume
  - Core-needle biopsy if needed; not if AFP elevated, radiographically teratoma
- Treatment
  - Teratoma: resection alone, no adjuvant therapy
  - Seminomatous: very radio- and chemo-sensitive (cisplatin-based). Residual disease is not resected.
  - Nonseminomatous: bleomycin, etoposide, and cisplatin chemotherapy. Residual disease is resected.

Middle Mediastinal Masses
Bronchogenic and Esophageal Cysts
- Bronchogenic
  - Most common mediastinal cyst, some malignant risk
  - Located anywhere along the course of lung development; most commonly in sub-carinal space
  - Most will eventually become symptomatic due to infection or mass effect; present with cough, wheezing, dysphagia, or airway obstruction
- Esophageal
  - Rare, attached to esophagus
  - Have epithelial tissue made up of some layer of gastrointestinal tissue
- Imaging
  - CT: homogeneous soft-tissue mass associated with tracheobronchial tree
  - MRI: hyperintense signal on T2-weighted imaging
  - Technetium pertechnetate scan: 50% of esophageal cysts have gastric mucosa
- Biopsy
  - Bronchogenic: transtracheal or transesophageal aspiration for mucoid material
  - Esophageal: avoid due to risk of infection
- Treatment: symptomatic or infected cysts should be resected

Pericardial Cysts
- Typically found at the right cardiophrenic angle or along diaphragm
- Imaging: MRI (differentiate from Morgagni hernia and pericardial fat pad)
- No malignant potential, rarely symptomatic
- Aspiration may be therapeutic but most cysts need no intervention

Other Masses
- Lymphadenopathy: most common middle mediastinal abnormality
  Metastatic disease: from lung, airway, esophageal, or head and neck
  Reactive: bacterial or viral infections or autoimmune disease (RA, SLE)
- Granulomas
  Sarcoidosis: noncaseating
  Infectious: histoplasmosis (Ohio or Mississippi River Valleys) or coccidiomycosis (San Joaquin Valley)

Posterior Mediastinal Masses
Principles
- Etiology: neurogenic tumors arising from peripheral nerves, sympathetic chain, or paraganglionic cells, slow growing
- **More likely to be malignant in children, benign in adults**
- Most tumors are located in the paravertebral sulcus
- Imaging: CT shows tumor characteristics and relation to adjacent organs, MRI if suspect extension into the spinal canal (10%)

Peripheral Nerve Origin: Schwannomas (aka Neurilemmomas) and Neurofibromas
- Most common posterior mediastinal mass, usually originating from nerve sheath of peripheral nerves (90%)
- Clinical presentation: typically asymptomatic
- Symptoms: pain, Horner's syndrome, brachial plexus compression, and paralysis (intraspinal)
- Imaging: well-circumscribed, round, smooth lesions usually in superior sulcus
- Histology
  - Schwannomas: S-100 positive; spindle cells or loose myxoid connective tissue
  - Neurofibromas: disorganized proliferation of all nerve elements, +/− S-100
  - Neurofibrosarcomas: rare (<5% of peripheral nerve tumors), more likely to invade and metastasize

Sympathetic Chain Origin: Ganglioneuroma, Ganglioneuroblastoma, and Neuroblastoma
- Typically in children and young adults, wide range of benign and malignant behavior
- Oblong, well-circumscribed lesions with frequent intraspinal extension
- Benign ganglioneuromas: can secrete VIP, causing diarrhea
- Ganglioneuroblastomas: typically encapsulated, more likely to have local invasion
- Neuroblastomas: mostly malignant and have intraspinal extension or local invasion at time of presentation

Paraganglionic Tissue Origin: Pheochromocytomas and Chemodectomas
- Most rare of posterior mediastinal tumors
- Typically unencapsulated, infiltrative, and vascular lesions

- Pheochromocytomas: <10% malignant
  - Hormonally active, symptoms from catecholamine release
  - Imaging: MIBG scan and CT
- Chemodectomas: highly vascular and may require embolization prior to resection; radiation therapy can be used when tumor is difficult to resect

Treatment
- Surgical resection with negative margins—VATS or thoracotomy
- If intraspinal extension: two-incision approach; posterior incision for laminectomy and freeing tumor from dura and neural foramina followed by intrathoracic resection
- Vagus and phrenic nerve injury can occur with tumors in superior thorax
- Adjuvant chemoradiation for malignant tumors with local invasion, lymph node involvement, or when the tumor crosses the midline

HEAD AND NECK

GEORGE A. SCANGAS • DAVID CARADONNA

17-1: NECK MASS—OVERVIEW

Epidemiology in Adults: Rule of 80s
- 80% of nonthyroid masses in adults are **neoplastic**
- 80% of neoplastic masses are **malignant**
- 80% of malignant masses are **metastatic**
- 80% of malignancies in adults are **squamous cell carcinoma (SCC)**
- 80% of metastases are from primaries above the clavicle
- 80% of parotid masses are **benign**
- 80% of minor salivary masses are **malignant**
- Risk factors: tobacco (chewing and smoking), alcohol, HIV+, and prior malignancy

Clinical Presentation
- Symptoms: hoarseness, dysphagia, pain, and time course
- Physical examination of mass: location, mobile vs. fixed, tenderness, drainage, moves with swallowing, and lymph node basins

Differential Diagnosis of Neck Mass by Location
• Midline: thyroglossal duct cyst, dermoid cysts, and pyramidal lobe thyroid
• Lateral: lymph node and branchial cleft cyst
• Submandibular: lymph node, parotid gland, and salivary gland
• Supraclavicular: lymph node
• Inflammatory (nodes): viral, Cat scratch, toxoplasmosis, TB, sarcoidosis, and lymphadenitis

Diagnosis
- **FNA** (SCC vs. adeno-CA) (Fig. 17-1)
- CXR
- CT face/neck +/– MRI
- Office: nasopharyngeal laryngoscopy
- **Operating room: panendoscopy of aerodigestive tract (rigid bronchoscopy, rigid EGD, and direct laryngoscopy)**
- **Biopsies of nasopharynx, base of tongue and pyriform sinus, tonsils**

Figure 17-1 Malignant lymph node algorithm. (From Fischer JE, Bland KI. *Mastery of Surgery*, 5th ed. Philadelphia, PA: Lippincott Williams & Wilkins, 2007.)

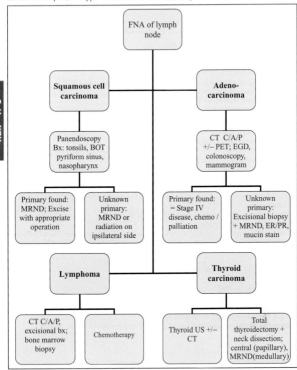

BOT: base of tongue
MRND: modified radical neck dissection

17-2: CONGENITAL MASSES

Thyroglossal Duct Cysts

Embryology
- Thyroid anlage from a stalk connecting the thyroid to anterior pharyngeal wall
- Secretion by remnant epithelium of the duct leads to thyroglossal duct cyst formation

Clinical Presentation
- Anterior, midline neck mass
- Mass rises with swallowing or protrusion of the tongue
- Typically within 2 cm of midline and over hyoid bone
  - Can be found anywhere along the course of the thyroglossal duct
  - Superiorly from foramen cecum at base of tongue to hyoid bone inferiorly
- Diagnosis: ultrasound

Surgical Treatment
- Sistrunk procedure
  - Cyst excised along with the entire length of thyroglossal duct
  - Dissect back to the foramen cecum including resection of the mid-hyoid bone
  - Delay surgery if active inflammation recurrence rate 5%

- Cystectomy alone: recurrence rate 25%
- Complications: bleeding adjacent to the upper airway can cause swelling of the mucosa which can result in respiratory distress and airway compromise
- Recurrence: usually within 1 year of procedure
  - Inflammation ± swelling of anterior neck or as draining sinus
  - Recurrence increased if inflamed/distorted tissue or rupture of cyst during surgery
  - Treat: reoperation via previous incision with wide excision

Branchial Cleft Cysts
Clinical Presentation
- Lateral neck mass or draining sinus
- Cysts: **typically located at the level of carotid bifurcation; appear after the first decade**
- Sinuses and fistulae: less common; present after first decade of life, 20% bilateral
  - External sinuses and fistulae: intermittent drainage from skin with external ostium located along anterior border of the SCM from the tragus of the ear to clavicle
  - Internal sinuses: empty into tonsillar fossa or pyriform sinus; presents as mass when outflow tract obstructs

Diagnosis
- Cysts: ultrasound (solid vs. cystic) + CT/MRI/FNA if solid
- Differential diagnosis of cystic masses without obvious associated sinuses or fistulae include metastatic lymph nodes of HPV+ SCC or papillary thyroid carcinoma
- Sinuses and fistulae: physical examination only

Surgical Principles
- **Probe any skin lesions with a lacrimal duct probe; dissect back to a blind ending in a sinus or to the tonsillar fossa for a fistula**
- **Utilize facial nerve monitoring for any tract in close proximity to the parotid gland as the facial nerve may course through or near the surgical field**
- Inclusion cyst: contains tract that can be identified leading from cyst to tonsillar fossa
- Neonates: delay surgical excision until 6 months old
- Evidence of infection: defer surgical excision and treat with antibiotics
- Recurrence: rare unless inflammation or infection is present

---

Branchial Cleft Anatomy

First Branchial Cleft and Cyst
- Opening at the angle of the mandible; passes near the facial nerve
- Normal development: external auditory canal, tympanic membrane, and middle ear
- Type 1: found inferior to the concha; runs parallel to the auditory meatus
- Type 2: originates in the anterior neck superior to the hyoid bone, passes posteriorly through the parotid gland, may involve the facial nerve, and ends in or directly adjacent to the auditory meatus

Second Branchial Cleft Cysts (90%)
- Opening at anterior border of SCM, generally at junction of lower and middle thirds Courses between internal and external carotid arteries, over cranial nerves IX, XII, and can end in or directly adjacent to the tonsilar fossae
- Typically found below the level of the hyoid bone and lateral to the carotid artery

Third Branchial Cleft Cysts and Sinuses
- Opening at the lower border of the SCM
- Courses between CN IX and XII, posterior to carotid artery to enter pyriform sinus

---

17-3: MUCOSAL TUMORS
Mucosal Tumors (Oral Cavity)
Epidemiology
- Mean age: 63; male: female = 2.4:1; **10% have a second primary tumor**
- **SCC: 80–90%**
- Risk factors: tobacco, alcohol, HPV (subtypes 16, 18), UV light, and immunosuppression
- Metastases: lung
- Prognosis: overall 5-year survival 60%

Clinical Presentation
- Symptoms: #1 nonhealing mouth ulcer, #2 persistent pain, mass, halitosis, and bleeding
- Late symptoms: loose teeth, lock-jaw, neck mass, dysphagia, and dysarthria

- **Sites: #1 floor of mouth** and **#2 lateral tongue**
- Physical examination: irregular ulcer, friable mucosa, and submucosal mass
- Thick white (leukoplakia) or red patch (erythroplakia) is a higher risk for malignancy

Diagnosis
- Physical examination of oral cavity, neck, and cervical lymph nodes
- Nasopharyngeal endoscopy and FNA biopsy/core-needle biopsy
- CXR, CT, and LFTs: assess for regional and metastatic disease

---

2002 American Joint Committee on Cancer TNM Staging System: Lip and Oral Cavity

T = tumor
- T0: no primary tumor
- T1: tumor <2 cm in the greatest dimension
- T2: tumor >2 cm but <4 cm in the greatest dimension
- T3: tumor >4 cm
- T4 (lip): tumor invades through cortical bone, inferior alveolar nerve, floor of mouth, or skin of face (i.e., chin or nose)
- T4a (oral cavity): tumor invades adjacent structures (e.g., through cortical bone, into deep [extrinsic] tissue of tongue, maxillary sinus, skin of face)
- T4b (oral cavity): tumor invades masticator space, pterygoid plates, or skull base and/or encases internal carotid artery

N = nodes
- N0: no positive regional lymph nodes
- N1: single ipsilateral lymph node ≤3 cm
- N2:
  - mets in single ipsilateral lymph node >3 cm but <6 cm
  - multiple ipsilateral lymph nodes, none >6 cm
  - bilateral or contralateral lymph nodes, all <6 cm
- N3: metastasis in a lymph node >6 cm in greatest dimension

M = mets
- Mx: distant metastases cannot be assessed
- M0: no distant metastases
- M1: distant metastases

Stage
- Stage 0: Tis N0 M0
- Stage I: T1 N0 M0
- Stage II: T2 N0 M0
- Stage III: T3 N0 M0, T1–3 N1 M0
- Stage IVA: T4a N0/1 M0, Any T N2 M0
- Stage IVB: Any T N3 M0, T4b Any N M0
- Stage IVC: Any T Any N M1

Treatment *(N Engl J Med. 2008;359(11):1143–1154)*
- Carcinoma in situ: excisional biopsy with clear margins; close primarily or allow granulation
- Stage I/II (tumors ≤4 cm): surgery and radiotherapy (5–6,000 rad) equally effective
  - Surgery generally recommended as the first line of treatment
  - Risks of micrometastases proportional to the tumor depth
    - SCC with >3 mm depth of invasion in the tongue has >20% chance of occult neck lymph node metastasis and normally modified radical neck dissection of levels I–III is recommended in these cases
- Combined therapy if microinvasion of margins, extracapsular extension upon pathologic examination of resected lymph nodes
- Stage III/IV: surgery + wide excision and neck dissection, radiation
  - May need to split lip or perform mandibulotomy for access
  - Free flaps may be needed for large wound closure to prevent scarring which can result in trismus and dysphagia
- 5-year survival: Stage I, 85–90%; Stage II, 70–80%; Stages III/IV, without nodes 50–60%
- **Survival rates cut in half with nodal involvement**

Mucosal Tumors, Site-Specific Issues
Lip
- Male: female ratio for SCC is 15:1
- Lower lip more common and requires bilateral neck dissection if advanced stage

- **Basal cell carcinoma: 99% upper lip (think sun)**
- **SCC: 95% lower lip (think tobacco)**
- Tumors of the commissure have the highest metastatic rate
- May perform Mohs surgery with plastic surgery referral for reconstruction

Floor of Mouth
- Larger lesions are at higher risk for cervical node metastasis
- Surgical issues: perform neck dissection even if clinically negative nodes; may need tracheostomy and/or gastrostomy tube; may require splitting the lip, mandibulotomy

Tongue
- Frequently has submucosal extension
- Larger cancers require multimodal treatment with surgery and radiotherapy
- >3 mm depth of invasion associated with >20% risk of occult neck metastasis and thus requires ipsilateral neck dissection
- Surgical issues: vertically excise lateral lesions; bilateral neck dissections for deep lesions. May need flap closure for larger lesions

Buccal Mucosa/Retromolar Trigone
- Smokeless tobacco users are at higher risk for forming buccal cancer
- Nodal metastases occur early
- Radiation and chemotherapy if bulky extension into tonsil or soft palate
- Surgical issues: large tumors may require a flap; transfacial approach can improve access

Hard Palate
- More nonsquamous cell cancers than in other oral cavity locations (think minor salivary glands)
- Many invade the underlying bone
- Thin lesions of the hard palate may be managed with wide local excision
- Larger lesion may require medial maxillectomy

Oropharynx (Base of Tongue and Tonsils)
- Important distinction between HPV+ and HPV− SCC
- Some types of human papillomavirus (HPV), especially HPV-16, are major risk factors for oropharyngeal SCCs involving the base of tongue or tonsils. The incidence of HPV+ oropharyngeal cancers is increasing, while the incidence of HPV− oropharyngeal cancers, normally related to factors such as smoking and alcohol use, is falling. HPV+ cancer are more radio- and chemo-sensitive and thus carry an overall better prognosis than HPV-tumors in the oropharynx.

Laryngeal Cancer
Risk factors: smoking, alcohol, age, environmental exposure (asbestos, nickel, and sulfuric acid mist), race (higher incidence in blacks), and sex (males 4:1 females)
   Clinical presentation: lump in throat, dysphagia, and change or hoarseness in voice

---

Anatomy of Larynx

- Supraglottis: tip of the epiglottis to the apex of laryngeal ventricle
- Glottis: laryngeal ventricle to approximately 5 mm inferior to true vocal cords
- Subglottis: starts 5 mm below free edge of true vocal cords to inferior edge of cricoid cartilage
- Spaces: pre-epiglottic and paraglottic (tumors spread between all regions of larynx)
- Muscle innervation and sensation
  - Superior laryngeal nerve: cricothyroid muscle and sensation superior to true vocal cords
  - Recurrent laryngeal nerve: all remaining laryngeal muscles and sensation at the level and inferior to the true vocal cords

---

Diagnosis
- Palpate for cervical lymphadenopathy
- CT or MRI of the neck
- Panendoscopy of upper aerodigestive tract
- Staging:
  - Primary tumor (T)
    - TX: primary tumor cannot be assessed
    - T0: no evidence of primary tumor
    - Tis: carcinoma in situ

- Supraglottis
- T1: tumor limited to one subsite of the supraglottis with normal vocal fold mobility
- T2: tumor invades mucosa of more than one adjacent subsite of the supraglottis or glottis or region outside the supraglottis (e.g., mucosa of base of tongue, vallecula, medial wall of pyriform sinus) without fixation of the larynx
- T3: tumor limited to the larynx with vocal fold fixation and/or invades any of the following: postcricoid area, pre-epiglottic tissues, paraglottic space, and/or inner cortex of thyroid cartilage
- T4a: (Moderately advanced local disease) Tumor invades through the thyroid cartilage and/or invades tissues beyond the larynx (e.g., trachea, soft tissues of neck including deep extrinsic muscle of the tongue, strap muscles, thyroid, or esophagus)
- T4b: (Very advanced local disease) Tumor invades prevertebral space, encases carotid artery, or invades mediastinal structures

- Glottis
- T1: Tumor limited to the vocal fold(s) (may involve anterior or posterior commissure) with normal mobility
- T1a: Tumor limited to one vocal fold
- T1b: Tumor involves both vocal folds
- T2: Tumor extends to the supraglottis and/or subglottis, and/or with impaired vocal fold mobility
- T3: Tumor limited to the larynx with vocal fold fixation and/or invasion of paraglottic space, and/or inner cortex of the thyroid cartilage
- T4a: (Moderately advanced local disease) Tumor invades the outer cortex of the thyroid cartilage and/or invades tissues beyond the larynx (e.g., trachea, soft tissues of the neck, including deep extrinsic muscle of the tongue, strap muscles, thyroid, or esophagus)
- T4b: (Very advanced local disease) Tumor invades prevertebral space, encases carotid artery, or invades mediastinal structures

- Subglottis
- T1: Tumor limited to the subglottis
- T2: Tumor extends to the vocal cord(s) with normal or impaired mobility.
- T3: Tumor imited to the larynx with vocal fold fixation.
- T4a: (Moderately advanced local disease) Tumor invades cricoid or thyroid cartilage and/or invades tissues beyond the larynx (e.g., trachea, soft tissues of the neck including deep extrinsic muscles of the tongue, strap muscles, thyroid, or esophagus)
- T4b: (Very advanced local disease) Tumor invades prevertebral space, encases carotid artery, or invades mediastinal structures

Early Stage Treatment: Single Modality (*J Clin Oncol.* 2006:24:3693)
- Radiation (tumor, neck, and superior mediastinum): for vocal cord, supraglottic larynx, and glottis
- Conservation surgery: vocal cord tumors with significant subglottic extension or tumors with vocal cord fixation and laryngeal cartilage invasion
- Transoral laser resection

Later Stage Treatment: Combined Modality (*N Engl J Med.* 2003;349(22):2091)
- Surgery (laryngectomy, thyroidectomy, and paratracheal node dissection) + radiation
- Chemoradiotherapy with surgical salvage of failures
- Organ preservation with concurrent chemoradiotherapy is an option

Indications for Complete Laryngectomy
- Advanced, resectable laryngeal cancer with base of tongue invasion or cartilage destruction
- Persistent or recurrent disease despite conservative treatment (surgical salvage)
- Chronic severe aspiration after chemoradiation and severe radionecrosis

Pharyngeal Cancer

Pharyngeal Anatomy

• Nasopharynx
   • Lateral walls: eustachian tubes
   • Anterior: posterior choanae and nasal cavity
   • Posterior: muscles of the posterior pharyngeal wall
   • Inferior: upper surface of the soft palate
 • Oropharynx: soft palate, base of the tongue, and tonsils
 • Hypopharynx: three subsites (posterior pharyngeal wall, pyriform sinuses, postcricoid area); hyoid to cricoid cartilage

Clinical Presentation
- Lump in throat, dysphagia, and change or hoarseness in the voice
- Unrelated to tobacco and alcohol use, risk factors include EBV exposure, Chinese ancestry
  - Diagnosis: check cervical lymph nodes, CT or MRI, panendoscopy
    - Staging: same as oral cancers (see above)

Treatment
- Nasopharynx: radiation (endoscopic laser excision for small superficial lesions)
- Hypopharynx
  - Small superficial lesions can be excised endoscopically with the laser (small defects can be allowed to granulate; larger ones may require flap closure)
  - Advanced tumors: surgery then radiation or chemoradiation with surgical salvage
- N2 or N3 neck disease: two options
  - Neck dissection + postoperative radiation to neck, definitive radiation to primary tumor, or planned neck dissection 4–6 weeks after radiation to primary tumor and neck
- Oropharynx

17-4: Salivary Tumors

Epidemiology
- Rare (0.5% of all malignancies)
- Risk factors: ionizing radiation, occupations involving rubber product manufacturing, asbestos, mining, plumbing, and some types of woodworking; most are idiopathic
- **Larger glands more commonly have neoplasms**
- **Neoplasms in smaller glands more likely to be malignant**
- Prognosis: gland of origin, grade, stage, involvement of facial nerve or fixation to the skin or deep structures
- Staging: same as oral cancers

Parotid Gland
Clinical Presentation
- Asymptomatic swelling
- Most common site of salivary neoplasms, most likely to be benign
- 20% malignant
Diagnosis: FNA biopsy, CT, or MRI

Benign
- Pleomorphic adenoma (77%): most common benign neoplasm, high recurrence
- Warthin tumor (22%): most common bilateral parotid neoplasm
- Treatment: superficial parotidectomy; if facial nerve involved, more likely malignant

Finding the Facial Nerve
• External auditory canal cartilage: forms a triangle that points to the facial nerve, 1 cm deep and inferior to the "tragal pointer"   • Styloid process: deep to the nerve   • Posterior belly of digastric muscle: superficial to nerve

Malignant
- Mucoepidermoid carcinoma: most common (30%), third to fifth decade of life
- Adenoid cystic carcinoma and adenocarcinoma
- Treatment
  - Total parotidectomy; try to spare facial nerve, but not at risk of leaving tumor
  - Neck dissection if clinically or radiographically positive nodes and/or high grade
  - Postoperative radiation
  - Consider chemo if T3/T4 or node-positive tumor, positive resection margins
- Surgical complication: Frey syndrome (gustatory sweating of skin over parotid)

Submandibular and Sublingual Glands

Epidemiology
- Sublingual: rare, but 80–90% malignant
- Most common neoplasm: pleomorphic adenoma
- Can be site of metastasis from breast, lung, GI tract, GU tract, head and neck cancers

Clinical Presentation
- Asymptomatic swelling
- Diagnosis: CT and Panorex

Treatment
- Surgery: submandibular triangle dissection
- High-grade tumors: post-op radiation to dissection site (entire ipsilateral neck to clavicle)
- Clinical N1: modified radical neck dissection (MRND) Type II (leave SCM and CN XI)
  Multiple positive nodes: postoperative radiation
  Single positive node: nothing further

17-5: Neck Dissection

Nodal Metastasis

Location of metastases is largely influenced by the location of primary
- Oral cavity: nodal levels I, II, and III
- Oropharynx, hypopharynx, and larynx: levels II, III, and IV
- Level V nodes: highest in primary oropharyngeal and hypopharyngeal neoplasms

Likelihood of metastases determined by tumor location, size, and histology
- Increased risk: increasing T/N stage, posterior location, and vascular/perineural invasion
- T1 tumor, 30% risk; T3 tumor, 70% risk
- Oral cavity tumors: lower risk
- Tonsil and base of tongue tumors: high risk
- Hypopharynx tumors: almost always present with nodal metastasis

Factors associated with worse prognosis
- **Extracapsular spread into surrounding soft tissue (mets and local recurrence)**
- **Metastases to level IV and posterior triangle nodes**

Comprehensive Neck Dissection

Radical Neck Dissection
- Level I–V nodes
- Identify and preserve mandibular and cervical branches of facial nerves
- Divide anterior facial vessels; ligate external jugular vein close to subclavian vein
- Identify and preserve the phrenic and brachial plexus nerves in the posterior triangle
- Divide the SCM and the omohyoid low behind the SCM
- Open the carotid sheath **to ligate the internal jugular vein** close to the clavicle
- **Take spinal accessory nerve, submandibular gland, and submaxillary duct**

Modified Radical Neck Dissection
- Level I–V nodes
- Type I MRND: spinal accessory nerve spared
  - Use: SCC of the oral cavity, oropharynx, and nasopharynx
- Type II MRND: spinal accessory nerve and sternocleidomastoid muscle spared
- Type III: spinal accessory nerve, internal jugular vein, and SCM spared
  - Use: metastatic thyroid carcinoma

Selective Neck Dissection
- Based on the assumption that primary neoplasms will metastasize in predicted patterns
- Use: SCC with clinically negative nodes (N0) if >15% chance of undiagnosed mets
  Spares the SCM, internal jugular vein, and spinal accessory nerve

Supraomohyoid Neck Dissection
- Use: SCC of the oral cavity with clinically negative nodes
  Levels I–III lymph nodes + submandibular gland

Extended Supraomohyoid Neck Dissection
- Use: SCC of the lateral tongue with negative nodes
  Levels I–IV + submandibular gland

Anteriolateral Neck Dissection
- Use: SCC of the pharynx and larynx with clinically negative nodes
  Levels II–IV nodes

Posterolateral Neck Dissection
- Use: primary melanoma or SCC of the posterior scalp
  Levels II–V lymph nodes + suboccipital and retroauricular nodes

Anterior Compartment Neck Dissection
- Use: thyroid carcinoma with disease limited to pretracheal and paratracheal nodes
- Lymph nodes in the prelaryngeal, pretracheal, and paratracheal regions

Cervical Lymph Node Anatomy

Figure 17-2 Memorial sloan kettering neck leveling system. (From Fischer JE, Bland KI. *Mastery of Surgery*, 5th ed. Philadelphia, PA: Lippincott Williams & Wilkins, 2007.)

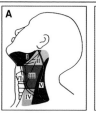 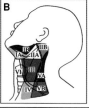 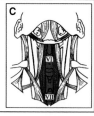

- Level I nodes: submental (IA) and submandibular (IB) triangles
- Superior: lower border of the mandible
- Posterior: posterior belly of the digastric muscle
- Inferior: hyoid bone
- Level II nodes
- Superior: base of skull
- Posterior: posterior border of the SCM
- Inferior: hyoid bone
- IIA inferior and IIB superior to spinal accessory nerve
- Level III nodes
- Superior: hyoid bone
- Posterior: posterior border of the SCM
- Inferior: cricothyroid membrane
- Level IV nodes
- Superior: cricothyroid membrane
- Posterior: posterior border of the SCM
- Anterior: anterolateral border of the sternohyoid
- Inferior: clavicle
- Level V nodes
- Posterior: anterior border of the trapezius muscle
- Anterior: posterior border of the SCM
- Inferior: clavicle
- VA superior and VB inferior to spinal accessory nerve
- Level VI nodes
- Superior: hyoid bone
- Inferior: suprasternal notch
- Lateral: medial border of the carotid sheath bilaterally
- Level VII nodes
- Superior: suprasternal notch
- Inferior: innominate artery

NASSRENE Y. ELMADHUN • PER-OLOF HASSELGREN

18-1: Thyroid

Surgical Anatomy and Physiology
Thyroid Cell Function
- Follicular cells: release T3/T4, responsible for regulation of metabolism
- Parafollicular cells: secrete calcitonin, responsible for decreasing serum calcium levels
- Hypothalamic–pituitary–thyroid axis: TRH from hypothalamus stimulates pituitary to secrete TSH, TSH from pituitary stimulates T4 synthesis and release, T4 provides a negative feedback loop to inhibit TRH release from hypothalamus

Hyperthyroidism
- Etiology: Graves' disease >> toxic multinodular goiter, toxic adenoma
- Clinical manifestation: tachycardia, anxiety, heat intolerance, sweating, and weight loss
- Labs: **elevated T3/T4, suppressed TSH**
- Treatment options
  - Propylthiouracil (PTU): inhibits organification of iodine and coupling of iodothyronine
    - Side effects: agranulocytosis; okay in pregnancy
  - Methimazole: inhibits organification of iodine and coupling of iodothyronine
    - Preferred over PTU due to longer duration of action; teratogenic
  - Radioactive iodine: repeat treatments often required
    - Contraindicated in pregnancy and in children; good option for elderly or patients with multiple comorbidities; often results in hypothyroidism
  - Total thyroidectomy: if medical management fails, large goiters causing mass effect
    - Preferred for women in the second trimester of pregnancy if PTU fails
    - **Current preferred treatment for Graves' disease**
    - Good solution for children and patients with severe exophthalmos
    - Consider in women who wish to become pregnant

Thyroid Cancer
Epidemiology
- 90% are well differentiated (papillary or follicular carcinoma) with favorable prognosis
- Occult thyroid cancer <1 cm in 3.6% of autopsies
- Risk factors
  - Personal or family history of thyroid cancer
  - **Head and neck irradiation**
  - Age: <20 or >60 years (indicates poor prognosis)
  - Male sex
  - MEN syndromes

Clinical Presentation
- Physical examination
- Incidental discovery during imaging for unrelated workup (carotid US, chest CT, and PET scan)
- Self-discovered palpable thyroid nodule
- Concerning: recent onset hoarseness, dysphagia, dyspnea

Diagnostic Workup
- Ultrasound: characteristics associated with malignancy
  - Nodule microcalcifications
  - Increased nodular central blood flow on Doppler
  - Hypoechogenicity
  - Gross local invasion
  - Irregular margins
  - Regional lymphadenopathy
- Fine needle aspiration (FNA)
  - 22 gauge needle/1.5 in length needle on empty 10-mL syringe
  - Use ultrasound guidance; repeat pass at least once
  - Expel contents on glass slides, smear with second slide, fix in 95% EtOH and dry
  - Sensitivity 65–98%, specificity 72–98%
  - False negative rates range from 2–10%, false positive rates 2%
  - Can confirm: papillary, medullary, or anaplastic thyroid cancer, lymphoma, and metastases

FNA Results/Response Algorithm—Bethesda Classification

Nondiagnostic (I)
- Repeat FNA

Benign (II)
- Essentially 0% of malignancy
- Repeat ultrasound in 6–12 mo
- DDx: colloid nodule, adenomatous hyperplasia, and thyroiditis

Atypia of Follicular Lesion of Undetermined Significance (III)
- 5–15% risk of malignancy
- Consider isotope scan, repeat FNA with genetic testing (Afirma), or surgery
  - If Afirma testing is suspicious for malignancy >> proceed with lobectomy

Follicular Neoplasm (IV)
- 10–30% risk of malignancy
- Repeat FNA with Afrima testing or Diagnostic lobectomy and isthmusectomy
- DDx: papillary carcinoma, follicular tumor, and Hürthle cell tumor

Suspicious (V)
- Lobectomy and isthmusectomy vs. total thyroidectomy
- >65% risk of malignancy
- DDx: papillary carcinoma, medullary carcinoma, anaplastic carcinoma, lymphoma, and metastatic carcinoma

Malignant (VI)
- Total thyroidectomy +/– node dissection
- Essentially 100% risk of malignancy
- DDx: papillary carcinoma, medullary carcinoma, anaplastic carcinoma, lymphoma, and metastatic carcinoma

- CT/MRI: no current guidelines
- FDG-PET: use if
  - Thyroglobulin positive with unknown tumor location
  - RAI negative (tumor does not show uptake on ^{131}I scan)

Papillary Thyroid Cancer (85–90%)
- Epidemiology
  - Rare hematogenous metastases, 30% positive lymph nodes
  - Multicentric (20–80%), bilateral (60–85%)
- Histology: cells in monolayer sheets, forming papillae and **psammoma bodies**
- Treatment
  - **Indications for total thyroidectomy:**
    - **Lesions >1 cm**
    - **Positive nodal disease**
    - **Multiple lesions**
    - **History of radiation**
  - Unilateral lobectomy with isthmusectomy if <1 cm
  - If enlarged lymph nodes, perform a central or lateral compartment dissection
- Prognosis
  - 10-year survival exceeds 90%
  - No relationship between the presence of nodal spread and long-term survival
  - Follow thyroglobulin level postop if total thyroidectomy for tumor recurrence
- Recurrence: up to 30% of patients
  - **Risk factors for poor prognosis:**
    - **Metastasis**
    - **Age at the time of diagnosis >45 years**
    - **Completeness of resection**
    - **Invasion (extra-thyroidal extension)**
    - **Size of tumor >1 cm**
    - **Pathologic subtype**
    - **Male gender**

Follicular Thyroid Cancer (5–10%)
- Epidemiology
  - 10–33% have distant metastasis at time of diagnosis: bone, lung, brain, and liver (hematogenous spread)
- Diagnosis: **need surgical specimen for definitive diagnosis**
  - 10–15% of patients with FNA showing follicular neoplasm have cancer

- **Cannot prove follicular cancer on FNA because must see vascular or capsular invasion**
- Treatment: thyroid lobectomy and isthmusectomy for diagnosis followed by completion thyroidectomy for positive pathology + radioactive iodine
- Prognosis: 85% 5-year survival
  - Follow thyroglobulin level postop if total thyroidectomy for tumor recurrence
  - Risk Factors: same as for papillary

Hürthle Cell Cancer (3%)
- Epidemiology
  - More aggressive than classic follicular neoplasms
- Risk factors: radiation, age, and familial Hürthle cell tumors
- Diagnosis: **need surgical specimen for definitive diagnosis**
  - **Cannot prove Hürthle cell cancer on FNA because must see vascular or capsular invasion**
- Treatment
  - Thyroid lobectomy and isthmusectomy for diagnosis followed by completion thyroidectomy for positive pathology
  - Total thyroidectomy if obvious malignant disease, contralateral nodular disease, or history of irradiation followed + radioactive iodine
  - Lymph node dissection for clinically or sonographically evident disease
- Prognosis: 10-year survival is 70%

Medullary Thyroid Cancer (7%)
- Epidemiology: 75% sporadic, 25% inherited
  - Associated with **RET proto-oncogene and MEN II syndromes**
  - Lymph node metastases in 70% of patients with palpable disease
  - Distant metastases to liver, lung, and bone
- Etiology: parafollicular cells
- Diagnosis: serum **calcitonin,** correlates with tumor bulk, nodal, and distant metastasis
  - **Need to exclude pheochromocytoma and parathyroid disease before proceeding to surgery (MEN II)**
- Treatment
  - Total thyroidectomy with central and lateral node dissections for sporadic cases
  - Prophylactic total thyroidectomy with central node dissection for familial syndrome or RET proto-oncogene positive
  - No role for post-operative iodine 131 therapy or chemotherapy
  - Radiation therapy may decrease local recurrence in high-risk patients
- Poor prognosis: high CEA, flushing, and diarrhea

Anaplastic Thyroid Cancer (1%)
- Epidemiology: more common in patients older than 60
  - 75% of patients have distant metastasis: lungs, bone, brain, and adrenal glands
- Clinical manifestation: fixed hard mass, tracheal compression, hoarseness, dyspnea, dysphonia, and dysphagia
- Treatment: usually palliative; diagnostic biopsy
  - Neoadjuvant and adjuvant radiation can increase longevity by months
  - Tracheostomy often required for tracheal involvement/compression
- Prognosis: almost always fatal within months

Lymphoma (1%)
- Epidemiology: female predominance, more common by age 70
  - Most commonly non-Hodgkin type
  - Associated with Hashimoto thyroiditis
- Clinical manifestation
  - Signs: painless, rapidly enlarging goiter, lymphadenopathy, and longstanding Hashimoto
  - Symptoms: tracheal compression/respiratory difficulty, dysphagia, and hoarseness
- Treatment: chemotherapy and radiation
- Poor prognosis: advanced stage, size >10 cm, mediastinal disease, and dysphagia

Metastatic Carcinoma
- Renal cell carcinoma: most common, 50% of isolated thyroid metastasis
- Lung cancer
- Breast cancer
- Malignant melanoma

Indications for ^{131}I Ablation After Total Thyroidectomy

- Invasive follicular and papillary tumors >1–2 cm
- All locally invasive tumors
- Regional lymphadenopathy
- Incomplete resection
  Timing: 4–6 wk after surgery
  Dose: 30–175 mci
  Post-ablation ^{131}I scan 1 wk later to look for metastases
  Recheck Tg, TgAb, TSH levels after ablation

Thyroid Surgery

Thyroid Surgery—Indications

- Malignancy—proven
- FNA: suspicious, follicular neoplasm or atypia (Bethesda III/IV), or three failed biopsies, Afirma testing suspicious for malignancy
- Local symptoms or marked cosmetic abnormality from an enlarged gland
- Lesions >4 cm
- Hyperthyroidism (failed medical therapy, desire to become pregnant, severe exophthalmus, mass effect)

Complications of Thyroid Surgery

Hematoma (1–2%)
- Can cause airway compromise
- Emergently open neck incision at bedside to restore airway
- Do not attempt intubation
- Majority occur within first 4–6 h

Recurrent Laryngeal Nerve Injury (0–2%, 5% in Reoperative Setting)
- One side: hoarseness (failure of complete vocal cord closure resulting in aspiration)
- Bilateral: airway emergency requiring tracheostomy (not universal)

External Branch Superior Laryngeal Nerve Injury
- Causes difficulty producing higher pitch sounds and loss of projetion
Hypocalcemia (7–30%)
- Most common complication; ranges from transient to permanent (2%)

Follow-up for Thyroid Cancer (in Conjunction with Endocrinologist)
- 4–6 weeks
  - Check thyroglobulin (Tg), anti-Tg antibody, and TSH level while hypothyroid
  - ^{131}I ablation for all high- and most intermediate-risk patients
- 6–12 months
  - Low-risk patient: Tg level with rhTSH (Thyrogen) stimulation and neck US
  - High-risk patient: Tg and anti-Tg antibody level with rhTSH, neck US, whole body iodine scan if levels are elevated or suspicious US; if negative, consider CT +/– FDG-PET
- First 3–5 years: annual Tg level and neck US for all patients
- Consider external beam radiation if locally advanced but unresectable disease
- Thyroxine suppression
  - Low risk and free of disease: keep TSH levels at 0.3–2 mU/L
  - High risk, clinically disease free: TSH levels at 0.1–0.5 mU/L for 5–10 years
  - Persistent disease: TSH levels <0.1 mU/L

18-2: PARATHYROID GLAND

Anatomy and Physiology
Embryology
- Superior gland: develops from branchial pouch IV
- Inferior gland: develops from branchial pouch III

Anatomy
- Generally four glands (30–50 mg); supernumerary glands in 13% of patients
- Superior gland: found in fat along posterior border of the thyroid gland 1–2 cm superior to inferior thyroid artery where the recurrent laryngeal nerve enters the larynx; **always in a plane posterior to the recurrent laryngeal nerve;** location more predictable

- Inferior: found on posterolateral surface of lower pole of the thyroid or at the tip of the cervical thymus or the thyrothymic ligament; location more variable
- Arterial supply: inferior thyroid artery

Parathyroid Hormone (PTH): Calcium Homeostasis
- Increases serum calcium
- Decreases serum phosphate
- Increases osteoclast and osteoblast activity
- Increases gastrointestinal absorption of calcium
- Increases renal bicarbonate excretion
- Increases renal hydroxylation of 25-hydroxy-vitamin D

Hypercalcemia—DDx
Calcium overdose
Hyperthyroidism, Familial **H**ypocalciuric **H**ypercalcemia
Immobilization/**I**atrogenic
Milk Alkali syndrome/**M**edications (thiazides, lithium)
Paget disease
Addisonian crisis
Neoplasm (metastatic to bone, PTHrp): lung > breast, head, and neck SCC, renal cell, medullary thyroid, parathyroid
Zollinger–Ellison syndrome
Excessive vitamin D
Excessive vitamin A
Sarcoidosis
• #1 cause general population: primary hyperparathyroidism
• #1 cause inpatient hospital setting: malignancy (65% of the time)
Symptoms of hypercalcemia
• Depressed mood
• Fatigue
• Muscle weakness
• Forgetfulness
• Constipation
• Kidney stones (15–20%)
• Osteoporosis (15%)

Hyperparathyroidism
Primary Hyperparathyroidism
- Epidemiology
  - 90–95%: sporadic, single hyperfunctioning adenoma
  - 5–10%: multigland disease
  - 2–3% double adenoma, remainder four-gland hyperplasia (3–4% MEN syndrome)
  - 1% carcinoma
- Pathophysiology: spontaneous loss of calcium-sensing receptors in parathyroid tissue leading to excessive secretion of PTH and therefore hypercalcemia
- Diagnosis: **elevated PTH, elevated calcium, Cl/PO₄ level >30**
- Preoperative workup
  - 24-hour urinary calcium to rule out familial hypocalciuric hypercalcemia
  - CXR to rule out tumors or bony metastasis
  - Ultrasound/technetium-99m sestamibi for localization of the affected gland
  - 4D CT scan

Guidelines for Surgery: Primary Hyperparathyroidism
Asymptomatic
• Serum calcium (> upper limit of normal) 1.0 mg/dL (0.25 mmol/L)
• Reduced bone mass (T-score <2.5 at lumbar spine, hip, distal radius) or vertebral fracture
• Renal:
• Creatinine clearance <60 mL/min
• 24-h urine for calcium >400 mg/day (>10 mmol/day)
• nephrolithiasis
• Presence of nephrolithiasis or nephrocalcinosis by radiograph, ultrasound, or CT
• Age <50 y
• Medical follow-up not feasible
Symptomatic
• Symptomatic hypercalcemia (muscle weakness, constipation, and polyuria)
• History of life-threatening episode of hypercalcemia

- Treatment
  - Medical: only treats symptoms, not cause
    - IV hydration > Lasix: first line
    - Bisphosphonates (7.5 mg/kg IV over 4 hours daily × 3 days)
    - Calcitonin (4 IU/kg q12h IM – effective only for first 48 hours)
    - Mithramycin (25 ug/kg IV over 6 hours × 3 days)
    - Calcimimetic (cinacalcet)
    - Hemodialysis
  - Surgery: gold standard, treats underlying cause
    - Bilateral neck dissection and identification of all four glands (for patients with negative imaging or increased activity in multiple parathyroid glands).
    - If preoperative imaging with US, sestamibi, 4D CT demonstrates adenoma:
      - Minimally invasive parathyroidectomy: unilateral neck exploration for single parathyroid adenoma with intraoperative PTH monitoring to biochemically confirm successful removal of offending gland
      - Minimally invasive radioguided parathyroidectomy (MIRP). Patients are injected with technetium sestamibi on the day of surgery and gamma probe is used to assist identification of the adenoma in the operating room.

Secondary Hyperparathyroidism
- Etiology: most commonly secondary to chronic renal failure
  - Other causes: sprue, chronic vitamin D deficiency, and aluminum toxicity from hemodialysis
- Pathophysiology: physiologic response to low serum calcium levels of non-parathyroid origin, i.e., "hungry bone syndrome"; in renal failure, elevated phosphorus levels and decreased production of calcitriol leads to decreased calcium absorption from nutritional sources
- Diagnosis: **elevated PTH, low to normal calcium levels**
- Treatment
  - Medical: calcium and vitamin D replacement, cinacalcet
  - Surgical: 3½-gland parathyroidectomy (four-gland if not a transplant candidate)
  - Indications: failure of medical management and severe symptoms
    - Renal osteodystrophy: bone pain, osteomalacia, pathologic fractures, and brown tumors
    - Calciphylaxis: painful deposition of calcium in the skin causing ulcerations; >50% mortality rate; very disabling

Tertiary Hyperparathyroidism
- Definition: hyperparathyroidism in patients with a history of kidney transplant
- Proposed pathophysiology: prolonged secondary hyperparathyroidism leads to autonomously elevated PTH concentrations due to loss of calcium-sensing receptors in parathyroid tissue, results in hypercalcemia (unproven)
- Treatment: surgery
  - 3½-gland or four-gland parathyroidectomy with forearm autotransplantation

Parathyroid Carcinoma
- Diagnosis: markedly elevated PTH and calcium levels
- Clinical manifestations
  - Kidney stones (>50%)
  - Severe bone disease (90%)
  - Palpable neck mass with features of invasion
  - Nodal metastasis in 30%
  - Histology: capsular/vascular invasion, cellular mitoses, thick fibrous bands separating lobules of tumor, and trabecular growth pattern
- Treatment: en bloc resection with overlying musculature and hemithyroidectomy
  - Re-operative surgery for any recurrence and localized distant metastasis
  - Minimal benefit with chemotherapy and radiation
- Prognosis
  - 5-year survival with treatment 60%
  - Recurrent hypercalcemia after surgery is usually local recurrence or metastasis

Parathyroid Surgery
Surgical Technique
- Four-gland disease:
  - Bilateral neck exploration: identify and biopsy all four parathyroid glands
- Adenoma seen on preoperative imaging:
  - Minimally invasive parathyroidectomy: unilateral neck exploration with intraoperative PTH monitoring to confirm successful removal of offending gland
  - Minimally invasive radioguided parathyroidectomy (MIRP)

Missing Parathyroid Glands

- Location
  - 40% neck, 20% mediastinum, 20% retroesophageal, 5% aortic arch area, 8% upper cervical area, and <2% in carotid sheath
- Inferior gland: inspect thyrothymic ligament, open the carotid sheath, and explore superiorly to the common carotid bifurcation; consider thyroid lobectomy on given side and/or transcervical thymectomy; explore retrolaryngeal space
- Superior gland: explore the tracheoesophageal groove from larynx to tracheal bifurcation; consider thyroid lobectomy on given side
- **Do not perform a sternotomy during initial exploration** if cannot find the adenoma
  - Close and reimage; repeat sestamibi, SPECT-CT, ultrasound
- Most common location for missed parathyroid adenoma is the normal anatomic position

Four-Gland Hyperplasia

- Subtotal parathyroidectomy: MEN patients, secondary and tertiary hyperparathyroidism
  - $3^{1}/_{2}$ glands resected, small remnant (40–50 mg) of a fourth, most normal looking parathyroid is left on its vascular supply;
- Total parathyroidectomy with forearm reimplantation
- Autotransplantation
  - Inadvertent removal or disruption of blood supply during thyroidectomy
    - Confirm that it is parathyroid gland by frozen section
    - Mince into very fine pieces and re-implant in ipsilateral sternocleidomastoid
    - Mark with clip or permanent suture so can easily find if re-exploration needed
- After four-gland parathyroidectomy
  - Use a portion of the most normal appearing gland
  - Mince gland and place in sternocleidomastoid muscle or in forearm muscle
  - Mark with clip or permanent suture so can easily find if re-exploration needed

Intraoperative PTH Monitoring

- Biochemical basis: half-life of PTH is 3–5 minutes
  - Collect PTH levels: before removing adenoma and 10–15 minutes after resecting the adenoma.
  - **If drop by >50% (and within normal limits),** operation considered successful and exploration is terminated
  - If PTH does not drop >50%, consider re-checking PTH level to see if the level continues to drop or continue neck exploration with identification of other parathyroid glands, recheck PTH level with each additional excised gland until all hyperfunctioning glands are removed.
- Results
  - Focused approach: 10-year disease-free rate 97%, similar to traditional four-gland exploration
  - Sensitivity 98%, specificity 96%, PPV 99%, NPV 90%, and overall accuracy 97%
  - Benefits: shorter operating time, lighter anesthesia, same day discharge, and cost savings

Minimally Invasive Radio-Guided Parathyroidectomy (MIRP)

- Technetium-labeled sestamibi is administered IV 1–2 hours preoperatively
- Gamma probe is used intraoperatively to locate area of highest radioactivity
- After suspected adenoma is removed, measure the radioactivity of the excised tissue and the post-resection surgical bed
- Successful if the ratio of the adenoma to background is >20%
- Can confirm with IPM and/or frozen section

Complications

- Hypoparathyroidism
  - Mild: perioral numbness and tingling in the fingertips
  - Severe: muscle cramping and spasm
  - Chvostek sign: twitching of facial muscles when zygomatic arch is tapped
  - Trousseau sign: elicited by inflating a sphygmomanometer above systolic blood pressure causing muscular contraction including flexion of the wrist, MCP joints, and palms with hyperextension of the fingers
  - Treat with calcium, vitamin D, and magnesium
- Recurrent laryngeal nerve injury

Anatomy and Physiology

Vascular Supply

- Arterial: multiple small branches of **inferior phrenic, aorta, and renal arteries**
- Venous: drained by a single vein
  - Right adrenal vein: empties into IVC, short = 1–1.5 cm, arises medially from gland
  - Left adrenal vein: empties into left renal vein, longer, arises inferomedially from the gland, and often joined by the inferior phrenic vein just before entering the renal vein

Hormones

- Adrenal cortex
  - Zona glomerulosa: mineralocorticoids (aldosterone)
  - Zona fasciculata: glucocorticoids (cortisone)
  - Zona reticularis: sex steroids (testosterone)
- Adrenal medulla
  - Catecholamines (epinephrine, norepinephrine, and dopamine)
- Ectopic tissue
  Sympathetic paraganglia along aorta: #1 = organ of Zuckerkandl at aortic bifurcation

Indications for Adrenalectomy

Unilateral Adrenalectomy

- Functional adenoma
  - Aldosteronoma
  - Cortisol-secreting adenoma (Cushing's syndrome or subclinical Cushing's)
  - Unilateral pheochromocytoma (sporadic or familial)
  - Virilizing or feminizing tumors
- Nonfunctioning unilateral tumor
- Size > 4–5 cm
- Imaging features atypical for adenoma, myelolipoma, or cyst
- Adrenocortical carcinomas
- Solitary unilateral adrenal metastases

Bilateral Adrenalectomy

- Bilateral pheochromocytomas
- Cushing syndrome secondary to:
  - Bilateral nodular adrenal hyperplasia
  - Ectopic ACTH-producing tumor unresponsive to primary therapy
  - Cushing's disease (pituitary tumor) unsuccessfully treated by surgery or radiation

Surgical Techniques

General Pearls

- Manipulate the adrenal by grasping the periadrenal fat or by gentle pushing
- Do not disrupt the capsule

Adrenalectomy

Right Adrenalectomy

- Mobilize and divide the right triangular ligament of the liver
- Develop the plane between the adrenal and IVC. Incise the peritoneum at the lateral border of the IVC and start dissecting at medial border of gland
- Roll the gland laterally to expose, clip, and divide the adrenal vein
- May have accessory right adrenal vein
- Dissect and divide all the inferior and posterior adrenal attachments
- Avoid the renal vessels inferiorly; visualize the superior pole of the kidney

Left Adrenalectomy

- Mobilize the splenic flexure; carry superiorly until the short gastric vessels
- Divide the splenorenal and splenocolic ligaments
- Develop the plane between the tail of the pancreas and kidney
- Visualize the splenic artery and vein, renal hilum and adrenal gland
- Dissect the medial, inferior, and lateral borders of the adrenal
- Clip and divide the adrenal vein close to the junction with the renal vein
- Divide the posterior and superior attachments to the gland
- Cannot find the adrenal? Find the phrenic vein on the left diaphragm and follow down to left adrenal vein

Laparoscopic Transperitoneal

- Now standard of care
- Lateral > anterior; most common approach

- Ports
  - Left: three to four; right: four (one for liver retraction in the most medial port)
  - Initial access: just medial to anterior axillary line two fingerbreadths below costal margin
  - Two to three additional ports from anterior to posterior axillary line. Keep a 5–7 cm distance between ports. Need 1–12 mm
- Pearl: stay medial to the kidney. Dissecting lateral can cause the kidney to fall medially and interfere with the operative field
- Prep and drape the patient across the midline in case of the need to convert

Indications for Open Adrenalectomy
- Large adrenal mass >8–9 cm
- Suspected or known malignancy
  - Wide resection including periadrenal fat, lymphatic tissue, and lymph nodes

Complications From Adrenalectomy
• Hemorrhage
• Vascular occlusion: i.e., inadvertent ligation of renal artery branch
• Diaphragm injury: tension pneumothorax (less in laparoscopy)
• Injury to pancreas, kidney, colon, stomach, liver, duodenum, and ureter

Adrenal Incidentalomas
Epidemiology (Arch Surg. 2008;393:121–126)
- Adults: benign, nonfunctional adenomas > functional adrenocortical adenoma > adrenocortical carcinoma > pheochromocytoma > metastases > ganglioneuromas
- Children: neuroblastoma > pheochromocytoma and adrenocortical tumors
- If >3 cm: up to 20% functional
- If no cancer history: 2/3 benign
- 25% of masses increase by 1 cm in size on follow-up
- Chance of malignancy doubles (from 5–10%) for tumors larger than 4 cm

Etiology
- Adrenal cortical tumors: most common (30–50%)
  - Adenoma >>> nodular hyperplasia > carcinoma (10%)
- Adrenal medullary tumors: pheochromocytoma (10%)
- Other adrenal tumors: myelolipoma (1%)
- Metastases (10%)

Benign Characteristics
- <4 cm in size
- CT: <10 Hounsfield units, smooth borders, round/oval, sharp margins, conform to shape of adrenal gland, homogeneous, no calcifications, and high lipid content
- MRI: signal drop on chemical shift imaging with an intensity similar to that of the liver on T2-weighted image

Diagnostic Pathway and Treatment (Fig. 18-1)

Figure 18-1 Management algorithm for adrenal incidentalomas. (From Fischer JE, Bland KI. *Mastery of Surgery*, 6th ed. Philadelphia, PA: Lippincott Williams & Wilkins, 2012.)

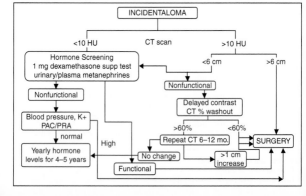

- FNA if
  - History of cancer and high attenuation >20 HU
  - Not surgical candidate and results will impact therapy
  - Must rule out pheochromocytoma before biopsy adrenal mass
- [^{11}C]metomidate (MTO)-PET: distinguish adrenocortical vs. noncortical adenomas

Surveillance
- First year: every 3 months
- Second year: every 6 months
- Three plus years: annual
- Mortality NOT related to adrenal mass but to other comorbid conditions

Cortical Neoplasms
Primary Hyperaldosteronism—"Conn Syndrome"
- Epidemiology
  - **Most common cause of secondary hypertension**
  - 5% of all hypertensive patients and 40% of hypertensive patients with hypokalemia
  - 2% of incidentalomas
  - 1–2 cm in size and rarely malignant
  - 50% patients will have a normal potassium
- Clinical presentation: Hypertension
  - Early onset
  - Difficult to control
  - Refractory to medical management
- Biochemical diagnosis: first
  - **High plasma aldosterone level**
  - **Low plasma renin activity:** inaccurate if taking spironolactone
  - Plasma aldosterone level/plasma renin activity >20–30; plasma aldosterone > 15–20 ng/dL
  - Confirm: 24-hour urine aldosterone level >12 ug after IV saline load
  - Urinary potassium excretion rate >30 mEq/24h
  - Captopril challenge: aldosterone and renin levels do not change
- Imaging: second
  - Thin cut CT/MRI
  - ^{131}I if localization studies equivocal
  - Adrenal vein sampling—for cortisol and aldosterone; rule out bilateral tumors/ hyperplasia; all patients over age 40–50
- Treatment
  - Aldosterone-producing adenoma (70%)
    - Surgical adrenalectomy
    - Blood pressure improves in 98%
    - Only 33% off all medications
  - Bilateral adrenal hyperplasia (25%)
    - Aldosterone-receptor antagonists (spironolactone)—90% effective
    - Na$^+$ and Ca^{2+} channel blockers
    - Glucocorticoid-remediable aldosteronism (<1%)—treat with steroids
- Prognosis: response to any antihypertensive predicts improved surgical outcome

Hypercortisolism—"Cushing's Syndrome"
- Epidemiology
  - 5–20% of incidentalomas are subclinical Cushing
  - Female >> male (9:1)
- Etiology
  - ACTH dependent: Cushing disease (70%)—pituitary tumor
  - Ectopic tumor (10%): lung, pancreas, thymoma, and bronchial carcinoid
  - **ACTH independent: cortisol-producing adenoma (10%)** of which 10% are bilateral adrenocortical carcinoma, adrenal hyperplasia
- Clinical presentation
  - "Classic" cushingoid habitus: truncal obesity, moon facies, hirsutism, abdominal striae, acne, buffalo hump, diabetes, and hypertension
- Imaging: CT/MRI
  - Should see contralateral gland atrophy
  - If >5 cm suspect carcinoma
  - Pituitary disease: MRI +/– inferior petrosal sinus sampling
  - Radioisotope scanning with NP-59

- Preoperative preparation
  - Subclinical hypercortisolism: perioperative glucocorticoids (wean over 1 month)
  - Cushing patients: steroids perioperative and for 6–18 months after
- Treatment

Laboratory Workup for Hypercortisolism/Cushing's Syndrome
• 24-h free cortisol level
• 1 mg dexamethasone suppression test
• Give dose at 11 pm, check cortisol level at 8 am
• Definite negative test = <1.8 mcg/dL (though most use <5 ug/dL)
• Positive test = >5 ug/dL
• **ACTH level**
• **Low or suppressed: adrenocortical disease → adrenal CT/MRI**
• **Elevated: pituitary/Cushing disease → pituitary MRI**
• **Very elevated: ectopic → torso CT/MRI +/– octreotide scan**
• **High-dose (8 mg) dexamethasone suppression test (over 24 h)**
• **Urinary free cortisol suppressed to <50%: pituitary disease**
• **Urinary free cortisol normal: adrenal adenoma and ectopic tumors**
• **CRH test: no change in ACTH in adrenal adenomas**

- Adrenal adenoma or carcinoma: unilateral adrenalectomy
- Pituitary (Cushing disease):
  - Medical therapy, transsphenoidal resection, and radiation
  - Bilateral adrenalectomy if the above fails
  - Metastatic disease or patient not a surgical candidate: mitotane
- Nelson syndrome
  - Complication of bilateral adrenalectomy (10%)
  - Elevated serum ACTH and MSH levels with hyperpigmentation
  - Progressively enlarging pituitary tumors, invasive; may develop into pituitary carcinomas (8–38%), increased if at an earlier age

Adrenocortical Carcinoma
- Epidemiology
  - Large, average 12 cm in diameter
  - 25% of tumors >6 cm
- Clinical presentation
  - Nonfunctional: abdominal or back pain, weight, malaise, and hematuria
  - Functional (60%): symptoms of Cushing syndrome, virilization, or both
- Imaging: MRI or CT
- Treatment
  - Surgical debulking including resection of kidney and continuous structures
- Prognosis: poor
  - 40% metastatic or advanced disease at presentation
  - Mean survival of 18 months and 16% 5-year survival

Metastases to Adrenal
- 75% of all incidentalomas in patients with history of malignancy
- Typical characteristics: bilateral, >3 cm
- Source: lung, breast, kidney, GI, melanoma, and lymphoma
- Imaging
  - PET/CT
  - CT-guided adrenal biopsy (only indicated to rule out metastatic disease to adrenal gland. Be certain that patient does not have a pheochromocytoma prior to biopsy adrenal mass)
  - Adrenal scintigraphy I-131 (NP-59): if >2 cm and has no uptake on PET
- Prognosis: some studies show 2- × 5-year survival for mets <4.5 cm vs. large lesions

Pheochromocytoma
Epidemiology
- Male = female

Rule of "10s"
• 10% malignant
• 10% bilateral
• 10% extra-adrenal
• 10% multiple
• 10% in children
• 10% hereditary

Clinical Presentation
- "Attacks" of: palpitations, sweating/flushing, anxiety, and headaches
- Precipitated by exercise, stress, and foods rich in tyramine
- Hypertension: uncontrolled, refractory, and young age of onset

Biochemical Screening
- **24-hour urine for VMA, metanephrine, and normetanephrine** (not on MAO inhibitor)
- Calcium and calcitonin levels (rule out MEN IIA)
- **Plasma metanephrines and normetanephrine**
- Chromogranin A
- Clonidine suppression test

Imaging
- CT abdomen/pelvis +/– mediastinum
- I-131 MIBG scan; PET/CT if negative
- Portosplenic vein sampling (if none or small bilateral lesions on imaging)
- **MRI: high signal on T2-weighted image**; no loss of signal on opposed phase T1
- Octreotide scan

Preoperative Management
- Start alpha-blocker 2 weeks prior to surgery
- Phenoxybenzamine 20 mg bid; increase by 20 mg/day until symptoms and blood pressure are controlled
- Then add beta-blocker as needed

Surgery: Special Considerations
- Aggressive excision of any recurrence or soft-tissue metastases
- Intraoperative hypertensive episodes
  - Marked catecholamine release from the tumor due to direct tumor manipulation or pneumoperitoneum
  - Have ready
  - **Neosynephrine**
  - **Lidocaine**
  - **Propranolol**
  - **Phentolamine**
- Bilateral: adrenal sparing surgery to preserve adrenocortical function if small

Postoperative Complications After Adrenalectomy
• Hypertension: tumor left behind, renal artery injury
• Hypotension: intravascular volume expansion due to preoperative α-blockade or shrunken blood volume no longer supported by vasoconstriction
• Hypoglycemia: loss of inhibition of insulin release after preoperative high levels of circulating catecholamines
• Bronchospasm: decreased β-2 activation after removal of pheochromocytoma
• Persistently elevated plasma catecholamines
• Wait 10–14 days after surgery before checking
• ^{123}I-MIBG if still high: MIBG uptake may have masked distant metastases preoperatively due to higher metabolic activity of primary tumor

Recurrence
- 5–10%
- Three-fold higher risk with a familial disease, R > L tumor
- 11-fold higher risk with extra-adrenal tumors

Surveillance
- First year: every 3 months tumor markers (urinary or serum metanephrines)
- Annual screening with imaging, tumor markers, calcium, PTH, and calcitonin

Malignancy
- Only reliable clinical criterion of malignancy is presence of distant metastases
- Metastases may appear years after removal of an apparently benign tumor
- Currently no certain way to predict which tumors will progress to malignancy
  - High 24-hour urinary dopamine levels and tumor dopamine concentration
  - High tumor weight
  - Post-operative persistent hypertension
- Prognostic factors
  - Large tumor size
  - Local tumor extension at the time of surgery

- DNA ploidy pattern–aneuploidy and tetraploidy more aggressive
- Absent or weak expression of inhibin/activin βB-subunit
- Molecular markers: human telomerase reverse transcriptase, heat shock protein 90, and secretogranin II-derived peptide

18-4: MEN SYNDROMES (J Clin Endo Metab. 2001; 86(12):5658–5671)

MEN I	MEN IIa	MEN IIb
Parathyroid (100%)	Parathyroid (25%)	Mucosal neuromas (90%)
Pancreas (35–75%)	Pheochromocytoma (50%)	Pheochromocytoma (50%)
Pituitary (15–55%)	Thyroid (medullary) (100%)	Thyroid (medullary) (100%)

MEN I "Wermer's Syndrome"

Genetics
- Familial MEN I definition:
  - At least one MEN I case + one first degree relative with one of the three main tumors
  - MEN I tumor + genetic mutation
- Autosomal dominant, near-complete penetrance, variable expressivity
- Inactivating mutations of protein *menin*
- Chromosome 11q13
- MEN I mutation in 20% of familial isolated hyperparathyroidism

Epidemiology
- Incidence 1/20,000 carry MEN I gene
- Peak incidence and first biochemical abnormalities in third decade
- **Most common presentation: PUD symptoms** with complications in fourth and fifth decades
- 2–4% of all patients with primary hyperparathyroidism have MEN I gene
- 35–45% of MEN I gene carriers died of MEN I-related causes of which >50% were malignant neuroendocrine tumors

Screening
- All family members of patients with gastrinoma or MEN I
  - Offer genetic testing for MEN I gene
  - If positive for a first-degree relative and genetic testing is not helpful: biochemical screening every 3 years
- All patients with pancreatic neuroendocrine tumors
  - Screen for hyperparathyroidism: Ca^{2+} and PTH levels
  - Screen for pituitary adenoma: prolactin level
  - Take family history for evidence of MEN I or VHL
- Sporadic case with two or more MEN I-related tumors: offer genetic testing

Screening for Known MEN I Carriers

• Annual biochemical tests
  • PTH and Ca: start at age 8
  • Prolactin +/– IGF-1: start at age 5
  • Gastrin, secretin-stimulation, gastric acid output: start at age 20
  • Fasting glucose and insulin: start at age 5
  • CgA, glucagons, and proinsulin: start at age 20
• Imaging: every 2–3 years
  • CT + somatostatin receptor scintigraphy (SRS): start at age 20
  • Brain MRI: start at age 5
  • Endoscopic ultrasound (EUS): if biochemical abnormalities but normal imaging

Treatment
- MEN I is a surgical disease

Order of Operations for MEN I
1. **Parathyroid** 2. **Pituitary** 3. **Pancreas**

Hyperparathyroidism: Treat First
- Epidemiology: most frequent and first manifestation of MEN I
  - 95% patients have gland over-activity by age 30
  - Earlier age of presentation, involvement of multiple glands, and a higher rate recurrence vs. sporadic cases (50% at 8–12 years post-op)
- Etiology: four-gland hyperplasia vs. multiple distinct adenomas
- Diagnosis: elevated calcium and PTH levels, sestamibi scan, and ultrasound
- Treatment: surgery
  Two choices of operation
- Four-gland parathyroidectomy with autotransplantation to forearm + transcervical bilateral thymectomy
- Subtotal parathyroidectomy + transcervical bilateral thymectomy
- Leave about 50 g in situ of the most normal gland with or without biopsy confirmation
- Most common first operation
- 50% recur after 10 years

Pancreatic–Duodenal Neuroendocrine Tumors
- Epidemiology: multifocal, malignant, and slow growing
- Pathophysiology: many are nonfunctional and produce pancreatic polypeptide
- Diagnosis: biochemical testing, CT/MRI, EUS, and octreotide scan
  - If persistent PUD in MEN I patient: workup for gastrinoma
- Treatment: **resect all functioning** enteropancreatic masses in an MEN I patient
  - Complete tumor resection while preserving as much normal pancreas as possible
  - Dissect the lymph nodes along the celiac trunk and hepatic ligament
  - Nonfunctioning tumors <2 cm can monitor
- Surgical options
  - Subtotal distal pancreatectomy + enucleation of tumors in head of pancreas/ duodenum
  - Whipple with enucleation distally
- Surveillance post-resection
  - First year: tumor markers, calcium, and CT scan every 3 months
  - Year one through three: biannual evaluation
  - Four plus years: annual evaluation

Gastrinoma
- Epidemiology: most common
  - 50% of MEN I patients
  - 25% of all gastrinoma patients have MEN I
  - 50% have metastases at diagnosis, 33% die from their tumor
- Location: **"gastrinoma triangle"**
  - **Junction second and third portion of duodenum ("sweep" of D3)**
  - **Junction head and neck of pancreas**
  - **Junction cystic duct and common bile duct**
- Clinical presentation: reflux, diarrhea, and abdominal pain
- Biochemical diagnosis
  - Elevated fasting serum gastrin: >130 suspicious, >1,000 with pH <2.5 diagnostic
  - High basal gastric acid output
  - Abnormal secretin stimulation test
- Imaging: tumor localization
  - CT scan +/– MRI
  - SRS
  - **Endoscopic ultrasound and intraoperative ultrasound**
- Systemic therapy for metastases: PPI, octreotide, streptozotocin, and 5-FU

Insulinoma
- Epidemiology: second most common, 30% of MEN I patients
- Biochemical diagnosis
  - **Fasting hypoglycemia <50 mg/dL**
  - Insulin : glucose ratio >0.3
  - C-terminal peptide (rule out exogenous use)
- Imaging: CT scan, EUS, +/– arteriogram, or MRI
- Surgical treatment: subtotal pancreatectomy with enucleation of head tumors
- Medical therapy: diet, diazoxide, and octreotide may help symptoms

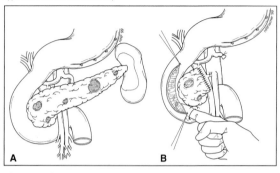

Operative Options for Resection of Gastrinoma (Fig. 18-2)

Figure 18-2 (From Fischer JE, Bland KI. *Mastery of Surgery*, 6th ed. Philadelphia, PA: Lippincott Williams & Wilkins, 2012.)

- Distal pancreatectomy
- Enucleation of any tumors in the head of the pancreas
- Duodenotomy and resection/enucleation of any duodenal tumors
- +/– lymph node dissection

Glucagonoma
- Epidemiology: 2% of tumors, mostly malignant
- **Diagnosis: elevated glucagon level, migrating rash**
- Imaging: CT + SRS, +/– EUS
- Pre-operative treatment: octreotide, anticoagulation, and IVC filter

Pituitary Adenomas
- Epidemiology
  - Most common functioning adenoma is prolactinoma > growth hormone
  - Larger and more aggressive vs. sporadic
  - First clinical manifestation of MEN I in up to 25% of sporadic cases
- Treatment: medical therapy (Bromocriptine) and trans-sphenoidal resection

Other MEN I Tumors
- Carcinoid: nonfunctional and aggressive
  - Foregut: most common
  - Thymus: male smoker
  - Lung: female
  - Stomach and duodenum
- Lipomas: 33% patients
- Cutaneous tumors: i.e., angiofibromas (40–80% patients)
- Adrenal cortical (20–40%): benign, nonfunctional, and bilateral hyperplasia
- Rarely adrenal pheochromocytoma
  - All unilateral, rarely malignant, hypertension from predominantly NE production

MEN II Syndromes
Genetics
- Autosomal dominant and incomplete penetrance
- Activating mutation of **RET** proto-oncogene
- Encodes a transmembrane tyrosine kinase receptor involved in the regulation of cell proliferation and apoptosis of the enteric nervous system progenitor cells, plus the survival and regeneration of sympathetic neural and kidney cells
- Chromosome 10q11.2
- MEN IIA: associated with Hirschsprung disease
- MEN IIB: 50% are spontaneous mutations

Epidemiology
- 1–7% of sporadic medullary thyroid carcinoma (MTC) patients have a *RET* mutation

Genetic Testing
- All patients with features of MEN IIB and no family history
- All patients with MTC
- All infants with Hirschsprung disease (*RET* exon 10 only)

Biochemical Testing
- Biannual levels: PTH, Ca^{2+}, epinephrine, and calcitonin
- Calcitonin: >80 ug/mL in women, >180 ug/mL in men after 3 days of omeprazole
- **Screen for pheochromocytoma**
  - **Before any surgical procedure**
  - All MEN II females before or early in pregnancy
  - Annual biochemical screen starting at an age that depends on familial pheochromocytoma pattern and codon mutation

Medullary Thyroid Cancer (100%)
- Epidemiology
  - Occurs 15 years younger in patients with MEN IIB vs. MEN IIA
  - More severe in MEN IIB; metastases found almost always at presentation
  - Almost always multifocal and bilateral
- Optimal age of thyroidectomy: based on the RET genotype (controversial)
  - High-risk mutations (codons 634 and 618) and all MEN IIB: 0–12 months of age
  - Intermediate-risk mutations (codons 790, 620, and 611): by 5 years of age
  - Low-risk mutations (codons 768 and 804): by 10 years of age
- **Surgical treatment: total thyroidectomy with central node dissection + lateral modified neck dissection if tumor palpable or >1 cm**
- Metastases: lymph nodes, lung, and liver
- Surveillance: pentagastrin-stimulated plasma calcitonin

Pheochromocytoma (50%)
- Epidemiology
  - Almost always within adrenal gland
  - 50% bilateral, asynchronous development
  - <5% malignant; if malignant is usually found in large tumor
  - 35% recurrence
- Clinical manifestation: early with palpitations, nervousness, anxiety, and headaches
- Diagnosis: urinary catecholamines and imaging with MIBG
- **Surgical treatment: treat first**
  - Unilateral adrenal tumor: laparoscopic adrenalectomy (40–60% recurrence)
  - Large bilateral adrenal tumors: bilateral laparoscopic adrenalectomy
  - Addisonian crisis in up to 35% with 3% mortality
  - Small bilateral tumors: unilateral laparoscopic adrenalectomy + contralateral cortical-sparing (subtotal) adrenalectomy
- Surveillance
  - First year: blood pressure and tumor markers every 3 months
  - Years 1–3: biannual
  - Four plus years: annual

Primary Hyperparathyroidism
- Surgical treatment
  - Hyperplasia: total parathyroidectomy and autotransplantation (implant 50 mg of the most normal parathyroid tissue in the nondominant forearm)
  - Single-gland disease (rare): single parathyroid gland excision after intraoperative biopsy of the other three glands. Mark all remaining parathyroid glands with a clip (because of high risk of persistence/recurrence)

HUZIFA HAJ-IBRAHIM • RANJNA SHARMA • MARY JANE HOULIHAN

Figure 19-1 Anatomy and surgical management of breast cancer

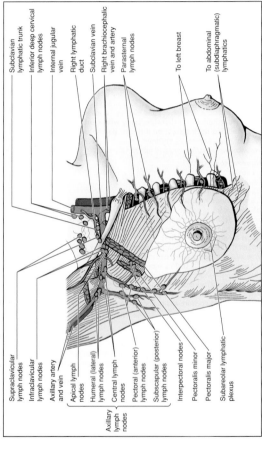

Subclavian lymphatic trunk
Inferior deep cervical lymph nodes
Internal jugular vein
Right lymphatic duct
Subclavian vein
Right brachiocephalic vein and artery
Parasternal lymph nodes
To left breast
To abdominal (subdiaphragmatic) lymphatics

Supraclavicular lymph nodes
Infraclavicular lymph nodes
Axillary artery and vein
Apical lymph nodes
Humeral (lateral) lymph nodes
Central lymph nodes
Pectoral (anterior) lymph nodes
Subscapular (posterior) lymph nodes

Axillary lymph nodes

Interpectoral nodes
Pectoralis minor
Pectoralis major
Subareolar lymphatic plexus

ANATOMY

Site

- Breast lies between the second and sixth ribs vertically, and between the sternal edge and the mid-axillary line horizontally also; projects into the axilla as the tail of Spence.
- Posteriorly, the upper portion of the breast rests on the fascia of the pectoralis major muscle
- Inferolaterally, it is bounded by the fascia of the serratus anterior muscle.

Structure of the Breast

- The breast is composed of skin, subcutaneous tissue, and breast tissue.
- The breast tissue includes epithelial parenchymal (10–15% of breast mass) and stroma
- Much of epithelial tissue found is in the upper outer quadrant which explains why it is the most common site of benign as well as malignant disease.
- Each breast consists of 15–20 lobes, each lobe has small structures called lobules, where milk is made.
- Ducts and lobules join together and form large ducts, connect together and ultimately becomes lactiferous duct (5–8) that exit the skin through tiny openings in the nipple called orifices.

VASCULAR SUPPLY

- Internal mammary artery/perforators accounts for 60% of blood supply of the breast.
- Lateral branches of the posterior intercostal arteries/veins
  - "Batsons plexus": network of veins which connect internal vertebral venous plexus with the deep pelvic veins and the thoracic veins. play a role of hematogenous dissemination of cancer
- Several branches of axillary artery: (highest) superior thoracic, lateral thoracic, and pectoral branches of the thoracoacromial artery; 30% of blood supply.
- Branches from the posterior intercostal arteries supply the remainder of the blood to the breast.
- Serratus anterior muscle: lateral thoracic artery/vein.
- Latissimus dorsi muscle: thoracodorsal artery/vein.

NERVE INNERVATION

- The fourth through sixth intercostal nerves (skin), long thoracic (serratus anterior), thoracodorsal (latissimus dorsi), and intercostobrachial nerves (skin of the upper half of the medial and posterior part of the arm)

LYMPHATICS

- Nodal station based on the relationship to the pectoralis minor muscle
  - Level I nodes: lateral to pectoralis minor
  - Level II nodes: deep to pectoralis minor
  - Level III nodes: medial to pectoralis minor
  - Interpectoral "Rotter nodes": between the pectoralis major and minor muscles
  - Internal mammary nodes: in retrosternal interspaces between the costal cartilages

Figure 19-2 Benign breast diseases

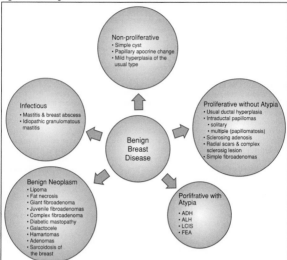

FIBROADENOMA

- Benign solid tumor.
- Most common solid breast mass in women between 15 and 35 years
- Clinical presentation: well circumscribed, painless, firm, mobile, and rubbery
- Pathology: normal ducts and lobules;
- Imagining: ultrasound for women under 30 years; ultrasound and mammogram for women >30 years old
- Management: imaging follow-up (ultrasound), tissue diagnosis with core needle or excisional biopsy
- Surgical excision if increasing size, pain, cosmetic deformity

FIBROCYSTIC CHANGES (PREVIOUSLY CALLED FIBROCYSTIC DISEASE)

- Unknown cause, influenced by hormonal function and fluctuation.
- More common in premenopausal age 35–50 than in postmenopausal women.
- Clinical presentation: painless or painful, solitary or multiple, large, small or cluster of small cysts.
- Classification: simple (no risk of malignancy), complicated (<1% risk) and complex (1–23% risk) cyst.
- Management: depends on classification, ranging from aspiration, core Bx, or excisional Bx

FAT NECROSIS

- Clinical presentation: firm, tender, ill-defined mass of superficial breast tissue, +/– skin/nipple retraction; history of trauma, breast surgery, or infection
- Treatment: **always rule out malignancy with imaging** +/– **CNB;** can observe only if clear history of trauma or prior surgery

Intraductal Papilloma *(Ann Surg. Oncol. 2013;20.6:1900–1905)*
- Papilloma is a benign lesion of papillary cells that grow from the wall of a cyst into the ductal lumen.
- Can be solitary or multiple lesions.
- Presentation: bloody nipple discharge or mass on imaging
- observation and interval imaging vs. perform wire-localized excisional biopsy to rule out adjacent carcinoma.

LIPOMA

- Present as soft, nontender, well-circumscribed masses.
- Diagnosis and treatment by excisional biopsy
- No increased risk of subsequent breast cancer

HAMARTOMA

- Present as discrete, encapsulated, painless masses
- Excision is recommended as coexisting malignancy can occur

GALACTOCELE

- Cystic collections of fluid, usually caused by an obstructed milk duct
- Present as soft cystic masses on physical examination
- Diagnosis is based on the clinical history and aspiration (Milky substance), drainage would increase the risk of formation Milk Fistula
- Excision is not necessary as there is no increased risk of subsequent breast cancer

RADIAL SCAR/COMPLEX SCLEROSING LESION

- Pathologic diagnosis, usually discovered incidentally when a breast mass or radiologic abnormality is removed or biopsied
- Microscopically: fibroelastic core with radiating ducts and lobules.
- Needs to be excised given risk for coexisting malignancy

MASTITIS AND ABSCESS

- Clinical presentation: painful, warmth, erythema, fever; 5% progress from mastitis to abscess
- Pathogen:
  - Nonlactating women: polymicrobial (Staphylococcus aureus, Bacteroides, Peptostreptococcus, and mixed flora); associated with ductal ectasia
  - Lactating women: Staphylococcus aureus, Staphylococcus epidermidis, Streptococcus, Diphtheroid, and MRSA.

Management of Breast Abscess

- **Broad-spectrum antibiotics plus NSAIDS**
- **OK to continue breast feeding**
- **Ultrasound-guided aspiration of abscess if fluctuant and does not improve with antibiotics**
- **Incision and drainage if fail aspiration**
- **Must role out inflammatory carcinoma if symptoms persist: dedicated breast imaging, core biopsy**

MONDOR DISEASE

- Definition: thrombophlebitis of the lateral thoracic vein and its branches
- Clinical Presentation: pain with palpable cord; history of surgery or trauma
- Treatment: often resolves spontaneously in 4–6 weeks. NSAIDS, warm compresses; if older than 35, get a mammogram

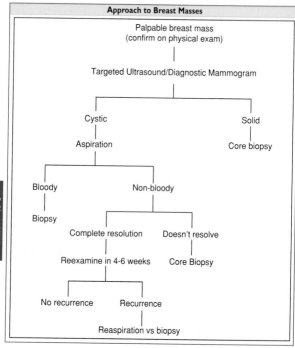

Approach to Breast Masses

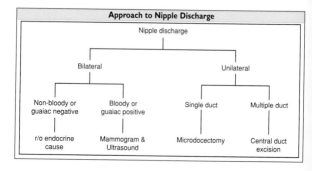

Approach to Nipple Discharge

19-3: BREAST ATYPIAS

Atypical Hyperplasia (AH)

1. Atypical ductal hyperplasia (ADH):
   - Usually found as target lesion on biopsy of mammographic microcalcifications.
   - Shares some features of ductal carcinoma in situ (DCIS)
   - Increase risk of breast CA
   - Majority diagnosed with core needle biopsy
   - Management: Wire localized excisional biopsy

2. Atypical lobular hyperplasia (ALH):
   - Characterized by proliferation of monomorphic, evenly spaced, dishesive cells filling part but not all of the involved lobules
   - Shares some features of lobular carcinoma in situ (LCIS)
   - Majority diagnosed with core needle biopsy
   - Management: Wire localized excisional biopsy vs imaging/clinical follow up
3. Flat epithelial atypia (FEA):
   - Mostly diagnosed with biopsy performed for microcalcification.
   - The risk of up grade to a concurrent malignancy ranges from 5–15%.
   - Managed by wire localized excisional biopsy.

Lobular Carcinoma in Situ (LCIS)
Epidemiology
- Most common in premenopausal women: 0.5–8.0% of all breast biopsies
- Bilateral in 50–90% of cases
- Twofold higher for developing invasive lobular than invasive ductal CA
- Ipsilateral breast has higher risk of developing CA than contralateral

Diagnosis
- No clinical or mammographic findings routinely associated with lobular carcinoma in situ.
- Incidental finding in breast biopsies preformed for other pathology.

Treatment
- Wire localized excisional biopsy
  - Close surveillance: clinical breast examination; mammography +/- alternating with MRI (younger women) on every 6-month schedule
  - Chemoprophylaxis: tamoxifen and raloxifene
    STAR trial: shown to reduce the risk of developing invasive carcinoma by 50% in women with lobular carcinoma in situ and other high-risk lesions

Gali Model (Risk Calculator)
- NSABP-P1 trial: (13,388 women at high risk of BC;826 had LCIS. A 7-year follow-up showed that the annual rate of development of invasive BC in the placebo group was 1.17% and was twice that of tamoxifen group 0.63%
- Candidate for chemoprophylaxis if Gail score >1.7% at 5 years (JAMA. 2001;286(18):2251–2256)
- Factors: race, age, first menarche, first-degree relative, number of previous biopesies, history of atypical hyperplasia, and age of first birth
- Bilateral mastectomy: considered for those with strong family history and other high-risk factors
- Genetic counseling and testing may be helpful decision making

19-4: MALIGNANT BREAST NEOPLASMS

Ductal Carcinoma in Situ (DCIS)
Epidemiology
- 14–44% of all new mammographically detected neoplasms
- Left untreated, DCIS will progress to invasive carcinoma in up to 75% of cases
- Pathology: clonal proliferation of malignant mammary ductal epithelial cells that do not cross the basement membrane

Clinical Presentation
- Mammographic abnormality (microcalcification) on screening mammogram
- Only 1–2% palpable on physical examination

Treatment

Principles of Breast Conservation Surgery (BCS)
• Mammographic needle localization of the lesion (if not palpable)
• Curvilinear incision placed along one of Langer lines of skin tension
• Need 2-mm margin
• Hemoclips applied along edges of biopsy cavity to mark it for boost of radiation therapy
• Orient the specimen for pathology (marking and/or inking)
• Consider postexcision mammogram to assure that all microcalcifications associated with the DCIS have been removed prior to initiating radiation therapy if calcifications were extensive

Contraindication to Breast Conservation	
Absolute	**Relative**
Extensive or multicentric disease	Local recurrence after partial mastectomy
Prior breast radiation	Larger lesion or small breasts (poor cosmesis)
Connective tissue disorder precluding use of radiation therapy	Close margins that cannot be re-excised
First or second trimester of pregnancy	

- Objective: prevent local recurrence and progression to invasive disease
- Surgical options
  - Breast-conserving therapy (BCT): partial mastectomy (lumpectomy) + radiation therapy (RT)
  - Total (simple) mastectomy (with or without immediate breast reconstruction)
- Adjuvant radiation therapy:
  - Utilized to decrease risk of local recurrence after BCS
  - Consider Van Nuys scoring system
    - Predicts local recurrence in DCIS without adjuvant radiation
    - Based upon size, margins, and histology

Endocrine Therapy
- Tamoxifen: all premenopausal woman
- Tamoxifen or aromatase inhibitor if postmenopausal woman

Surveillance
- Diagnostic mammogram to establish a new baseline
- Clinical breast examination and bilateral mammography semiannual, then yearly

INVASIVE BREAST CANCER

Epidemiology
- Second most common cause of cancer death in women.
- Genetic aberrations account for <10% of all breast cancers

Risk Factors for Breast Cancer
Demographics
100 times more frequently in women than in men
Risk increases with age
Ethnicity: white > Black > Asian American/Pacific Islands > Hispanic/Latina > American Indian/Alaska natives
Prior history of breast cancer
• 1% per year risk in contralateral breast for premenopausal
• 0.5% per year risk in contralateral breast for postmenopausal
• Lifetime risk 10–20% historically
Lifestyle: alcohol consumption, tobacco use, and high-fat diet
Reproductive (duration of hormone exposure)
• Early menarche (<12 y of age)
• Late menopause (>55 y)
• Oral contraceptives
• Nulliparity or age >30 at first pregnancy
• Exogenous hormones use
Family History
• Positive family history reported by 15–20% of women
• >Two first-degree relatives, higher if relatives are premenopausal
Genetic Risk
• BRCA1 or 2 (mutation with impaired DNA repair)
• Ataxia-telangiectasia
• Li-Fraumeni (p53 tumor suppressor mutation)
• Cowden syndrome (PTEN mutation)

Pathology
- Infiltrating ductal carcinoma: most common (85%)
  - Mammography: cluster of pleomorphic microcalcifications, speculated mass, or architectural distortion
  - Ultrasound: solid mass, may have echogenic foci (calcifications)
  - Includes medullary, mucinous, papillary, tubular, and colloid carcinoma

- Invasive lobular carcinoma (13%)
  - Vague, ill-defined distortion due to infiltrating pattern
  - less commonly well-defined on mammogram

Clinical Presentation
- Mammographic abnormality
- Palpable mass: firm, dense, irregular +/– tethering or fixation to overlying skin or underlying muscle
- nipple retraction
- Less common: nipple discharge
- axillary lymphadenopathy if locally advanced

Screening
- Average risk patient: begin at age 40–45 with annual breast examination and mammogram
- High-risk patient: begin screening 10 years before age of diagnosis in youngest first-degree relative
- BRCA1 and 2: monthly self-examination, biannual physician examination, alternate yearly mammogram and MRI at 6 month intervals, and yearly pelvic ultrasound after age 30

Genetics
- BRCA1: chromosome 17
  - Associated with ovarian (20–40%), endometrial, prostate, and colon cancer; more aggressive
- BRCA2: chromosome 13
  - Associated with male breast cancer (6%), ovarian (only 10–20%), prostate, colon, melanoma, stomach, pancreas, and biliary cancers
- Li Fraumeni syndrome: chromosome 17, mutation in p53 tumor suppressor gene
  - Associated with leukemia, osteosarcoma, brain, and adrenal cancers

Indications for BRCA Gene Testing: (NCCN Guideline Version 2.2016)
- Non-Ashkenazi Jewish women
  - Two first-degree relatives with breast cancer, one diagnosed age of 50 or younger
  - Combination of three or more first or second- degree relatives with breast cancers; regardless of age at diagnosis
  - Combination of both breast and ovarian cancer among first- and second-degree relatives at any age.
  - First-degree relative with bilateral breast cancer
  - Combination of two or more first- or second-degree relatives with ovarian cancer, regardless of age at diagnosis
  - History of breast cancer in male relative
- Women of Ashkenazi Jewish descent
- Diagnosed <60 y with a triple negative breast cancer.

SURGICAL MANAGEMENT
- Preoperative work-up: bilateral mammogram (if not already done), core biopsy

Staging (TNM Staging System)
- Primary tumor
  - T is: Carcinoma in situ (Intraductal, lobular, or Paget disease with no tumor)
  - T1: ≤2 cm
  - T2: ≥2 cm but ≤5 cm
  - T3: ≥5 cm
  - T4: any size with direct extension to chest wall or skin
- Regional lymph nodes
  - N0: no regional lymph node metastases
  - N1 clinical: moveable ipsilateral lymph nodes
  - N1 pathologic: 1–3 axillary lymph nodes and internal mammary lymph + microscopic disease detected by sentinel lymph node only
  - N2 clinical: ipsilateral axillary nodes fixed or matted, or clinically + ipsilateral internal mammary nodes without clinically + axillary nodes
  - N2 pathologic: 4–9 axillary lymph nodes, or clinically + internal mammary nodes without axillary lymph node metastases
  - N3 clinical: ipsilateral internal mammary lymph
  - N3 pathologic: ≥10 axillary nodes, or in supraclavicular nodes

- Distant metastases
  - M0: no metastases
  - M1: Distant metastases s
- Stage grouping
  - Stage I: T1 N0 M0
  - Stage IIA: T0–2 N1 M0
  - Stage IIB: T2 N1 M0; T3 N1/2 M0
  - Stage IIIA: T0–2 N2 M0; T3 N1/2 M0
  - Stage IIIB: T4 any N M0; any T N3 M0
  - Stage IV: any T any N M1

- Stages I and II
  - Breast conservation: partial mastectomy + radiation +
    - SLNB for clinically negative axilla
    - Axillary node dissection (ALND): positive SLNB or clinically positive axilla
    - If SLNB is positve, can perfor ALBD or give RT (axillary tangents).
- Mastectomy with SLNB and/or (ALND)
- **NCI Consensus Conference 1991: breast conservation should be considered the preferred local surgical therapy in early-stage breast cancer (see "Contraindications to Breast Conservation")**
- Stages IIIa and IIIb
  - Step 1: neoadjuvant chemotherapy; decreases locoregional cancer burden and tumor size
  - Step 2: breast conserving surgery with SLNBx/ALND or modified radical mastectomy (MRM)
  - Step 3: adjuvant chemotherapy (if NeoAdj ChemoTx not given) and radiation therapy if BCT

Adjuvant Systemic Therapy
- Goal: reduce risk of subsequent systemic disease
- Benefits majority with early-stage breast cancer, most if node-positive disease
- **Three factors determine need and type of therapy:**
  - Her 2-neu status, ER/PR receptor status, and axillary lymph node status
- Oncotype DX: 21 gene assay
  - Node negative, ER +
  - Determine 10-year risk of recurrence and potential benefit of chemo and/or endocrine tx

Treatment	
Recommendations for Adjuvant Therapy	
Patient Group	**Recommended Treatment**
Node Negative, Low Risk	
Tumor <1 cm	No treatment or endocrine therapy if ER+
Special histologic types 1–2 cm, grade 1, ER+	
Node Negative, Higher Risk	
ER+	Endocrine therapy OR chemotherapy + endocrine therapy
ER–	Chemotherapy
Any HER2+	Add trastuzumab to chemotherapy
Node Positive	
ER+	
Premenopausal	Chemotherapy + endocrine therapy
Postmenopausal	Chemotherapy + endocrine therapy OR endocrine therapy alone
ER–	Chemotherapy
Any HER2+	Add trastuzumab to chemotherapy

ER+, estrogen receptor positive; ER–, estrogen receptor negative.

©2009–2014. The Surgical Council on Resident Education Inc. All rights reserved.

Radiation (N Eng J Med. 2010;362(6):513–520)
- Primary role: adjuvant setting with breast conserving surgery
- Traditional regimen: 50–66 gy in divided doses to breast and axilla if >4 lymph nodes

- Other regimens: partial (shortened course), intraoperative breast irradiation
- **Indications for postmastectomy radiation**
  - Locally advanced: >5cm, tumor extending into skin or underlying muscle
  - Aggressive biology: high-grade, extensive lymphatic vessel invasion
  - Young women
  - Positive nodes or one node >2 cm
  - Extracapsular nodal involvement
  - Positive margins
  - Inflammatory cancer

Complications of Breast Surgery + Radiation Therapy	
Lymphedema	Breast edema
Erythema	Increased risk of contralateral breast cancer
Pneumonitis	Recurrent breast cellulitis
Rib fractures	Sarcoma

Management of Locoregional Recurrence
- Risk of a postmastectomy locoregional recurrence is slightly lower than that after breast-conserving therapy
- Need to restage patient with CT scan and bone scan
- Pervious mastectomy: either in residual breast tissue or dermal lymphatics (metastatic)
  - Surgical re-resection and reconstruction as needed
  - Chemotherapy and/or hormonal therapy if indicated
  - Radiation therapy if the chest wall not previously radiated
- Previous breast conservation surgery RT and adjuvant drug Rx
  - Mastectomy +/− reconstruction
  - Chemotherapy and/or hormonal therapy
- Recurrent disease involving the axillary lymph nodes
  - ALND
  - Adjuvant chemotherapy and/or hormonal therapy
  - Axillary radiation therapy if no prior RT to the axillary nodes

Prognosis
- 5-year survival based on nodal status
  - Stage I, 80%
  - Stage II, 60%
  - Stage III, 20%
- Metastases: bone, lung, and liver most common
  - Radiation: bone metastases, local recurrence (chest wall)
  - Surgical resection: isolated, single liver/lung metastases, if primary tumor controlled
  - If ER/PR+: tamoxifen, aromatase inhibitors, androgens, or LHRH
  - Chemotherapy should be strongly considered, doxorubicin or taxol based

Prognostic Factors in Cancer
- Nodal involvement
- Tumor size
- Tumor grade
- ER/PR status
- Her 2 neu status
- Presence of other tumor markers

INFLAMMATORY BREAST CANCER

Epidemiology
- 1–4% of all breast carcinoma
- 17–36% present with distant metastases
- 3-year survival, 40–70%

Clinical Presentation
- Peau d'orange of the skin
- Diffuse induration, erythema, and warmth
- Diffuse firmness with ill-defined mass
- Often present with axillary lymphadenopathy

Diagnosis
- Punch or incisional biopsy of reddened area including an area of normal skin (so you can also get receptor status): shows dermal lymphatic invasion
- Mammogram and US, with core bx

- Consider MRI
- Metastatic work-up: CXR, CT head/neck/ab/pelvis, bone scan +/– PET

Treatment
- Induction chemotherapy: three cycles of cytoxan/adriamycin followed by a taxane (alternative: taxane/Cytoxan); add Herceptin if HER 2-neu positive
- Re-evaluation of the breast: if good response, MRM. If no response, chest wall radiation and then MRM
- Postmastectomy RT
- Antiestrogen therapy: either tamoxifen or an aromatase inhibitor if ER positive

Breast Cancer During Pregnancy (Facts Views Vis ObGyn. 2009I; 1.2:130)
Management of breast cancer during pregnancy should be defined in multidisciplinary setting depends on which trimester patient is in when diagnosis is made:
- If first trimester: mastectomy with nodal evaluation (SNLBx with radioactive tracer/axillary dissection)
- Second trimester: neoadjuvant chemotherapy therapy with breast conservation vs. mastectomy with nodal evaluation
- Third trimester: breast conservation vs. mastectomy with nodal evaluation, radiation therapy after delivery
- No XRT
- No chemotx in first trimester
- Can give adriamycin/cytoxan after first trimester
- Can give XRT after patient delivers

DAVID C. TOMICH • NICHOLAS E. TAWA, JR

20-1: MELANOMA

Background
Epidemiology
- The fifth most common cancer in men, the sixth most common in women in the United States
- The second most important cause of cancer death in young women (age 20–40)
- Most die if disease metastatic without systemic therapy ("years of life lost")

Risk Factors
- Ultraviolet light exposure (blistering sunburns in childhood, 75% increase in melanoma incidence if tanning booth use before age 35)
- Predisposing phenotype (Caucasian, blue–green eyes, blond-red hair)
- Atypical or dysplastic nevi, dysplastic nevus syndrome (>100 atypical nevi)
- Family history of melanoma (10% of patients)
- Genetic syndromes: Li-Fraumeni (p53 gene), familial retinoblastoma (Rb gene), Lynch, xeroderma, BRCA2
- Melanoma-specific mutations: CDKN2A, PTEN, BRAF (70% of cutaneous, not mucosal), MITF (red heads), NRAS

Pathogenesis
Melanocytes arise in embryonic neural crest
- Diffusely distributed in adult tissue
- Accounts for unusual primary sites of origin (eye, vagina, GI tract, anus)

Progression to melanoma
- Benign nevus: a cluster of normal melanocytes
- Dysplastic nevus: premalignant lesion with dysplastic cells
  - Driven by oncogenic mutations
- Melanoma: in situ (epidermis only, Clark I, no potential for spread) or invasive

Growth phase concepts of Wallace Clark (no longer used in staging)
- Radial growth phase: cells spread laterally
- Vertical growth phase: cells grow primarily vertically
  - Superficial spreading melanoma: both radial and vertical
  - Nodular melanoma: all vertical, small surface profile, deeply invasive
- Clark Level I: epidermis only—all cells above basement membrane
- Level II: invasion into the papillary dermis
- Level III: invasion to the junction of the papillary and reticular dermis
- Level IV: invasion into the reticular dermis
- Level V: invades subcutaneous fat ("subcutis")

Metastasis
Lymphatic: "local-regional" or Stage III disease.
- Increases risk for progression to stage IV by 20–80%)
- May be to dermal lymphatics ("in transit" or "satellite" metastasis) or to a regional lymph node, or both.

Hematogenous: stage IV disease, fatal in 95% without systemic therapy

Diagnosis and Staging of Melanoma
Clinical Presentation: ABCDE
A—asymmetry
B—border irregularity
C—color variability
D—diameter greater than 6 mm
E—evolution (change in any variable over time)
- Exceptions: 50% of melanomas arise de novo (no nevus), 50% arise in nonsun-exposed areas, some melanomas are "amelanotic" (no pigment)

Histologic Classification
Note: The histologic subtype of melanoma is less important for predicting outcome than the patient's formal staging (see following page)

Histologic Classification of Melanoma		
Melanoma in Situ • Confined to epidermis • No metastatic potential • May be geographically pervasive **Superficial Spreading Melanoma (70%)** • Any site or age • Radial and vertical growth • ABCDE criteria fit well	**Nodular Melanoma (15–20%)** • Any site or age • All vertical growth • Often de novo, no pre-existent nevus • Late diagnosis with ulceration, growth rapid • May not follow ABCDE criteria	**Lentigo Maligna (5–7%)** • Elderly patients • Flat, slow-growing lesion which is black or brown • Terminology confusing, most are melanoma in situ • Limited metastatic potential as at worst superficially invasive
Desmoplastic Melanoma 1% of all melanomas • Often amelanotic • Perineural invasion common • Increased rate of local recurrence • Postoperative XRT may be helpful	**Acral/Lentiginous Melanoma** • Most common form of melanoma in non-Caucasians • Anatomic locations: fingers (subungual), palms (palmar), and soles (plantar) • Often neglected (e.g.. subungual melanoma mistaken for trauma)	**Primary Mucosal Melanoma** • 5% of all melanomas. BRAF wild-type, not responsive to kinase inhibitors • Locations: vulva, anus, oral cavity, and nasopharynx • Often neglected (e.g., anal melanoma confused for hemorrhoid)

Biopsy of the Primary Lesion
- Shave: most common method for dermatologists, rarely underestimates depth
- Punch: use instrument 3–10 mm wide, gives full-thickness depth, may be subject to sampling error
- Excisional: for larger, more complex lesions where depth uncertain.
  - Large incision may theoretically alter pattern of lymphatic drainage, make sentinel node less accurate.
  - Orient incision along the axis of the extremity to facilitate future wide local excision and wound closure
- If subungual, remove, for example, the proximal nail to allow punch biopsy

Biopsy of a Suspected Metastasis
- Intransit or satellite lesion: punch biopsy
- Subcutaneous mass, bulky node, deep occult metastasis on imaging
  - Fine needle aspiration: cytology very sensitive for melanoma
  - Core needle biopsy
  - Excisional biopsy
- Unexplained anemia: endoscopic biopsy

Important Concepts for Melanoma Staging and Prognosis
- Tumor thickness, ulceration, mitotic rate, and sentinel node status most important
- In-transit or satellite metastases carry the same negative prognostic significance as two positive nodes.
- The size and number of nodal metastases are predictive.

TNM Staging of Melanoma

T—largely determined by tumor thickness ("Breslow depth")
• Tis: in situ disease
• T1: ≤1.0 mm
• T2: 1.01–2.0 mm
• T3: 2.01–4.0 mm
• T4: > 4.0 mm
  • For all T: "a" = without ulceration, "b" = with ulceration
  • For T1 lesions only: if visible mitoses, also "b"
 	
N—nodes
• N0: no lymph node metastases
• N1: one positive
• N2: two to three positive
• N2c: any intransit or satellite metastasis, normal nodes
• N3: four or more positive nodes, matted nodes, or any positive node with an in-transit or satellite metastasis
• "a" micrometastases, "b" macrometastases

M—metastases
- M0: no metastases
- M1a: distant skin, subcutaneous, or lymph node metastases, normal LDH
- M1b: lung metastases, normal LDH
- M1c: All other visceral metastases, normal LDH. Or, any metastasis with an elevated LDH.

Stage Groupings

Stage Groupings of Melanoma	
Stage 0	TisN0
Stage I	IA: T1aN0
	IB: T1bN0
Stage II	IIA: T2b/T3a N0
	IIB: T3b/T4a N0
	IIC: T4b N0
Stage III	IIIA: T1–4a N1–2a M0
	IIIB: T1-T4a or b N1–2b or T1-T4a/bN2c M0
	IIIC: T1–4bN1–2b or T1–4a/bN3 M0
Stage IV	M1a: mets to distant skin, subcutaneous layer, distant LN; LDH normal
	M1b: lung mets; LDH normal
	M1c: mets to vital organs other than the lungs, LDH normal; or any distant mets + elevated LDH

Survival by Stage in Absence of Systemic Therapy
- I: >90–100%
- IIA: 80%, IIB: 60–70%, IIC: 50–60%
- IIIA: 80%, IIIB: 50%, IIIC: 15–20%
- IV: 5% (spontaneous remission)

Initial Staging Workup
Imaging
- Reserved for stage III or high-risk stage II (e.g., IIC)
- FDG-PET-CT most sensitive but misses lesions less than 5 mm in size
- If not PET, then Torso CT
- Head MRI
- Role of serial imaging for surveillance in stage III or IV is unclear

Laboratory Studies
- No specific marker for melanoma
- LDH: rises with necrotic tumor burden, worse prognosis if elevated in stage IV
- CBC: anemia may indicate occult GI primary or metastasis
- If suspected metastasis is found, image guided or office fine needle aspiration cytology or core biopsy usually sufficient

Treatment
Management of the Primary Lesion
- Local control of melanoma requires wide excision down to the deep fascia with a margin of normal skin

Surgical margins for excision (retrospective, some limited prospective data)
- Melanoma in situ: 0.5-cm margin
- T1 invasive: <1 mm thick—1-cm margin
- T2: 1–2 mm thick—1–2 cm margin
  - 1 cm acceptable in anatomically restricted areas (neck, face, distal extremities)
- T3 or 4: >2 mm thick—2-cm margin or greater
- Anal melanoma: local excision; APR almost never indicated due to high rate of metastatic disease
- Digits, toes: avoid amputation as long as the required soft tissue margin is obtained (skin graft, local flaps)
- Major extremity amputation only in extreme palliative circumstance
- Skin grafts preferred to complex flaps if difficult wound closure
  - Easier margin identification if re-excision required

Sentinel Lymph Node Biopsy
Nodal status is an important prognostic factor for progression to stage IV and survival

Indications
- Anticipate at least 5% will be positive as a threshold to offer the procedure
  - Any primary melanomas thicker than 1.0 mm (all T2 and above)
  - Less than 1.0 mm thick but visible mitoses or ulcerated (T1b)

- Early T1b lesions (<0.7 mm, rare mitoses only) may show less than 5% positivity and a selective approach may be allowable (elderly, anticipated diffuse drainage pattern)
- No palpable nodes or clinically or radiographically apparent metastases should be present

Technique
- Pre-op lymphoscintigraphy: inject radio-labeled colloid around the primary tumor
- Intra-operative gamma probe to find node, vital dyes used only rarely in present era
- Mapping most important for tumors with ambiguous drainage pattern (e.g., trunk)
- An "interval node," e.g., a node found between the primary and the nodal basin is as important as a basin node for biopsy

"Completion" or Regional Lymph Node Dissection for Melanoma
If sentinel node is negative: no further surgery

Little Prospective Data for Outcomes Following Major Lymphadenectomy
- Over 90% with a positive sentinel node will have no additional positive nodes
- Multicenter Selective Lymphadenectomy Trial I (John Morton):
  - Removal of a positive sentinel node by itself may confer a survival advantage

Completion Lymphadenectomy
- Recent data (MSLT-II and European studies) show no survival benefit for completion lymphadenectomy following a + SN biopsy
- Best means for local-regional control of residual disease
- Serial ultrasound examination of the nodal basin following a + SN biopsy to monitor for recurrence a new paradigm
- Remains best means to control bulky metastasis

Pelvic Nodal Metastasis (external iliac chain)
- If a positive Cloquet's node (femoral canal in thigh), 50% will eventually show disease in the pelvis.
- Usually perform pelvic lymphadenectomy only if metastatic disease found on imaging.
- Pelvic disease often heralds higher level of future lymphatic involvement or progression to true stage IV.
  - New immune therapies may be an alternative to surgery.

In-Transit Disease
Definition: dermal lymphatic metastases located between the primary tumor site and the draining regional lymph node basin (N2c disease).

Treatment Options
- Excision: preferred, until frequency unreasonable
- Systemic therapy alone: as adjuvant (stage III) or if not "surgically manageable," as for stage IV
- Isolated limb perfusion: 50–80% response rate, usually not durable. Newer immune therapies now often preferred
- Radiotherapy: no data, brachytherapy may be useful

Local Recurrence (At Site of Primary Excision)
- Risk factors: high T-stage, satellite metastases in initial wide excision specimen, inadequate initial margins
- Poor prognosis as often heralds onset of additional metastatic events
- Treatment: re-excision, possible radiation. Re-staging imaging studies should be performed

Management of Stage III and IV Patients
Surgical Resection
- Best outcomes in M1a patients (oligometastatic, nonvisceral metastases)
- May prolong disease-free interval, unlikely to influence overall survival
- Usually palliative (GI bleeding or obstruction, brain met, bulky nodal recurrence)

Radiation Therapy
- Prospective data only for CNS metastases
- "Cyberknife" highly targeted XRT best for isolated metastases (e.g., brain)
- Often given postoperatively for bulky nodal disease or for extracapsular lymph node extension, but only retrospective data to support
- Can markedly worsen post-operative extremity lymphedema

Chemotherapy
- For stage IV patients with no other treatment options
- Dacarbazine: alkylating agent that disrupts DNA; response rates 10%

- Temozolomide: improved penetration across blood–brain barrier
- Thalidomide: anti-angiogenic agent

Tyrosine Kinase Inhibitors
- For stage IV patients with fulminant disease or who have failed immunotherapy
- Usually acquire resistance within months
- Vemurafenib: inhibits only "mutated" BRAF, present in 70% of truncal melanomas
- Trametinib: inhibits MEK kinase, in combination with BRAF inhibitors up to 75% response rate
- Sorafenib and other agents: Broad spectrum inhibitor of MAP kinase and others. Anti-angiogenic, inhibits vascular endothelial and platelet-derived growth factor receptors

Immunotherapy
Vaccines: currently no melanoma vaccine has shown efficacy but genetically engineered patient-specific lymphocyte approaches are encouraging (Steven Rosenberg)
Interferon: for adjuvant therapy of stage III disease
- 20% improvement in disease-free interval, no clear survival benefit
- Remains most common therapy for stage III
- Biology of response complex, some patients will benefit
Interleukin-2: limited role for stage IV
- 20–50% response rate, only 5% durable, high toxicity
- Immune checkpoint inhibitors and TK inhibitors superior
Immune checkpoint inhibitors: remove immune-suppressive effects of tumor.
- Most important development in overall cancer care in decades.
- Up to 70% response rates, many durable (e.g., potentially curative).
- Major toxicities are autoimmune events (colitis, arthritis, uveitis, etc.)
Ipilimumab: anti-CTLA-4 monoclonal antibody; increases T-cell activation.
- For adjuvant treatment of stage III or for stage IV.
Pembrolizumab, Nivolumab: monoclonal antibodies block tumor-induced apoptosis of effector T-cells ("anti-PD1" antibodies)
- For stage IV, in clinical trials for stage III

20-2: OTHER SKIN TUMORS

Squamous Cell Carcinoma
Risk Factors
- Risk of developing squamous cell carcinoma (SCC) is a function of number of lesions and duration
- Exposure to ultraviolet radiation, light skin, outdoor occupation
- Ionizing radiation exposure
- Human papillomavirus ("verrucous" SCCs)
- Arsenic or other toxic chemical exposure
- Immunosuppression: HIV, concurrent CLL, immunosuppressive Rx for arthritis, organ transplant
- Chronic inflammation (infection, injury, burns)
  - "Marjolin ulcer," long 10–30 year lead time
- Prior treatment with psoralens and UVB light (PUVA) for psoriasis

Benign Precursor Lesions
- Actinic keratosis: most common precursor of SCC, scaly pink macules
- Bowenoid papulosis: associated with HPV 16 and 18; hyperpigmented papules
- Epidermodysplasia verruciformis: widespread flat warts, usually genital
- Keratoacanthoma: volcano-like lesion with central keratin—extruding papule, may rapidly progress to SCC

Carcinoma in Situ
- Bowen's disease: can appear in nonsun-exposed areas or mucosa; sharply demarcated and erythematous, usually in elderly and slowly progressive
- Erythroplasia of Queyrat: on glans penis of uncircumcised men or vulva, smooth erythematous plaques, may be HPV-related

Invasive SCC
- Most common in head and neck, secondarily trunk and extremities
- Clinical presentation: papules or plaques, smooth or scaly, variable color, often pruritic, may bleed if ulcerated
- Verrucous carcinoma (HPV-associated subtype)

TNM Staging of SCC

T—largely based on diameter
- Tis: in situ disease ("SCCIS"), tumor confined to the epidermis
- T1: tumor ≤2 cm diameter, less than 2 "high-risk factors"
- T2: tumor greater than 2 cm
  - Or T1 with 2 or more high risk features (>2 mm thick, Clark level IV or V, perineural invasion, poor differentiation, ear or lip)
- T3: invasion into facial bones
- T4: invasion into axial or appendicular skeleton or skull base

N
- N0: no lymph node metastases
- N1: single node <3 cm
- N2: single node >3 cm or in multiple nodes or contralateral basin node
- N3: node >6 cm

M
- M0: no metastases
- M1: distant metastases present

Stage 0: TisN0
Stage I: T1N0
Stage II: T2N0
Stage III: T3N0 or T1 to 3N1
Stage IV: any T any N M1 or T1 to 3 N2 M0 or any T N3 M0 or T4 any N M0

S&ST 20-6

Management of the Primary Lesion
No mandatory margin for excision, any microscopically negative sufficient

Mohs micrographic surgery
- Usually for anatomically restricted areas (face, neck, smaller lesions)
- Excised with real-time frozen section analysis by specially trained dermatologist

Surgical excision:
- For larger lesions (trunk, extremities)
- Use measured margin for reporting, 0.5–1 cm usually adequate

Cryosurgery: most appropriate for in situ SCC

Electrodessication and curettage: most appropriate for in situ SCC

Topical chemotherapy (5-fluorouracil): for superficial lesions or poor surgical risk

Imiquimod: most appropriate for in situ SCC
- Topical modulator of innate immune response (activates toll-like receptor 7)

Photodynamic therapy: for SCC in situ
- Photosensitizing compounds activated by UV light, cause cell damage via reactive oxygen

Topical retinoids

Radiotherapy: to reduce local recurrence when perineural invasion is found; may be primary therapy in high risk patient

Role of Lymphatic Surgery
- Sentinel node biopsy
  - No data concerning outcomes or survival benefit
  - Usually perform for any T2 or above (10% positive) or high risk T1
- Complete node dissection: for clinically evident disease or following + SN biopsy
  - Local–regional control the primary rationale, no proven survival benefit

Prognosis
- Excellent for early disease with negative nodes (T1 and most T2): cure rates >90%
- Poor if metastatic disease
  - Regional lymph node involvement only (stage III): 20% survival at 10 years
  - Distant metastases (stage IV): <10% survival at 10 years

Basal Cell Carcinoma

Epidemiology
- Causation: driven by Hedgehog signaling pathway
  - Mutations in SMO or PTCH1 genes
    - Such mutations underlie "nevoid basal cell carcinoma syndrome"
- Vismodegib: inhibitor of SMO receptor
  - Some efficacy in familial BCC syndromes
  - Used for locally advanced or metastatic disease, efficacy unproven
- Location and risk factors
  - As described for SCC earlier
- Natural history: usually slow growing; if left untreated can deeply invade surrounding structures; hematogenous or lymphatic metastasis rare but can occur (<0.5%)

Classification
- Nodular: "pearly" nodule, telangiectasias, some ulcerated
- Superficial: erythematous, scaly, flat macules
- Morpheaform/infiltrative: may be white or yellowish; indurated but flat and infiltrative
- Mixed histopathology most common
- "Eccrine de-differentiation": BCC acquires appearance of secretory glands

Staging: same as for cutaneous SCC

Treatment: approach to local control similar to cutaneous SCC

Lymphatic Surgery: no data, sentinel node biopsy may be appropriate for lesions with eccrine dedifferentiation

Merkel Cell Carcinoma

Epidemiology
- Rare neuroendocrine tumor that originates in dermis
  - Unclear if tumor arises from sensory (light touch) mechanoreceptor "Merkel" cell
  - Causative role for Merkel cell polyomavirus (MCPyV) controversial
  - Classically CK20 + (low–molecular-weight keratin)
- Must rule out metastatic lesion to skin
  - Small-cell lung cancer (will be TTF1 +)
  - Ewing's sarcoma
  - Abdominal neuroendocrine primary tumor
- Risk factors: UV exposure, immunocompromised state
- Location: head and neck 40%, extremities 40%, trunk 15%
- Aggressive lesion: high rate of local and distant recurrence

Diagnosis
- Workup analogous to melanoma
  - Tissue biopsy
  - Sentinel node biopsy for all patients with primary lesion
  - FDG-PET-CT scanning very sensitive for staging

Treatment

Wide Local Excision and SN Biopsy
- No agreed minimal margin, 1–2 cm preferred
- Postoperative RT

Completion Lymph Node Dissection
- For + SN or clinically evident disease
- Best rationale at present is local control of disease

Radiation Therapy
- Postoperative radiotherapy to the primary site of excision, even when negative margin, is standard and reduces local recurrence
- Irradiate nodal basin following lymphadenectomy for metastasis

Systemic Therapy
- For stage IV hematogenous metastatic disease, unclear role for node + alone
  - Conventional chemotherapy: platinum-based, as for small-cell lung cancer
  - Newer immunotherapies (anti-PD1) and kinase inhibitors show promise

Adnexal Skin Tumors

- Neoplasms arising in structures imbedded in normal skin (sweat glands, apocrine glands)
- Histology shows epithelial differentiation (a carcinoma), cytokeratin positive
- Large variety of lesions with overlapping terminology
  - Eccrine carcinoma, digital papillary carcinoma, hidradenoma, poroma/porocarcinoma, etc.
- Must rule out adenocarcinoma hematogenously metastatic to skin
  - Breast (ER+), prostate (PSA+), GI tract (CEA+)
  - Possible imaging workup to rule out occult primary or additional metastases
- Predicting benign or malignant behavior may be difficult, metastasis rare
- Treatment: excision to negative margin
  - Role of sentinel node biopsy unclear but usually perform for malignant lesions

Extra-Mammary Paget's Disease

- Most common in elderly, groin/scrotum/vulva most common sites, indolent in most
- A low grade, usually in situ adenocarcinoma of skin, often weeping and superficially ulcerated. Must rule out metastatic lesion.
- May be geographically pervasive and difficult to control surgically
- Treatment: aggressive wide excision or topical imiquimod, and/or local radiotherapy

Lymphadenopathy
- Nodes may appear outside of established basins and mimic other masses
- FNA cytology often sufficient to assess for metastatic lesions
- Lymphoma suspected: excisional bx preferred, or multiple core needles
  - Send fresh: flow cytometry, immunohistochemistry, DNA analysis
  - Microbiology for TB, Bartonella

Epidermal Inclusion Cysts/Pilar Cysts of Scalp
- Origin unclear, inverted skin growth at hair follicle?
- Have self-perpetuating capsule, rarely contains squamous carcinoma
  - If prior history of rupture/abscess/I&D, excise widely with normal fat

Pilonidal Sinuses/Cysts
- Multiple causes plausible: "field defect or embryonal" vs. inverted hair growth
- Treatment
  - Antibiotics (quinolone +/− anaerobic coverage) and soaks
  - Surgical excision
    - Primary closure has high rate of abscess formation but can heal quickly
    - Marsupialization more reliable but can give chronic nonhealing wound
    - Recurrence common

20-3: SOFT TISSUE SARCOMA

Background

Clinical presentation: usually painless mass; may be large and occult if intraperitoneal

Pathology
- Heterogeneous group of mesenchymal tumors arising from embryonic mesoderm
- Immunohistochemistry and genetic analysis of the tumor (chromosomal rearrangements, fusion proteins) often critical for classification
- Nomenclature reflects tissue of origin, often benign and malignant variants (lipoma/liposarcoma)

  Most important prognostic factors for survival: degree of differentiation (grade) and achieving negative histologic margin (R0) at surgery

Risk Factors for Occurrence
- Prior ionizing radiation therapy (e.g., for breast CA, lymphoma, sarcoma)
  - 8–50 × increased incidence
  - Latency period long (>10 years)
  - Often rapidly progressive
- Viral infection
  - Epstein–Barr virus: perhaps in some leiomyosarcomas
  - Human herpes virus 8: spontaneous Kaposi sarcoma
- Chronic lymphedema: lymphangiosarcoma (Stewart–Treves syndrome)
- Chemical exposure (vinyl chloride, arsenic): hepatic angiosarcoma

Genetic Associations
- Neurofibromatosis (NF): neurofibrosarcoma (NF type 1), meningioma (NF type 2), malignant peripheral nerve sheath tumor (malignant Schwannoma (NF 1 and 2))
- Gardner syndrome in familial polyposis coli: desmoid tumors, retinoblastoma, soft tissue sarcoma
- Li–Fraumeni syndrome (p53 mutations): breast cancer and soft tissue sarcoma

Subtypes of Sarcoma		

Pleomorphic undifferentiated sarcoma (formerly termed malignant fibrous histiocytoma, 40%)
 • Trunk and extremities
 • All are high grade
 • Metastatic potential high (lung)
	Liposarcoma (25%)
	 • Often MDM and CDK amplified on FISH
	 • Five subtypes
	   • Well-differentiated
	   • Myxoid
	   • Round cell
	   • Dedifferentiated
	   • Pleomorphic
		Leiomyosarcoma
		 • From smooth muscle, e.g., vascular elements within unrelated tissue
		 • Typical locations
		   • Uterus: may have distinct genetic profile
		   • Abdominal viscera
		   • Urologic structures
		   • Extremities (e.g., intramuscular)
		 • May have associated venous tumor thrombi

Synovial cell sarcoma
- Two recognized types: monophasic (epithelial and fibroid) and biphasic
- Common chromosomal translocation diagnostic
- Typical locations
  - Acral
  - Ligaments
  - Near joints, tendons
- Metastatic potential high (lung)
- Lymphatic metastasis in up to 10%

Alveolar soft part sarcoma
- Found in fascial planes
- Slow growing
- Metastases may appear late (20–40 y)
- Metastasis to brain and diffuse sites

Malignant peripheral nerve sheath tumor
- Benign variant = Schwannoma
- Most common in NF type-1
- PET scanning may help differentiate benign from malignant lesion if multiple tumors present
- R0 resection may involve sacrifice of critical nerves, vessels

Typical locations
- Retroperitoneum
  - Diffuse distribution, achieving R0 margin difficult, may require en bloc resection (kidney, colon)
  - Extremities
- Metastasis: predicted by grade, usually to lung. Myxoid and round cell more diffuse pattern.
- "Atypical lipoma"
  - Well-differentiated, superficial location
  - R0 margin not justified if morbid procedure, low rate of recurrence

Rhabdomyosarcoma
- Common pediatric tumor, also arises in adults
- Five subtypes
  - Embryonal: 60–70%
  - Alveolar: 31%
  - Botryoid
  - Pleomorphic
  - Anaplastic
- Painless mass, may arise in association with rib
- Diffuse site of origin: head/neck, chest, pelvis, extremities
- Lymphatic metastasis in up to 10%
- Chemo-sensitive tumor, role for neoadjuvant therapy

Angiosarcoma (rare lesion)
- Risk factors: chronic lymphedema, prior irradiation (e.g., after mastectomy)
- Surgical margin clearance difficult
- High-rate local recurrence
- Wide variety of additional vascular tumors, variable metastatic potential

- Metastatic potential (lung) predicted by grade
- Cutaneous variant no longer considered a true sarcoma

Kaposi's sarcoma
- Elderly people of Mediterranean descent (genetic basis?)
- Spontaneous cases HHV-8 virus associated
- Common malignancy in poorly controlled HIV
- Pink–brown–black patches/nodules
- Oral mucosa, skin, GI tract (may cause GI bleed), extremities
- Wide range of indolent vs. aggressive disease
- Excise or primary XRT to site

Epithelioid sarcoma
- Location: extremities
- Lymphatic metastasis in up to 10%
- Metastasis predicted by grade

Solitary fibrous tumor
- Arise in pleura, abdominal cavity (pelvis)
- Slow growing, metastatic potential unclear

Staging of Sarcoma

T
- T0: No evidence of tumor
- T1: ≤5 cm. T1a, superficial to fascia; T1b, deep to the superficial fascia
- T2: >5 cm. T2a, superficial; T2b, deep

N
- N0: no lymph node metastases
- N1: regional lymph nodes involved

M
- M0: no distant metastases
- M1: distant metastases present

G (Histologic Grade)
- GX: indeterminate grade
- G1: well-differentiated
- G2: moderately differentiated
- G3: poorly or undifferentiated

S&ST 20-10

Stages

- Stage I: T1–2a or b N0M0 G1
- Stage II: T1–2a or b, N0M0 G2
- Stage III: T1–2a or b, N0M0 G3
- Stage IV: any T N1M0 or any T N0M1, any G

Note: The TMN staging system for sarcoma is not well predictive, and tumor grade is the most important variable.

Management of Soft Tissue Sarcoma

Biopsy: A Critical Initial Event

- Prefer image guided technique to avoid sampling error (tumors often heterogeneous)
- Results allow subclassification, indications for preoperative XRT
- Meticulous technique: if hemorrhage occurs, may up-stage patient (violates fascial planes)
- Core needle biopsy most common
  - Excision of needle tract ideally at time of definitive surgery, need not well defined
- If extremity lesion and "open" surgical biopsy
  - Orient incision longitudinally ("axial") along the extremity
  - Gives the greatest latitude for subsequent definitive resection

Imaging in Sarcoma

Magnetic Resonance Imaging

- Modality of choice for any soft tissue lesion
- Shows internal heterogeneity of tumor (striations, focal nodularity, contrast enhancement)
- Helps decide benign vs. malignant (e.g., lipomatous neoplasms)
- Helps determine site for needle biopsy

CT Scanning

- Of lung and at times torso, for initial staging and subsequent metastatic surveillance
- Useful to determine anatomic relationships for retroperitoneal sarcomas

FDG–PET–CT Scanning

- Uncommon modality, expensive, limited by not all sarcomas having predictable affinity for glucose

Ultrasound

- Generally not useful for diagnosis
- May help determine blood flow for benign AVMs, use for guiding biopsy needle

Treatment of Sarcoma

Surgery: most important modality (see below)

External Beam Radiotherapy: A mainstay in modern sarcoma management

- Improves local tumor control when combined with surgery
- "Sterilization" of tumor periphery allows closer margins and sparing of vital structures
- Most commonly performed prior to surgery
  - Presence of tumor allows better targeting
  - Preoperative RT will increase wound complication rate
  - No difference in survival pre- vs. postoperatively
- Decision to pursue is dependent on tumor grade, location, and histology

Brachytherapy

- Limited role (Kaposi's, palliation for extremity lesions)

Chemotherapy (anthracycline based)

- Neoadjuvant: prior to surgery
  - Limited applicability for sarcoma: rhabdomyosarcoma and Ewing's most common
  - In combination with preoperative chemotherapy may allow closer margin of resection in critical locations (e.g., to spare sciatic nerve)
- Adjuvant: stages I–III: no benefit for disease-free or overall survival
- Systemic (stage IV): poor efficacy

Isolated Limb Perfusion Chemotherapy
- May use as neoadjuvant prior to definitive resection, role unclear
- Palliation for patients who would otherwise require amputation

Extremity or Truncal Sarcoma
- Wide excision
  - Ideally to a 1–2 cm margin
  - Any microscopically negative margin, esp. when combined with preoperative RT
  - Close but negative (mm) margin gives higher rate of local recurrence, similar survival
- Mark site (clips, fiducials) if XRT to be performed later
- Can resect arteries and reconstruct with vein or conduit
- Consider amputation when resection cannot be achieved or poor-predicted functional outcome

Retroperitoneal Sarcoma
- Often poorer prognosis than extremity lesions
  - Reflects delayed presentation, large size, higher incidence of positive margins after resection
  - Higher rates of local recurrence following surgery (80% in the first 2 years)
- En bloc resection frequent (tumor, colon, kidney, etc.)
- Surgery often not longlasting or technically unfeasible for recurrent disease
- Liposarcoma by far most common lesion

Sentinel Node Biopsy in Sarcoma
- May pursue for synovial, epithelioid, rhabdo (up to 10% incidence)
- Role of lymphatic surgery unclear as node positive disease often lethal

Resection of Metastases
- Will almost always be palliative vs. curative
- Surgery common for lung metastasis, repeated VATS procedures acceptable

Surveillance and Prognosis for Sarcoma
- Overall 5-year survival rate: localized disease 90%, metastatic disease: <15%
- No clear guidelines for frequency of postoperative surveillance
  - Usually every 6-month imaging, e.g., MRI to wound bed and chest CT for 5 years, then annually
  - Every 3–6 month exam for the first 5 years, then annually

20-4: Skin and Soft Tissue Infections

Cellulitis
- Bacterial infection of skin which spares deep fascia
- Most commonly Group A streptococci and *S. aureus* unless immunocompromised
  - Human bite requires coverage for anaerobic peptostreptococci

Uncomplicated Cellulitis
- Superficial, skin only, resolves rapidly
- Gram + coverage, IV or PO (nafcillin, penicillin, kefzole, dicloxacillin, quinolones, bactrim)

Complicated Cellulitis
- May involve subcutaneous fat, more edema, slower to clear
- Lymphangitis may occur: infection of subdermal lymphatics
  - Tender erythematous "streaks"
- Often recurrent
  - Risk factors: prior lymphadenectomy, radiation therapy
- Treatment: Prolonged antibiotics, elevation
  - Broad coverage for resistance, as for necrotizing infection (below)

Variants of Cellulitis
- Impetigo: epidermal infection
  - Blisters/bullae
  - Beta-hemolytic streptococci usually
- Erysipelas: dermal layer infection
  - Raised, erythematous, and painful lesion
  - Streptococcal species, especially *Streptococcus pyogenes*
  - Treatment: penicillin
- Folliculitis: superficial hair follicle infection; *Staphylococcus aureus*
- Hidradenitis: infection of apocrine glands

Severe Soft Tissue Infections

Necrotizing Fasciitis
- Infection of deep fascia, rarely muscle, may spread rapidly via fascial planes
- Life threatening: early diagnosis and intervention key
- Clinical presentation
  - Symptoms: pain, fever, elevated WBC
  - Signs: ecchymotic necrosis, blisters, crepitus
  - Differentiating from complicated cellulitis often difficult
- May require open tissue/fascial biopsy for diagnosis

Microbiology
- Type I: polymicrobial
  - At least one anerobe (*Bacteroides, Clostridium, Peptostreptococcus*)
  - With mixed aerobes (*Escherichia coli, Klebsiella, Proteus*, gram-positive cocci)
- Type II: monomicrobic, usually group A Streptococcus
  - *S. aureus/MRSA* also common
  - *Vibrio vulnificus* in seawater

Role of Diagnostic Imaging: CT vs. MRI
- Most specific indicator of necrotizing fasciitis is the presence of air
- CT more sensitive than MRI and is usually sufficient
- Edema in fascial planes and soft tissues often nonspecific
- MRI more sensitive than CT for edema
- False positive/ "over-read" may lead to excessively aggressive treatment

Treatment of Necrotizing Infection
- Broad-spectrum antibiotics (e.g.,vancomycin + zosyn +clindamycin + ciprofloxacin initially)
- Aggressive and early surgical debridement (often needs to be repeated)
- Hyperbaric oxygen
- Intravenous immune globulin

Diabetic Foot Infection
- Causes: trauma; nonhealing ulcer, ischemia
- Physical examination and plain film/ MRI for osteomyelitis/ assess perfusion
- Pathogens often mixed, use broad-spectrum therapy, debridement

Other Soft Tissue Lesions

Meleney's "Synergistic Gangrene" or Ulcer
- Indolent necrotizing wound infection suggested to occur following operation
- Caused by synergistic interaction of microaerophilic streptococci and *S. aureus*

Fournier's Gangrene
- Necrotizing infection of the male perineum
- May begin as small area of discoloration on scrotum and rapidly progress to full-thickness necrosis
- Treatment: emergent wide excision, marsupialization of testicle, delayed skin graft

Pyoderma Gangrenosum
- Necrotizing soft tissue process often confused for infection
- Etiology unclear: autoimmune, reaction to injury
- Usually recurs and expands geographically after surgical excision
- Preferred treatment: assess for inciting cause, topical or systemic steroids

21-1: RENAL TRANSPLANTATION

Goals of Renal Transplantation (Arch Intern Med. 2004;164:1373–1388)
- Transplant decreases mortality and has an improved quality of life
- Transplantation is more cost effective than dialysis

Indications
- End-stage renal disease or chronic kidney disease with expectation of need for dialysis in the near future (**pre-emptive transplantation**) in patients who can tolerate the operation and demonstrate appropriate psychosocial support
- Most common etiologies: hypertension and diabetic nephropathy

Patient Evaluation
- Referral to transplant center when glomerular filtration rate (GFR) is less than 20–25 mL/min
- Age-appropriate routine health care and cancer screening: mammography, Pap smear, colonoscopy, prostate-specific antigen
- Assessment for peripheral vascular disease, coronary artery disease, cancer, chronic infections, hypercoaguable state, urologic dysfunction
- Psychosocial evaluation to assess family support, substance abuse/sobriety, financial support/stability, likelihood of compliance with posttransplant medications and care

Organ Allocation (www.optn.transplant.hrsa.org)
- System updated in 2014 to prioritize using organs with the longest predicted survival in the youngest/healthiest recipients, to increase the likelihood of highly sensitized patients to be transplanted, and to facilitate placement of the lowest quality organs
- Top 20% of kidneys preferentially allocated to the healthiest/youngest 20% of recipient pool with considerations for highly sensitized recipients, prior organ donors, zero-antigen mismatch for HLA between donor and recipient
- Separate consent for bottom 15% of kidneys with expedited placement of these organs to minimize cold ischemic time
- Donor organ score (Kidney Donor Risk Index) reflects age, height, weight, race, history of hypertension or diabetes, cause of death, serum creatinine, hepatitis C status, donor after cardiac death status
- Recipient score (Estimated Posttransplant Survival score) reflects candidate age, time on dialysis, current diagnosis of diabetes, prior transplant
- Live donor considerations
  - No history of renal disease nor significant family history of diabetes or hypertension
  - GFR >80 mL/min, 24-hour protein <150 mg
  - Risk of perioperative death 3/10,000 (JAMA. 2010;303:959)
  - Risk of long-term renal failure higher than evaluated/approved donors who did not donate but still much lower than the general population (Kidney Int. 2014;86:162)

Outcomes (OPTN & SRTR Annual Data Report 2012. www.srtr.transplant.hrsa.gov)
- Deceased donor kidneys graft survival: 1-year: 97%, 5-year: 74%; half-life: 10 years
- Living donor kidney graft survival: 1-year: 97%; 5-year: 83%; half-life: 14 years
- Complications
- Early posttransplant complications (first 6 months)
  - Vascular thrombosis, bleeding
  - Ureteral stricture or leak
  - **Delayed graft function** (need for dialysis in the first week after transplant): 5% for living donor grafts; 22% for deceased donor grafts
  - Acute rejection: 10% at 1 year
  - Medication effects, toxicity of immunosuppression
  - Infection (wound, urinary, blood, viral, fungal)
  - Early recurrence of primary disease
  - **Primary nonfunction of graft** (recipient remains on dialysis at 3-months posttransplant): ~1%
- Late posttransplant complications (beyond 6 months)
  - Chronic allograft nephropathy
  - Noncompliance/rejection
  - Recurrent and de novo renal disease

- Related to immunosuppression: infection, CMV, BK nephropathy, malignancy (non-melanoma skin cancers, posttransplant lymphoproliferative disease, cervical cancer)

Early Graft Dysfunction	
Evaluation of Early Graft Dysfunction	**Differential Diagnosis**
• H&P, review of meds • CBC, chemistries, immunosuppression levels • Urinalysis • Renal US (vessels, urinary obstruction, perinephric collection) • Consider CT, MRI/MRA, nephrouretero-gram, biopsy	• Delayed graft function • Acute rejection • Dehydration • Medication effect (calcineurin toxicity) • Vascular thrombosis • Urinary tract infection • Ureteral stricture or leak • Urinary retention/obstruction • Lymphocele, hematoma

21-2: PANCREAS TRANSPLANTATION

Goals of Pancreas Transplantation
- Restore autonomous control of blood glucose
- Prevent ongoing complications of diabetes (hypoglycemic unawareness, cardiac and vascular disease, gastroparesis, retinopathy, nephropathy)

Indications
- Type 1 diabetes mellitus with uremia (**simultaneous pancreas–kidney, SPK**)
- Type 1 diabetes mellitus without uremia but with significant complications
  - **Pancreas transplant alone** (PTA) most commonly for severe hypoglycemic unawareness
    - Must balance risk of surgery and immunosuppression against ongoing risk of diabetic complications
  - **Pancreas after kidney** (PAK) most commonly for patients who have already received a living donor kidney
- Type 2 diabetes mellitus with uremia, BMI <28 for SPK only
- Secondary diabetes (i.e., after traumatic or surgical loss of native pancreas)

Patient Evaluation
- As for kidney transplant with special emphasis on cardiac, cerebrovascular and peripheral vascular disease given increased burden of disease in the diabetic population
- Outcomes (OPTN & SRTR Annual Data Report 2012. www.srtr.transplant.hrsa.gov)
- Best pancreas outcomes for SPK possibly due to improved detection of early rejection in evaluation of increased creatinine and relative ease of kidney biopsy compared to pancreas biopsy
- Complications of diabetes may stabilize but not necessarily improve; risk of cardiac and vascular complications may decrease at long-term follow-up

Graft Survival Rates		
Type of Pancreas Transplant	**1-Year Graft Survival**	**5-Year Graft Survival**
SPK	85%	73%
PAK	83%	65%
PTA	75%	53%

Complications
- Pancreas graft thrombosis: ~10% at 1 month, thought to be due to venous thrombosis
- Leak: 5–21% for bladder-drained grafts; 4–9% for enteric-drained grafts
  - Leak from enteric-drained graft may be successfully repaired but may require graft removal
- Bleeding: 15–30% due to increased use of systemic anticoagulation due to increased risk of graft thrombosis
- Pancreatitis: may be due to ischemia/reperfusion injury, peripancreatic collection or infection, urinary reflux in bladder-drained grafts
  - Treat with supportive case, drainage of collections, antibiotics
- Nonspecific symptoms: prolonged hospitalization or re-admission for fever, nausea, vomiting very common, and may reflect pancreatitis or underlying gastroparesis
  - Treat with NGT decompression, antiemetics, prokinetics, IV fluids
- Evaluation for complications includes: H&P, CBC, chemistries, amylase, lipase, immunosuppressive levels, urinalysis, US/CT/MRI, biopsy

21-3: LIVER TRANSPLANTATION

Goals of Liver Transplantation
- Improved survival for patients with complications of end-stage liver disease or acute liver failure

Indications
- Chronic liver disease with evidence of decompensation
  - Most common etiologies: hepatitis C, hepatitis B, alcoholic cirrhosis, nonalcoholic steatohepatitis (NASH), cholestatic diseases (PBC, PSC), autoimmune hepatitis, metabolic disorders, Budd–Chiari syndrome; biliary atresia and metabolic disorders in pediatric patients
  - Decompensation in the form of hepatic encephalopathy, GI bleeding from varices, intractable ascites/spontaneous bacterial peritonitis, edema, jaundice, development of early yet unresectable hepatocellular carcinoma (HCC)
- Acute liver failure with concern for imminent death (<7 days) without transplantation
  - Development of acute liver failure: presence of **hepatic encephalopathy** within 8 weeks of onset of jaundice in absence of underlying liver disease
  - Most common etiologies: acetaminophen toxicity, cryptogenic, idiosyncratic drug reactions, mushroom poisoning, acute fatty liver disease of pregnancy, Budd–Chiari syndrome, HSV, HBV, EBV, acute autoimmune hepatitis, acute Wilson's disease
  - High risk of cerebral edema and herniation with need for intensive monitoring and treatment to prevent cerebral herniation prior to transplant

Patient Evaluation
- Age-appropriate routine health care and cancer screening: mammography, Pap smear, colonoscopy, prostate-specific antigen
- Assessment for uncorrectable cardiac or pulmonary disease, extrahepatic cancer, chronic or uncontrolled infections, hypercoagulable states
  - Echocardiogram to assess cardiac function and pulmonary artery pressure
    - Mean pulmonary artery pressure >45 mm Hg excludes candidate
  - CT or MRI imaging to assess for presence, extent of hepatocellular carcinoma
  - **Milan criteria** define extent of HCC that will still receive exception points
    (N Eng J Med. 1996;334:693)
    - Single tumor less than 5 cm in diameter
    - Up to three tumors, each less than 3 cm in diameter
    - No extrahepatic spread or vascular invasion
- Psychosocial evaluation to assess family support, substance abuse/sobriety, financial support/stability, likelihood of compliance with posttransplant medications and care
  - Most centers require a period of 3–6 months of documented sobriety from substances prior to listing a candidate with a history of alcohol or other substance abuse
- Assessment for technical/anatomic barriers including extensive portal vein/SMV thrombosis
- Specific considerations for various etiologies of liver disease

Specific Considerations for Various Etiologies of Liver Disease	
Etiology	**Considerations**
Hepatitis C	• Debate over treatment with direct acting antivirals before or after transplant (i.e., if treat after transplant, can use HCV-positive donor and be transplanted sooner)
Hepatitis B	• Require peritransplant treatment with HBIg and life-long treatment with antivirals to prevent reinfection
PSC	• Increased risk of cholangiocarcinoma (CCa) • Selected hilar CCa can be treated with transplant as part of the **Mayo protocol** (pretransplant radiation, chemo) *(Liver Transpl. 2000;6:309)*

Acute Liver Failure	• Considered **fulminant liver failure** if progress from insult to encephalopathy within 1 week
	• **King's College Criteria** may predict poor outcome without transplant *(Gastroenterology. 1989;97:439)*
	  • For acetaminophen overdose: arterial pH <7.3 after resuscitation or PT >100, Cr >3.3, and grade III encephalopathy
	  • For other etiologies: PT >100 or 3 of the following: age <10 or >40, jaundice to encephalopathy >7 days, bilirubin >300 mmol/L, PT >50, or due to drug effect, non-A/non-B, or halothane-induced hepatitis

Non-alcoholic steatohepatitis (NASH)	• Rapidly increasing indication for liver transplantation in the United States • Need to consider recipient weight/BMI • Increased likelihood of other metabolic complications (DM, CAD, CVA, PVD)
Alcoholic Cirrhosis (Laennec's)	• Often in combination with HCV or HBV or NASH • Various requirements for period of sobriety and need for relapse-prevention counseling prior to listing for transplant

Organ Allocation (www.optn.transplant.hrsa.gov)

- Priority on the liver transplant waiting list is determined using the MELD-Na score
  - Formula using bilirubin, INR, creatinine, and sodium with scores ranging from 6–40
  - MELD exceptions–extra points for specified disease processes in an attempt to model added mortality (HCC, hepatopulmonary syndrome, portopulmonary hypertension, primary hyperoxaluria, cystic fibrosis, cholangiocarcinoma)
  - MELD-Na score can be used to estimate likelihood of 3-month survival
- Status 1 priority for recipient candidates with predicted mortality within 1 week
  - Acute liver failure, primary nonfunction of a transplanted liver, hepatic artery thrombosis within 1 week of transplant, acute Wilson's disease
  - Status 1 candidates go to the "top" of the list, above MELD-Na scored candidates
- Live donor considerations
  - Living donors can donate left lateral section (usually to a pediatric recipient), right or left lobe (usually to an adult)
  - Anatomic issues (hepatic arteries, portal veins, bile ducts) and graft size are paramount for donor safety and suitability of graft for transplant
  - Not all recipients are suitable for living donor grafts due to need for full graft or anatomic considerations in the recipient (i.e., portal vein thrombosis)
  - Risk of morbidity for the donor 40% (bile duct issues, bleeding, liver failure/need for transplant, infections, renal failure, re-operation); donor mortality ~1/200–400 donations (Am J Transplant. 2012;12:1208)

Outcomes (OPTN & SRTR 2012 Annual Data Report. www.srtr.transplant.hrsa.gov)

- Deceased donor 1-year survival: 85%; 5-year survival: 70%
- Living donor 1-year survival: 85%; 5-year survival: 72%
- Complications
  - Bleeding (transfusion, return to OR); infection (wound, blood, urine, deep space, viral), acute kidney injury, prolonged ventilatory support, cardiac complications
- Hepatic arterial thrombosis (HAT, 5–10%)
  - Attempt thrombectomy in OR/IR
  - Recipient will likely require re-transplant if HAT occurs in the first 2 weeks due to biliary necrosis, acute liver failure
  - Consider arterial stenosis/thrombosis if bile leak develops
- Portal vein stenosis/thrombosis (PVT, 1%)
  - Attempt thrombectomy in OR/IR vs. observation
  - If untreated, recipient may develop sequelae of portal hypertension
  - Increased in recipients with pretransplant PVT, use of split or living donor grafts, portal venous conduits
- Biliary leak or stenosis (10–20%, increased in split or living donor grafts, donors after cardiac death)
  - Suspect stenosis if rising alkaline phosphatase and bilirubin
  - Suspect leak if bilious drain output, new subhepatic collection
  - ERCP or T-tube studies to diagnose and treat with balloon dilation (stenosis) or stent (leak or stenosis); if large leak, consider Roux-en-Y hepaticojejunostomy
- Rejection (15–20% in first year)
  - Most commonly acute cellular rejection which may be treated with increased baseline immunosuppression, steroid bolus, antibodies (i.e., antithymocyte globulin)
  - Increasing understanding that acute or chronic humoral rejection may play a role in long-term graft failure
- Recurrence of disease
  - Prior concern for recurrent infection with HCV leading to recurrent cirrhosis, graft failure and need for re-transplantation
    - Rapidly progressive **fibrosing cholestatic hepatitis** could lead to cirrhosis within a year of transplant
    - New direct-acting antivirals result in high likelihood of cure of HCV
  - Relapse with alcohol or recurrence of autoimmune hepatitis can lead to recurrent cirrhosis

Immunology

- HLA (human leukocyte antigens) and blood group antigens are important in transplantation
  - ABO-compatible transplants are preferred for all organs
  - Protocols for ABO-incompatible transplants exist but with increased risk of complications due to increased immunosuppression and risk of rejection

ABO-Compatible Donor & Recipient Combinations

Blood Typing for Transplant	
Recipient Blood Type	Acceptable Donor Blood Types
O	O
A	A, O
B	B, O
AB	O, A, B, AB

- HLA are encoded within the major histocompatibility complex
  - Class I (A, B, C) and Class II (DP, DQ, DR) are most important
  - Zero-mismatch kidney transplants have no mismatches in these classes and receive some priority in kidney allocation; also important for pancreas transplant
  - HLA matching not considered in liver transplantation
- Potential recipients can be screened for preformed antibodies to HLA
  - **Sensitization** (development of antibodies to foreign HLA) can occur due to blood transfusion, prior transplantation, or pregnancy
  - Traditionally, a panel reactive antibody (PRA) test was performed
  - Single-antigen beads can now determine specific antibodies in recipient blood
- Cross-matches are performed between potential donor cells and recipient serum
  - Positive cross-match demonstrates pre-formed antibodies in the recipient
  - Transplantation generally does not take place following a positive cross-match; however, special protocols may allow **desensitization** (removal of antibodies and increased immunosuppression to prevent reformation)

Types of Rejection

Types of Rejection			
Type	Mechanism	Time Frame	Treatment
Hyperacute	Preformed antibodies	Minutes	Removal of organ
Acute Cellular	Activated T-cells	Weeks to months	Steroids, increased baseline immunosuppression, antibody therapies
Acute antibody–Mediated (Humoral)	Reactivation of low-level preformed antibodies or newly developed (*de novo*) antibodies	Weeks to years	Plasmapheresis, IVIg, steroids, increased baseline immunosuppression, antibody therapies
Chronic (*Likely not just an immune-mediated process)	Multiple pathways including antibodies, cell-mediated, possible toxicity due to immunosuppression	Months to years	Poorly responsive to specific medication changes Avoid acute rejection episodes

Induction immunosuppression: initial immunosuppression at time of transplant

- Antibodies to specific components of the immune response
  - Depleting: destroy immune cells (i.e., anti-thymocyte globulin, alemtuzumab, OKT3)
  - Nondepleting: block specific receptors in immune response (i.e., basiliximab)
  - Side effects include SIRS-type reactions, hypersensitivity
- Steroids alter genetic expression of cytokines and T-cells activation
  - Prednisone and methylprednisolone most commonly used
  - Steroids can also be part of maintenance immunosuppression regimens
  - Side effects include weight gain/central obesity, wound healing complications, development of glucose intolerance, moon facies, osteoporosis, hypertension
- Some agents may also be used to treat rejection

- **Maintenance Immunosuppression:** ongoing, long-term medication regimen
  - Started at time of transplant or shortly after; usually given in combination of 2–3 agents
  - Calcineurin inhibitors (CNIs) bind to immunophillins and blocks release of IL-2
    - Tacrolimus and cyclosprine are the main agents in use
    - Side effects include nephrotoxicity, hypertension, hyperlipidemia, diabetes, tremor, headache, hyperkalemia
  - Mammalian target of rapamycin (mTOR) inhibitors block cell cycling of IL-2 stimulated T-cells
    - Rapamycin and everolimus are the main agents in use
    - Side effects include poor wound healing, leukopenia, anemia, oral ulcers
  - Antimetabolites inhibit *de novo* synthesis of guanosine nucleotides
    - Myophenolic acid, mycophenolate mofetil, azathioprine are common agents
    - Side effects include leukopenia, nausea, vomiting, diarrhea

Risks of Immunosuppression
- Specific agents' side effects/toxicities as above
- Increased risk of viral infections and more severe manifestations of viral disease including CMV, BK virus, EBV, HSV, HPV, JC virus
- Increased risk of nonmelanoma skin cancers
  - Counsel sun avoidance
  - Annual visit with dermatologist for skin examination
- Posttransplant lymphoproliferative disease
  - EBV-driven lymphoma
  - Highest risk in EBV-negative recipients who receive organs from EBV-positive donors
  - Treatment can range from decreasing immunosuppression to systemic chemotherapy

DRE M. IRIZARRY • SAMUEL LIN

22-1: Reconstructive Ladder (Fig. 22-1)

Figure 22-1 (From Fischer JE, Bland KI. *Mastery of Surgery*, 5th ed. Philadelphia, PA: Lippincott Williams & Wilkins, 2007.)

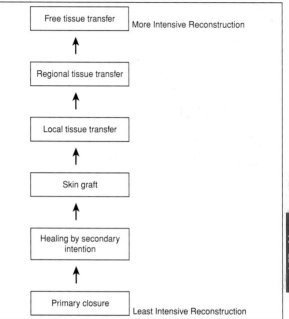

22-2: Skin Grafts

Indications
- To close defects that cannot be closed primarily
- To accelerate rate of healing compared to healing by secondary intention

Biology
- Recipient bed vascularity essential to provide nutrients for grafted skin
- *Imbibition*: displacement of one fluid by another immiscible fluid (plasma supports graft survival for first 24–48 hours; fibrin helps fix graft to tissue)
- *Inosculation*: vascular budding and branching (graft supported by a true circulation after days 4–7)
- **Contact of graft to wound bed is critical for survival**
  - Tension = bad
  - Fluid (hematoma, serum, and pus) between wound bed and graft = bad
  - Movement (shearing forces) = bad
- **Recipient tissues that cannot support grafts require tissue flaps for closure:**
  - Bone without periosteum
  - Cartilage without perichondrium
  - Exposed tendon
  - Infected wounds ($>10^5$ per gram of tissue)

Split-Thickness Skin Graft
- Definition: contain epidermis and portion of dermis (0.01–0.25 inches thick)
- Common donor sites: abdomen, buttocks, and thigh
- Advantages: large supply of possible donor sites, ease of harvesting, availability of reharvesting from same donor site in 10–14 days, coverage of large surface area, storage, and decreased primary contracture
- Disadvantages: "Cobblestone" appearance after healing if meshed, inferior cosmetic appearance, friability, pigment changes of donor site after healing, and secondary contracture

Full-Thickness Skin Graft
- Definition: epidermis and entire thickness of dermis; no subcutaneous tissue
- Used for coverage of wounds on face and hand
- Advantages: better appearance once healed, improved durability, and decreased secondary contracture compared to split-thickness grafts
- Disadvantages: increased primary contracture, fewer donor sites, and less available tissue

Composite Graft
- Definition: contains multiple tissues, e.g., cartilage, fat, fascia, and bone (fingertips, ear, and nose)
- Superior results and improved take in younger population
- Needs good recipient blood supply

Procedures
- Harvest devices
  - Drum dermatome (Reese): fixes epidermis to drum with glue
  - Electrical dermatome (Padgett, Brown): rapidly oscillating blade
  - Full-thickness skin grafts (FTSG) with scalpel: defatted after harvest to leave only dermis and epidermis
- Donor site care
  - Split-thickness skin grafts (STSG) sites: meshed gauze is incorporated into wound; dressing dries, is incorporated into scab, and falls off in 1–2 weeks; semipermeable membranes form fluid layer rich in leukocytes, hastens epithelialization
  - FTSG donor sites: usually closed primarily with sutures; occasionally require STSG to cover donor site
- Recipient site care
  - Hemostasis is critical to ensure contact between wound site and graft; avoid shearing forces that would sever and impair vascular bud formation
  - Meshed grafts/fenestrations allow for improved drainage, hence improving graft take between donor graft and recipient site
  - Graft fixed to recipient site by sutures/bolster dressing, vacuum-assisted device (sponge), or open method (especially in burn wounds where daily inspection is critical)
  - FTSG often secured using a bolster

22-3: FLAPS

Definition: unit of tissue transferred from one site to another while maintaining blood supply; useful in treating defects that require thicker tissue then provided by skin grafts

Classification Schemes
- Component parts: cutaneous, myocutaneous, fasciocutaneous, and osseocutaneous
- Relationship to defect: local, regional, and distant
- Nature of blood supply: random and axial
- Nature of movement: advancement, pivot, transposition, and free

Skin Flaps
- Random
  - Blood supply from nondominant contributions from dermal–subdermal plexus
  - Flap length-to-width ratio is critical to flap survival
  - Useful for coverage of small defects
  - Types: Z-plasty, V-Y advancement, rotation, and transposition
- Axial
  - Based on reliable, anatomically defined vascular territory
  - Vessels oriented longitudinally within flap, extends beyond flap base

- Can obtain greater length but has a limited topographic arc of rotation
- Types: forehead flaps, groin flaps, and deltopectoral flaps

Muscle (Myocutaneous) Flaps (Classification by Mathes and Nahai)
- Based on patterns of circulation or pedicles that enter muscle between its origin and insertion
- Provides increased blood supply to area
- Used to cover exposed bone, tendons, or cartilage
- Often used to reconstruct lower extremities and irradiated tissue

Fasciocutaneous Flaps
- Definition: transfer of skin, subcutaneous tissue, and underlying fascia with an anatomically distinct artery
- No undermining of muscle leading to less functional morbidity

Free Flaps
- Definition: native blood supply completely severed, tissue is transplanted to separate body area
- **Requires microvascular anastomosis**
- Can be used to provide function (such as for facial palsy)
- Examples: free transverse rectus abdominis myocutaneous (TRAM) flap, deep inferior epigastric flap, and anterolateral femoral fasciocutaneous flap
- Uses
  - Wound closure of areas with poor vascularity such as bare bones, nerves, tendons, and irradiated tissue
  - Facial reconstruction
  - Areas where padding/thick tissue is needed such as ischial tuberosity, over large vessels, or exposed nerves or tendons

---

22-4: BREAST RECONSTRUCTION

Terms
- Micromastia: small breasts
- Macromastia: large/hypertrophic breasts
- Ptosis: drooping of the breast
- Gynecomastia: enlargement of male breast tissue

Augmentation With Prosthetic Implant
- Implant location
  - Subglandular: between breast tissue and pectoralis major (less favorable long-term cosmetic outcomes)
  - Submuscular: underneath pectoralis major
- Complications: rupture, hematoma, infection, and capsular contracture (subglandular)
  - Symptoms: discomfort, asymmetry, and deformity ("double bubble" sign)
  - Clinical presentation of implant rupture
  - Silicone implant: frequently no visible change in appearance of breast
  - Saline implant: deflates over a period of days as saline reabsorbs
  - **Diagnosis**
  - **Ultrasound: "snowstorm" appearance of silicone in breast tissue and "Stepladder" sign of linear echoes**

Breast Reconstruction Following Mastectomy
- Alternative to the use of prosthetic devices; immediate or delayed reconstruction

Options
- Immediate reconstruction with implant
- Tissue expander followed by implant: Silastic "balloon" is gradually expanded with saline to increase tissue envelope
- Latissimus dorsi myocutaneous flap: alone or in combination with prosthetic implant
- TRAM: superior epigastric vessels
- Free flaps (*Figs. 22-2 and 22-3*)
  - Rectus abdominis myocutaneous free flap (free TRAM): deep inferior epigastric pedicle
  - Deep inferior epigastric perforator—free flap: spares rectus abdominis
  - Superior gluteal artery perforator: women who have inadequate abdominal tissue for reconstruction
- Nipple–areola reconstruction: often times done as a second stage, most common with local flaps, skin graft, and tattooing to increase pigmentation

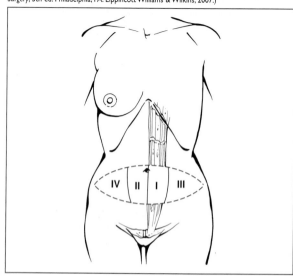

Figure 22-2 Location of free TRAM flap harvest. (From Fischer JE, Bland KI. *Mastery of Surgery*, 5th ed. Philadelphia, PA: Lippincott Williams & Wilkins, 2007.)

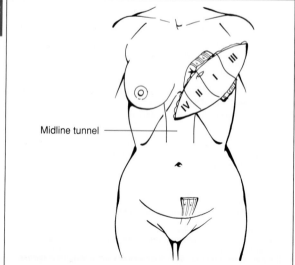

Figure 22-3 Location of free TRAM flap for postsurgical breast reconstruction. Note the severed abdominis muscle. (From Fischer JE, Bland KI. *Mastery of Surgery*, 5th ed. Philadelphia, PA: Lippincott Williams & Wilkins, 2007.)

Midline tunnel

22-5: ABDOMINAL WALL RECONSTRUCTION

Indications
- Numerous causes: trauma, operative, previous hernias, and previous repairs
- Defects <5 cm usually managed with local tissue rearrangement (e.g., abdominal wall advancement)
- Defects >6 cm (e.g., "loss of domain") may require reconstruction with autologous tissue, with or without synthetic material

Options for Reconstruction

Component Separation Surgical Technique for Midline Hernias
Midline incision
⇩
Elevate soft tissues off the fascia until linea semilunaris is visualized If needed, flaps can extend laterally as far as the posterior axillary line
⇩
Incise external oblique fascia parallel to the linea semilunaris; this should be 1 cm lateral to the linea semilunaris which releases the external oblique muscle/fascia
⇩
Develop the plane between the external oblique fascia (deep) and the internal oblique fascia (superficial); take dissection to the mid-axillary line or further to the posterior axillary line as needed. Expected yields: 8 cm at the waist, 4 cm in the upper abdomen, 3 cm in the lower abdomen (violation of internal oblique fascia can damage rectus abdominis innervation or Spigelian fascia)
⇩
If additional advancement is needed, consider releasing the rectus muscle from the posterior rectus sheath for an additional 2 cm of mobility
⇩
If flaps still do not meet in midline (e.g., obese patient with loss of domain) or are too attenuated (e.g., very thin patients), consider mesh to supplement
⇩
Place surgical drains between superficial soft tissues and external obliques + external obliques and internal obliques. Drains should exit laterally through separate stab incisions, remove when output <30 cc/24-h period
⇩
Close anterior rectus fascia with large, nonabsorbable suture. Close Scarpa's fascia to minimize dead space

- Synthetic material risks: infection, extrusion, and enterocutaneous fistulae
- Autologous tissue options
  - Component separation
  - Free flaps: tend to atrophy leading to recurrent weakness/herniation, risk of flap loss (partial or complete), and donor site morbidity

---

22-6: BURN SURGERY

Initial Assessment
- Determine% body surface area affected: rule of nines
- Determine burn depth
  - First degree (epithelium intact): no risk of scarring
  - Second degree (dermis damaged): superficial or deep
  - Third degree (full dermal thickness): "Leathery" appearance; needs surgery
  - Fourth degree (tendon or bone involvement): **extremities at risk** (Fig. 22-4)

Figure 22-4 Determination of degree of body burned. In adults, arms are each 9% of body area. Head is 9%. Legs are each 18%. Chest and back are each 18%. Pediatric patients are slightly different, with larger heads and smaller legs. (From Fischer JE, Bland KI. *Mastery of Surgery*, 5th ed. Philadelphia, PA: Lippincott Williams & Wilkins, 2007.)

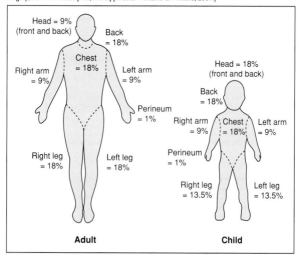

Parkland Formula
Fluid resuscitation in burn patients Fluid for first 24 h (mL) = 4 × patient's weight in kg × %BSA burned • Give first half of replacement volume in first 8 h • Give the remaining half in the next 16 h • Goal is to maintain end-organ perfusion while minimizing soft tissue edema and joint stiffness

- **Inhalation injury present?** If yes, intubate; airway edema can develop rapidly and prevent intubation. **Be wary of undiagnosed carbon monoxide poisoning**
- Transfer criteria: most burn injuries can be managed on outpatient basis; burn centers improve patient outcomes, but the cost of transport can exceed the cost of treatment in certain scenarios; discuss transfer with the burn team
  - When transferring a patient, wrap wounds in dry gauze. Do not delay transfer for antimicrobial or moist dressings

Surgical Indications
- Circumferential burns require escharotomy
- Second- and third-degree burns should be excised within 2–3 days: minimizes septic complications and hypermetabolic response

Surgical Technique
- Sequential, tangential excision until healthy tissue (subcutaneous tissue, tendon, bone) is encountered
- Patients will lose 3.5–5% of blood volume for every 1% of body surface area excised
- Minimize blood loss with local epinephrine, electrocautery, tourniquet, and early excision
- Closure: close primarily when possible to decrease systemic response; can be covered with autograft (best option), allograft, or synthetic skin
- Autografts: FTSG are suboptimal; meshed STSG maximize coverage area and allow for fluid drainage but leave patients with meshed appearance
- Other considerations
  - **Topical antibiotics are effective prophylaxis**
  - Systemic antibiotics not indicated without signs of bacteremia or sepsis; overuse will only select for resistant organisms
  - Organisms: *Staphylococcus aureus, Pseudomonas, Acinetobacter*

Paronychia

- Definition: mixed bacterial infection of soft tissue fold around the fingernail
- Etiology: break in the barrier between the nail fold and the nail plate (e.g., trauma, nail biting, hang nails, and manicures)
- Most can be managed by primary care physicians
- Diagnosis: based on examination, no radiographs, and no serum studies needed
- Medical treatment: 2–3 warm water (or dilute Betadine) soaks +7–10 days of PO antibiotics + hand elevation
- Surgical treatment: incision and drainage of abscess and send pus for culture
- Recurrent or complicated infection
  - Incise and elevate the perionychium: pus under the nail plate requires partial or complete removal of the nail plate by separating it from the underlying nail bed (e.g., with a Freer elevator) or eponychial marsupialization
- Key points: tailor the nail plate removal to only the affected area; avoid injuring the nail bed; tell patients that nail plate deformity can occur

Felon

- Definition: rapidly developing subcutaneous abscess of the distal pulp of finger; palmar pad must be involved; and strict definition requires compartment syndrome of the fingertip pulp
- Mechanism: vertical septations of the pulp lead to multiple abscesses that compromise venous return
- Risks: bone necrosis secondary to ischemia, osteomyelitis, involvement of tendon sheaths (see "Tenosynovitis"), obliteration of distal digital arteries resulting in pulp necrosis, and sinus tract formation
- Treatment
  - Early: antibiotics, elevation, and warm soaks (see "Paronychia")
  - Surgery: fluctuance on examination
- Surgical principles
  - Preserve fingertip function (sensation, stable pad for functional pinch)
  - Preserve digital arteries and nerves
  - Do not enter flexor sheaths
  - Do not cross DIP flexion crease
- Operative technique: digital block, tourniquet, incision (selection based on examination), debridement of necrotic tissue, irrigation, culture, and 2–5 days of wound drainage

Tenosynovitis

- Definition: closed-space infection (**S. aureus and beta-hemolytic Streptococcus**) of the flexor tendon sheath, usually with a history of penetrating trauma
- Complications: obliteration of flexor gliding mechanism, adhesion development, and loss of finger range of motion
- Diagnosis via Kanavel signs
  - Fusiform swelling
  - **Pain with passive extension** (most sensitive and reproducible sign)
  - Maximal pain along flexor tendon sheath (midline)
  - Finger held in partial flexion
- Nonoperative management: elevation, splint in the neutral resting position, broad IV antibiotic coverage; inadequate except for early, mild presentations; and inappropriate for diabetic and immunocompromised patients
- Surgical technique
  - Expose the tendon sheath through mid-axial incision, dorsal to Cleland ligament
  - Open sheath proximally and distally, minimizing exposure to limit damage to gliding structures and to limit postoperative scar formation
  - Sheath irrigation with an angiocatheter
  - Place wick or consider extended (24–72 hours) irrigation via a drainage catheter (e.g., pediatric feeding tube)

BHARATH NATH • THOMAS HAMILTON

23-1: GI TRACT ABNORMALITIES

Esophageal Atresia and Tracheoesophageal Fistula (TEF)
Epidemiology
- **50% have associated malformations in other organ systems**
- **VACTERL (vertebral, anorectal, cardiac, tracheoesophageal, renal, limb)**
- Higher incidence in trisomy 18 and 21

Classification

Figure 23-1 Types of tracheoesophageal fistula and esophageal atresia.

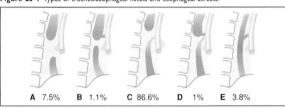

A 7.5%   B 1.1%   C 86.6%   D 1%   E 3.8%

Type A—esophageal atresia, without fistula; "pure esophageal atresia" (10%)
Type B—esophageal atresia with proximal TEF (<1%)
Type C—esophageal atresia with distal TEF (85%)
Type D—esophageal atresia with proximal and distal TEFs (<1%)
Type E—TEF without esophageal atresia; "H-type fistula" (4%)
Type F—congenital esophageal stenosis (<1%)

Clinical Presentation
- Excessive salivation at birth
- **Failure to pass NGT**

Imaging
- Prenatal US: small or absent gastric bubble +/– polyhydramnios (low sensitivity)
- **Plain film: NGT in superior mediastinum (within upper pouch)**
  - GI gas signifies distal tracheoesophageal fistula (TEF)
  - "Gasless abdomen" signifies isolated esophageal atresia or proximal TEF
- Echo: identifies structural cardiac anomalies prior to operative planning

Surgical Treatment and Perioperative Care
All patients need surgical repair
- Bronchoscopy: identify entry site of TEF and assess tracheomalacia
  - Can also place Fogarty catheter into fistula to occlude and prevent air leak into GI tract
- Esophagoscopy: define length of upper esophagus and identify upper pouch fistula
- Right thoracotomy approach
  - Mobilize proximal and distal esophageal segments, may divide azygous vein
  - Divide TEF, primarily close tracheal fistula site
  - End-to-end esophageal anastomosis if gap length <2 vertebral bodies
- If delayed operation is preferable (long-gap atresia, difficulties with anesthesia) consider TEF ligation and G-tube placement

Pyloric Stenosis
Epidemiology
- 4:1 male to female, familial association
- Gastric outlet obstruction due to hypertrophy of circular pyloric musculature

Clinical Presentation
- **Projectile non-bilious emesis between the second and sixth weeks of life**
- **Palpable mid-epigastric mass or "olive" (90%)**
- **Contraction alkalosis: hypokalemia, hypochloremia, and "paradoxic aciduria"**

- **Abdominal US:** >4 mm muscle thickness and >16 mm channel length
- Upper GI (if US nondiagnostic): pyloric "string sign," distended stomach, and GERD

Surgical Treatment and Perioperative Care (*Lancet.* 2009;373:390–398)
- **The treatment of pyloric stenosis is a medical, not a surgical emergency.**
  - Metabolic derangements can be severe and life threatening
  - Surgical correction should never proceed until electrolyte abnormalities are corrected to acceptable levels and hence can sometimes happen a few days after admission
  - NGT should be avoided as suction can worsen alkalosis
- Weber–Ramstedt pyloromyotomy (Fig. 23-2)
  - RUQ incision (Robertson), periumbilical incision, or laparoscopic approach
    - Incise long axis of serosa and muscle on avascular mid-anterior surface, from 2 mm proximal to pyloric vein to 5 mm onto the lower antrum
    - Watch for mucosa becoming thinner on the antral side
    - Open circular muscle bluntly with Benson retractor, spread to achieve pyloromyotomy
    - Laparoscopic approach: umbilical camera port, two stab ports, one to grasp the stomach or duodenum and the other to perform the pyloromyotomy
    - If mucosa is violated, defect is closed in layers and pyloromyotomy repeated on opposite side
    - Leak test can be performed by insufflating air and looking for bubble
    - *Adequate repair: protrusion gastric mucosa + free movement muscle edges*

Figure 23-2 Weber–Ramstedt pyloromyotomy. **A:** Incise serosa along long axis. **B:** Incise muscle along long axis, on mid-anterior surface. **C,D:** Open circular muscle with Benson retractor. **E:** Allow for protrusion of gastric mucosa. (From Fischer JE, Bland KI. *Mastery of Surgery,* 5th ed. Philadelphia: Lippincott Williams & Wilkins, 2007.)

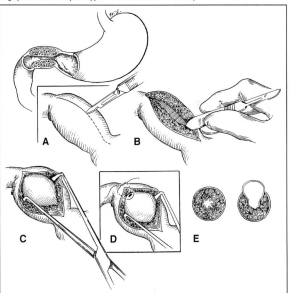

A B C D E

PS 23-2

Intussusception
Epidemiology
- Age: 3 months to 3 years
- 80% ileocolic location

Pathophysiology
- Telescoping of one portion of small bowel or colon into another
- **Most common cause is idiopathic, related to hypertrophic Peyer's patches; often a history of URI or gastroenteritis is elicited.**
- **The most common *nonidiopathic* cause of intussusception is a Meckel's diverticulum**
- Other causes can include polyps, lymphoma with bowel involvement, or inspissated secretions/stool (e.g., in cystic fibrosis).
- Intussusception of mesentery causes venous obstruction and subsequent bowel wall edema; if uncorrected, arterial insufficiency and ischemic/necrotic bowel may result

Clinical Presentation
- **Colicky abdominal pain: typical story is multiple episodes of child writhing in pain inconsolably and then 30–60 minutes later appearing pain-free**
- Back arching, stiffening, pulling up legs to abdomen, and writhing
- **Vomiting**, which may become bilious
- **Lethargy** is a less common but important alternate presentation
- Stool: normal → blood-tinged → dark red mucoid, "currant jelly" (ischemia)
- Physical findings: "sausage-like" mass, distension, blood-stained rectal mucus

Imaging
- Plain film: mass, abnormal gas and fecal pattern, air fluid level (obstruction)
- Abdominal US: essentially 100% sensitive and specific for ileocolic intussusception in this age group
  - Target lesion: two rings of low echogenicity separated by hyperechoic ring
  - Pseudokidney sign: superimposed hypo- and hyperechoic layers on longitudinal US
- CT abdomen: intraluminal mass with layered appearance within the mass or in continuity with adjacent mesenteric fat. Typically only considered if ultrasound nondiagnostic or if patient outside of typical age range of disease

Nonoperative Management (Diagnostic and Therapeutic)
- Hydrostatic enema reduction
  - Advance pliable catheter (Foley) rectally and tape buttocks firmly together
- Pneumatic enema reduction: higher rates (75–94%) of successful reduction
  - Maximum air pressure 80 mm Hg (younger) or 110–120 mm Hg (older infants)
- Reduction attempts may be repeated multiple times

Operative Management
- Indications: peritonitis, free intraperitoneal air, shock, incomplete reduction after multiple nonoperative reduction attempts, residual intraluminal filling defect with terminal ileal reflux, and radiologic evidence of pathologic lead point
- Preoperative NGT placement
- Gentle pushing (not pulling) of lead point back toward its normal position
- Resection and primary anastomosis required IF:
  - Serosal tearing upon attempted manual reduction
  - Questionable viability or necrosis of reduced bowel
  - Pathologic lead point

Complications
- Perforation during nonoperative hydrostatic/pneumatic reduction
  - Can cause massive insufflation of abdomen causing cardiopulmonary collapse
  - Treatment is urgent needle decompression (14-gauge Angiocath through umbilicus) and carry to operating room
- Recurrent intussusceptions: 2–20% (one-third occurs within the first day, majority in 6 months)
  - Usually no lead point; less likely following surgical reduction
  - Follow same treatment

Midgut Volvulus and Intestinal Rotation Abnormalities ("Malrotation")
Definition
- Malrotation and other intestinal rotation abnormalities refer to failure of the bowel to follow normal developmental rotation patterns. This can be asymptomatic, but places the bowel at risk for *midgut volvulus.*
- *Midgut volvulus* in this context refers to twisting of the bowel around its own blood supply causing ischemia and eventually necrosis

Epidemiology
- 70% of patients present in first year of life, of which 70% present in the first month of life
- Associated with other disorders (omphalocele, gastroschisis, and diaphragmatic hernia)

Pathophysiology
- Malrotation is often associated with a thin mesentery with a narrow, mesentery as opposed to the normal broad mesentery
- This narrow mesentery can act as an axis around which the bowel can twist.

Clinical Presentation
- **Sudden onset bilious vomiting**, if progress to bloody vomit: necrosis, shock
- **Bilious emesis in an infant or a child is a surgical emergency** because of the potential diagnosis of malrotation with midgut volvulus; necrosis may be complete in as little as 4 hours from onset
- **Abdominal distention** common, tenderness varies depending on how far into the disease process the patient has progressed; bloody stools on rectal examination (28%)
- If peritoneal signs are present, go directly to OR

Diagnostic Studies
- **Upper GI with water-soluble contrast (preferred test)**
  - Malposition of **ligament of Treitz to right of spine;** "Bird's beak" obstruction
- **If upper GI is positive for malrotation with likely volvulus, no further diagnostic testing is required and urgent laparotomy is indicated**
- Barium enema: determine cecal location (not test of choice)
- Plain film: **"double bubble" sign (duodenal obstruction);** gasless abdomen
- Duplex US: determine blood flow in SMA and relationship of SMA/SMV

Surgical Treatment
- **Emergent laparotomy through supraumbilical transverse incision for all patients**
- Laparoscopic approach is possible, mostly in setting of incidentally discovered malrotation

---

Ladd Procedure

- Evisceration and reduction of volvulus through counterclockwise rotation ("turn back the hands of time")
- Divide Ladd bands to widen the mesenteric base between duodenum and colon and abdominal sidewall
- Appendectomy due to abnormal position in RUQ post procedure
- Open anterior mesentery to expose mesenteric vessels and broaden mesentery
- Place small bowel in RLQ, cecum to left of midline and colon in LLQ
- Only resect frankly necrotic bowel; in 48 h, even bowel that looks nonviable (but not necrotic) may reperfuse and remain viable
- If resection performed, total bowel length remaining should be carefully measured
- Close and come back for "second-look" laparotomy if ischemic bowel

---

Necrotizing Enterocolitis
Epidemiology (Pediatr Perinat Epidemiol. 2006;20(6):498–506; N Engl J Med. 2011 20;364(3):255–264)
- **90% cases in preterm infants, 15% in-hospital mortality**

Pathophysiology (Pediatr Surg Int. 2006;22(7):573–580)
- Idiopathic: inadequate gut perfusion allowing for infectious processes, usually following onset of PO intake
- Preemies: immature bowel mucosa is not an adequate barrier to intraluminal flora. Early feeding may precipitate bacterial translocation
- Risk factors: **prematurity, low birth weight**, congenital heart disease, perinatal asphyxia/hypoxia, hypotension, umbilical artery catheter, gastroschisis, and indomethacin exposure (isolated intestinal perforation)

Clinical Presentation
- **Classically, symptoms manifest after first feeding in a premature baby**
- Fever, apnea, bradycardia, and lethargy
- Ileus, vomiting, **abdominal distention,** and gastrointestinal bleeding **(bloody diarrhea)**
- Sepsis, shock, acidosis, and thrombocytopenia

Imaging
- Plain film: bowel dilatation, pneumatosis intestinalis and portal venous air (pathognomonic), pneumoperitoneum (perforation)

Indications for Surgery
- **Absolute indications: perforation, pneumoperitoneum, and clinical deterioration**
- Relative indications: bowel necrosis, RLQ palpable mass, and fixed loop bowel on x-ray

Nonoperative Management
- NPO, NGT, broad-spectrum antibiotics (7–14 days), and TPN
- Serial abdominal examinations, plain films, and laboratory values (q6h until stable)
- Enteral nutrition (after complete antibiotic course and resolution of any signs of NEC)
- Can advance if there is no feeding intolerance or clinical deterioration

Operative Management
- **In general, laparotomy is preferred if clinical status permits.**
- Multicenter randomized trial data has shown comparable survival between drain placement and subsequent laparotomy vs. laparotomy alone, but worse survival with drain placement alone. (Ann Surg. 2008; 248:44–51)
- In extenuating circumstances (unstable for transport to OR; extremely low–birth-weight preterm infants) drain can be considered as a temporizing measure, with OR to follow once clinical status permits
- Bowel resection and ostomy
  - Preserve bowel length as much as possible
  - Second look operations usually indicated (bowel ischemia and unknown viability). Multiple ostomies sometimes needed

Duodenal Atresia
Epidemiology
- Pathophysiology: failure of recanalization from solid cord stage

Clinical Presentation
- **Polyhydramnios** (neonatal duodenal obstruction)
- **Bilious vomiting,** subtle upper abdominal fullness, and dehydration

Imaging
- Prenatal US: all pregnancies with polyhydramnios; look for obstructive pattern
- **Plain film: "double-bubble" sign** (prestenotic dilatation of stomach and proximal duodenum with no distal bowel gas)
- Upper GI: if suspicious for intestinal volvulus
- Echo: examine for associated cardiac anomalies prior to OR

Surgical Treatment and Perioperative Care
- **All obstructing duodenal atresias need operative repair**
- Preoperative cardiac workup to detect associated cardiac anomalies
- Surgical treatment
  - Resect duodenal membranes through a duodenotomy with Mikulicz closure
  - If complete atresia or annular pancreas:
    - Perform Kocher maneuver and duodenoduodenostomy (Kimura procedure) diamond shape—proximal transverse to distal longitudinal incisions
  - Do not divide pancreas; preserve ampulla of Vater
  - **Before closure, test distal patency** (3% have second web) **and evaluate for other atresias** by distal passage of a soft red rubber catheter and saline injection

Jejunoileal Atresia
Incidence
- Common cause of bowel obstruction within the first days of life
- Pathophysiology: **intrauterine vascular insults**

Clinical Presentation
- Polyhydramnios (prenatal ultrasound)
- SBO (bilious vomiting, distention, high-pitched bowel sounds, or visible peristalsis)
- Jaundice and electrolyte imbalance
- Failure to pass normal amounts of meconium in first 48 hours of life, peritonitis
- Types of intestinal atresia (Grosfeld classification) Fig. 23-3
  - Type 1: mucosal atresia
  - Type 2: fibrous cord but continuous mesentery
  - Type 3a: v-shaped mesenteric defect with complete atresia
  - Type 3b: "apple peel" deformity
  - Type 4: multiple intestinal atresias

Figure 23-3 Types of intestinal atresia.

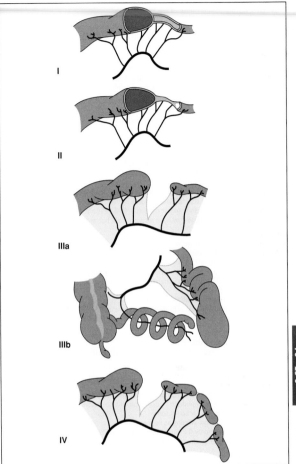

I

II

IIIa

IIIb

IV

Imaging
- Prenatal US: polyhydramnios
- Plain film: proximal dilated bowel with air–fluid levels, distal gasless bowel loops, and calcifications are sign of intrauterine perforation (12%)
- Barium enema: evaluate for microcolon, colonic atresia, and position of cecum

Surgical Treatment and Perioperative Care
- Extent of proximal bowel dilatation + length remaining bowel determine strategy
  - Resect atretic segments and taper the dilated proximal segment
  - If distal microbowel, place diverting double lumen enterostomy and feed distally
  - Evaluate the bowel for additional atresias as above
- TPN until bowel function is restored; sweat chloride test (10% cystic fibrosis)

Colonic Atresia
Pathophysiology
- In utero vascular compromise of the mesentery

Clinical Presentation
- Failure to pass meconium in the first 24 hours, abdominal distention, and bilious vomiting

Diagnostic Studies
- Plain film: dilated intestine with air–fluid levels and pronounced dilated segment at the point of obstruction; pneumoperitoneum if perforated
- Contrast enema: confirms diagnosis by showing blind distal end of microcolon

Surgical Treatment and Perioperative Care
- Right-sided and transverse colonic atresias can be primarily anastomosed, temporary colostomy if colonic ends have large size discrepancy or sigmoid atresia
- Inspect bowel for other atresias

Meckel Diverticulum
Epidemiology
- **Most common cause of painless lower GI hemorrhage in children**
- **Rule of 2's: 2% population, 2 years old, 2 feet from ileocecal valve, 2 cm diameter, and 2 inches long**
- **True diverticulum of persistent vitelline (omphalomesenteric) duct**
  - On antimesenteric border of ileum, usually not attached to abdominal wall
- **Heterotopic tissue:** gastric (most common, 60%). Pancreatic (second most common), jejunal, and colonic mucosa also possible but more infrequent

Clinical Presentation
- Usually asymptomatic, can go undiagnosed for many years
- Three main presentations
  - **Hemorrhage (40–60%): painless rectal bleeding; intermittent and self-limited, most common presentation in young children**
  - **Obstruction (25%): intussusception; volvulus—most common presentation in older patients**
  - **Inflammation/diverticulitis** (10–20%): most common presentation in teenaged patients periumbilical pain with migration across abdomen
  - Rarely, Meckel's can incarcerate in an inguinal hernia (Littre's hernia)

Imaging
- Plain film: obstructive pattern
- Technetium-99m: ectopic gastric tissue; poor sensitivity (negative scan cannot rule out)

Surgical Treatment
- Indications for surgery
  - Symptomatic, narrow-necked, or gastric mucosa containing diverticula
  - Incidental diverticula in pediatric population due to lifelong risk of complications
- Laparoscopic or open diverticulectomy
  - Retrograde inspection starting at ileocecal valve
  - Simple diverticulectomy for thin diverticula or ileal resection for wide-based diverticula where bleeding source likely on mesenteric border

Meconium Ileus
Epidemiology
- Pathophysiology: obstruction from inspissated meconium within terminal ileum
  - Less water content, increased protein: viscid, thick, and dehydrated meconium

Clinical Presentation
- **Failure to pass meconium within 24–48 hours of life**
- Obstructive symptoms: feeding intolerance, abdominal distention, and bilious emesis
- "Doughy" abdomen on palpation; anus and rectum typically narrowed
- Possible family history of CF and/or maternal history of polyhydramnios (20%)
- 50% associated complications: intestinal volvulus, bowel necrosis/perforation, intestinal atresia, meconium peritonitis from degrees of perforation +/– closure

Meconium Plug Syndrome (1:500 Neonates)
- More tenacious cap to meconium mass than normal that causes colonic obstruction
- Pathologic causes: CF, small left colon syndrome, Hirschsprung disease, congenital hypothyroidism, maternal narcotic addiction, and neuronal intestinal dysplasia

Imaging

- Prenatal US: hyperechoic abdominal mass, dilated bowel, polyhydramnios, peritoneal calcifications
- Plain film: +/– air–fluid levels, dilated loops of bowel, "soap-bubble" appearance of air mixed with meconium in RLQ, and intra-abdominal calcifications if perforation
- **Water-soluble contrast enema (diagnostic and therapeutic)**

Nonoperative Management

- NGT/OGT decompression, empiric antibiotics
- Sweat chloride test for CF
- **Gastrografin enema (80% diagnostic and 80% therapeutic)**
  - Hyperosmolar, water-soluble contrast hydrates and softens meconium; rapid passage of semi-liquid meconium proceeds for 24–48 hours
  - Serial plain films to confirm evacuation and rule out late perforation

Operative Management

- Inadequate evacuation: manual disimpaction aided by intraoperative Gastrografin/N-acetylcysteine irrigation (per NGT/OGT, per rectum, per enterostomy). If resection and primary anastomosis, complete evacuation necessary
- Complicated meconium ileus or perforation postenema: resect necrotic bowel, pseudocysts, remove inspissated meconium, diverting ostomy, correct any identified volvulus, atresia, and obstruction
- Postoperative enteral nutrition as tolerated
- Vigorous pulmonary monitoring and therapy

Hirschsprung Disease

Epidemiology

- **Genetic mutations: familial trait; associations with *RET* proto-oncogene**
- **Congenital aganglionic megacolon: absence of functional myenteric nervous system**
- Affected colon: rectum and sigmoid colon (70%) > long colonic segment (15%) > total colon (10%) > + small bowel (5%) > ultra-short/anorectal achalasia (1%)

Clinical Presentation

- Chronic constipation plus fecal soiling (older children)
- Neonatal intestinal obstruction: distention, bilious or feculent vomiting, and dehydration
- Failure to pass meconium within 48 hours
- Shock (enterocolitis or toxic megacolon) and possible perforation with sepsis

Imaging

- High index of suspicion: neonatal diagnosis 50%, most before 2 years
- Plain film: distal bowel obstruction or free air
- Unprepared water-soluble enema: up to 96% accurate (lower in newborns)
- Rectal manometry: absence of reflexive internal anal sphincter relaxation induced by rectal dilation (not necessarily sensitive in preemies or full term younger than 12 days)
- **Rectal or colonic suction or full-thickness biopsy**
  - Biopsy can be negative (+ ganglion cells) if past transition point
  - AChE increased, hypertrophied nerves in the myenteric plexus

Surgical Treatment

- Indications: most cases elective; emergent repair if obstructive symptoms, peritonitis/perforation, and sepsis
- Preoperative care
  - Decompress colon with large caliber soft tube, followed by serial irrigation with saline to prevent Hirschsprung enterocolitis
  - Broad-spectrum antibiotics and fluid resuscitation (if emergent)
- Operation
  - One- or two-staged repair with or without preliminary colostomy
  - Take biopsies to determine the definite extent of the disease
  - Definitive pull-through procedure performed 6–12 months later
  - If unstable, perform urgent leveling colostomy with the level determined by the presence of ganglion cells on frozen section
  - Swenson: combined abdominoperineal; open or laparoscopic
  - Dissect colon and splenic flexure, resect diseased bowel; then pull-through with anastomosis to distal rectum, 1–2 cm above dentate (0.5 cm newborns)
    - Duhamel: retrorectal pull-through with creation of rectocolonic pouch between aganglionic rectum and ganglionic colon

- Soave: endorectal pull-through of colon through muscular rectal cuff with anastomosis 1 cm above dentate line
- Mondragon: transanal one-stage endorectal pull-through; relies on mobilization of the rectum via the perineum
- Incise rectal mucosa circumferentially 5 mm proximal to dentate line
- Develop submucosal plane until the peritoneal cavity is reached
- Incise posterior muscle wall linearly and pull bowel with mesenteric vessels ligated under direct vision

Complications
- Anastomotic leak
- Constipation
- Anal stenosis: treat with serial rectal dilatation
- **Fecal incontinence common (>50%); greatly improves by adolescence (<10%)**

Imperforate Anus
Epidemiology
- High/intermediate anomalies: 2:1 male to female, 60% GU malformation or reflux
- 95% females have low anomalies
- **Associated anomalies (60%): duodenal or esophageal atresia, vertebral anomalies (i.e., tethered cord), renal anomalies, heart disease, and VACTERL**
- Pathophysiology: disruption of the normal cloacal cavity to differentiate into the urogenital cavity, opening and the anorectal cavity

Clinical Presentation: discovered on physical examination at birth
- Imperforate anus without fistula (complete anal atresia): 50% + trisomy 21
- Imperforate anus with fistula
  - Male (90% with fistula): perineal, anocutaneous, rectourethral, and rectovesicular
  - Female (95% with fistula): perineal, rectovestibular, persistent cloaca, and complete anal atresia

Preoperative Care
- All neonates: perineal US to delineate fistulae + VACTERL workup
  - Perineum: flat perineum indicates poor sphincter and levator muscle development
- If fistula visible, dilate to facilitate passage of meconium
  - Anoplasty deferred until clinically stable and other comorbidities evaluated
- If no fistula visible: NGT for decompression, perineal US, and urinalysis
  - Wait for 24 hours to allow gas and meconium to progress toward perineum
- If no clinical diagnosis possible (<20% cases)
  - Perform cross-table plain film in prone position
  - If rectal gas above the coccyx or rectal gas <1 cm from skin (suggests imperforate anus without fistula), consider diverting colostomy

Surgical Management
- **All imperforate anus must be surgically repaired, but not all need to be addressed in OR right away**
- If stool is able to be passed with dilations of fistula tract, and baby is able to feed and grow, can often bring baby back as an outpatient in 3–6 months
- Posterior sagittal anorectoplasty
- Perform stimulation to identify sphincter location
  - Midline incision through all posterior musculature
  - Identify rectal pouch and incise into the posterior inferior wall of the rectum
  - If present, identify and close rectourethral fistula from rectum and continue mobilizing the rectal pouch
  - Close striated muscle complex anteriorly and posterior musculature over rectal pouch
  - "Double diamond" anoplasty to promote sensation and avoid stricture

Postoperative Care
- If no laparotomy, oral feedings begin within hours
- Foley catheter for 5–7 days if rectourethral fistula
- Anal dilatation at 2 weeks postoperatively (may need to continue for months)
- Once correct size dilator achieved, colostomy reversed

Common Causes of Pediatric GI Hemorrhage

Upper GI Hemorrhage	Lower GI Hemorrhage
Neonates, infants/toddlers: • Esophagitis • Gastritis • Gastroduodenal ulcer • Foreign body ingestion (infant/toddlers)	Neonates: • Swallowed maternal blood • Anorectal fissure • NEC • Malrotation with midgut volvulus • Hirschsprung disease • Coagulopathy
Adolescents: • Peptic ulcers • Gastritis • Mallory–Weiss tears • Varices • Dieulafoy lesions • Pill esophagitis	Infants/toddlers: • Anorectal fissure • Allergic colitis • Intussusception • Meckel diverticulum • Hemolytic uremic syndrome • Henoch–Schonlein purpura • Lymphonodular hyperplasia • Intestinal duplication
	Adolescents: • Infectious gastroenteritis/colitis • Juvenile polyps • Inflammatory bowel disease

23-2: BILIARY TRACT ABNORMALITIES

Biliary Atresia

Pathophysiology
- Etiology unclear
  - Fetal vascular accident vs. malunion of pancreatic and biliary ductal systems
  - Majority are sporadic, but a small group (10–15%) are syndromic
  - Viral infection (CMV, group C rotavirus), congenital association, autoimmune
  - Biliary ductal obstruction leads to progressive periportal fibrosis and cirrhosis, obstruction of the intrahepatic portal veins, portal hypertension, and ascites
- Left alone, most die before 20 months from pneumonia, sepsis, and portal hypertension
  - Classification depends on location of atresia: Type 1 involves common bile duct, Type 2 involves common hepatic duct, and Type 3 extends to porta hepatis

Clinical Presentation
- Often a full-term baby who develops progressive jaundice and acholic stool
- Rapidly developing jaundice with mild anemia (icterus praecox) within first 36 hours
- Prolonged icterus (>8 days, >14 days preemies), acholic stool, and dark brown urine
- High conjugated bilirubin (>25% of total bilirubin) and elevated alkaline phosphatase
- Hepatosplenomegaly after 4 weeks and ascites after 4 months
- Cardiac malformations are most common in sporadic BA; in syndromic biliary atresia, associated anomalies can be disorders of rotation (malrotation, preduodenal portal vain, situs inversus) or others including anorectal malformations, atresias, and GU abnormalities

Imaging and Workup
- Imaging and lab tests to exclude other causes of neonatal hyperbilirubinemia, CF, hypothyroidism, metabolic disorders
- RUQ US: absence of gall bladder (~70% sensitive); triangular cord sign
- HIDA (technetium-99) scan: 98% sensitive, but only 70% specific
- Other preoperative workup can included MRCP or ERCP depending on center expertise
- Percutaneous or operative cholangiogram is undertaken in most cases to confirm diagnosis prior to proceeding operative repair
- Liver biopsy can be done but important to note that multiple cholestatic processes can have similar appearance on biopsy

Treatment
- **Indication for surgery: progressive cholestasis (all patients)**
- Laparotomy or laparoscopy before 8 weeks
- Preoperative evaluation should evaluate the extent of liver dysfunction, severe dysfunction should prompt a transplant workup

- Start with diagnostic cholangiography, liver wedge biopsy
  - Elevate all tissue anterior to portal vein and hepatic artery as an intact flap from the duodenum to the hilum of the liver; completely dissect the hilum
- **Roux-en-Y portoenterostomy (Kasai procedure)**
  - Ligate the fibrous common bile duct distally
  - Identify fibrous cone at portal plate and transect to completely remove extrahepatic biliary structures
  - Construct Roux-en-Y limb with 40-cm limb and pass retrocolic
  - Perform single-layer anastomosis between fibrous transected cone and jejunum

Choledochal Cyst
Background and Epidemiology
- High union of pancreatic and bile ducts causes reflux of pancreatic enzymes into biliary system, damaging ductal walls, leading to cystic transformation in utero
- All types have malignant potential towards cholangiocarcinoma or gallbladder carcinoma
- Wide range of incidence from 1:150,000 in western population to 1:13,000 in East Asian populations; strong female predilection

Classification
- **Type I (>85%): cystic dilatation of CBD; antenatal obstruction of ampulla of Vater**
- Type II: diverticular malformation of the common bile duct
- Type III: intraduodenal (more common) or intrapancreatic choledochocele
- Type IV: multiple intrahepatic and extrahepatic cysts
- Type V: single or multiple intrahepatic cysts; normal extrahepatic biliary system; Caroli disease if liver fibrosis present

Clinical Presentation
- Obstructive jaundice, conjugated hyperbilirubinemia, and elevated alkaline phosphatase
- <6 months old with complete biliary obstruction and jaundice
- >2 years old with recurrent icterus, RUQ abdominal pain, recurrent cholangitis, and possibly palpable mass

Imaging
- **Abdominal US: best; shows ductal dilatation in biliary and pancreatic system**
- HIDA: demonstrates biliary obstruction or abnormal drainage
- MRCP without breath holding: images of hepatopancreaticobiliary ductal systems
- Invasive studies are somewhat center specific but can include percutaneous transhepatic cholangiography or endoscopic retrograde cholangiopancreatography; unlikely to yield more information than MRCP

Treatment
- Indications for surgery: cholestasis, prevention of malignant transformation
- Objective: complete excision of choledochal cyst and/or mucosectomy
- **Operation: cyst resection and Roux-en-Y hepaticojejunostomy (preferred)**
- If anatomy unclear, intraoperative cholangiography can be performed to further delineate biliary tree
- Cystoduodenostomy and Roux-en-Y cystojejunostomy (higher morbidity): recurrent cholangitis and anastomotic stricture
- Types III–V: individual resection strategy, possible hepatectomy +/– pancreatectomy
- Prognosis better for patients with extrahepatic cysts post-resection

Complications
- Retained choledochal cyst or residual mucosa leading to malignancy (15%)
- Cholangitis (10%): patients with intrahepatic ductal ectasia
- Biliary stricture

23-3: ABDOMINAL WALL DEFECTS
Omphalocele
Clinical Presentation
- **Central abdominal wall defect (>4 cm) at the umbilicus**
- **Covered by thin membrane or sac, which may rupture upon delivery**

- Usually contains midgut, liver, and possibly spleen/gonads

Pathophysiology: failure of the lateral embryonic folds to fuse in the midline

Associated Anomalies
- Historic mortality of 30–40% has greatly improved, with >80% survival of giant omphalocele, and >90% for all patients with isolated omphalocele
- Cardiac (40–50%): pentalogy of Cantrell—omphalocele, defective sternum, ventral diaphragmatic defect, intrinsic cardiac abnormality, and anterior pericardial deficiency
- Schisis association: omphalocele, neural tube defects (anencephaly, encephalocele, and spina bifida cystica), oral clefts (cleft lip +/– palate and posterior cleft palate), congenital diaphragmatic hernia—high mortality
- OEIS syndrome: omphalocele, bladder exstrophy, imperforate anus, and spinal defects
- Beckwith–Wiedemann: omphalocele, macroglossia, visceromegaly, and hypoglycemia
- Intestinal malrotation
- Trisomy 13, 18, and 21

Imaging
- Amniocentesis: elevated alpha fetoprotein (AFP)
- Prenatal US: determines liver status of omphalocele; **detects 95%** of omphaloceles

Treatment
- **All omphaloceles should be repaired**
- Operative details
  - **Perform closure or coverage of intact membrane within 24 hours**
  - Circumferential skin incision several millimeters away from the sac
  - Large defects require staged closure
    - Suture Silastic pouch or silo to fascial edges to contain viscera
    - Serially reduce the pouch from anterior to posterior (maintain abdominal pressure <20 cm H_2O; paralyze the infant)
    - When pouch at level of fascia (~1 week), close fascia and remove pouch (pulmonary monitoring to monitor abdominal pressure)
- Very large omphaloceles unlikely to achieve fascial or skin closure can epithelialize via serial dressing changes (rotate bacitracin, Silvadene, and Betadine)

Complications
- **Life-threatening hypothermia secondary to insensible losses**
- **Abdominal compartment syndrome** and/or torsion of hepatic veins upon premature fascial closure or overaggressive reduction of intra-abdominal contents

Gastroschisis
Clinical Presentation
- **Central abdominal wall defect (4 cm) to the right of the umbilicus**
- **No covering membrane**
- Usually only midgut is herniated
- Exposed gut initially normal appearing, but will develop edema, matting, and thick peel

All babies with gastroschisis have IUGR, but most will catch up with their peers by age 2

Epidemiology
- Second most common cause of intestinal failure (after NEC)
- Incidence has approximately doubled in last twenty years
- Risk factors include young maternal age, smoking, drug use, GU infections, and others
- In US, >90% of gastroschisis is diagnosed with prenatal ultrasound
- Simple, low-risk gastroschisis has nearly 100% survival, but complex, high-risk gastroschisis (associated with other anomalies, ischemia, thick rind) can have up to 13% mortality (largely due to respiratory failure of prematurity)
- Associated anomalies: intestinal malrotation, intestinal atresia (15%), and NEC

Pathophysiology
- Failure of the umbilical coelom to form
- Peritoneal cavity too small to contain growing GI tract
- Possible vascular compromise of umbilical vein or omphalomesenteric artery

Imaging and Laboratory Studies
- Amniocentesis: elevated AFP (also in maternal serum) and acetylcholinesterase; **100% of pregnancies with gastroschisis have elevated AFP and 80% with acetylcholinesterase** in some studies
- Prenatal US: small defect and large mass of eviscerated bowel

- **All gastroschisis should be repaired**
- **Early repair preferred; avoids induration and edema of exposed bowel over time**
- Preoperative care
  - In the delivery room, place cellophane bowel bag with drawstrings cinched under the arms in order to prevent evaporative and heat losses
  - NGT/OGT, IVF, and antibiotics
  - Rectal examination to stimulate meconium passage
- Operative details: reduction and primary closure if possible
  - Hold umbilical cord up and reduce bowel loop by loop
  - Evacuate meconium by anal dilatation
  - Place mattress sutures through all layers except skin, test before tying
  - Leave umbilicus intact; divide umbilical vessels and urachus at peritoneal level after trimming cord
  - Examination for atresia not performed with initial reduction (matted, edematous bowel may appear atretic when actually normal)
  - If immediate reduction of the bowel is unlikely, a silo is placed.
  - When in a silo, the bowel will reduce into abdominal cavity by gravity and with daily or twice daily cinching and tying of the silo to push bowel into the belly
  - Excessive pressures can cause ischemia

Congenital Diaphragmatic Hernia
Pathophysiology
- Etiologic theories
  - Failed closure of the embryonic pleuroperitoneal canal
  - Malformation of the primordial diaphragm or pleuroperitoneal fold
- Persistent fetal circulation causes right to left shunting
- Survival directly related to the degree of associated pulmonary hypoplasia

Classification
- **Bochdalek hernia (85–90%):** posterolateral hernia; 20% hernia sac present
- Morgagni hernia (2–6%): retrosternal hernia—located in anterior diaphragm posterior to xiphoid; associated with trisomy 21 (35%) and congenital heart anomalies
- 20% associated congenital defects (mostly cardiovascular)

Clinical Presentation
- Bochdalek hernias
  - Symptoms may not develop until several hours after birth ("honeymoon period")
  - Decreased breath sounds + respiratory distress, improves by lying on affected side. Scaphoid abdomen; heart sounds on contralateral side, and paradoxical breathing
  - The vast majority are on the left side
- Morgagni hernias: generally asymptomatic
  - Incidental findings on CXR in adolescents and adults
  - Recurrent respiratory infections, epigastric pain, emesis, and bowel obstruction

Imaging
- Prenatal US: 50–60% diagnostic but up to 93% in tertiary care centers
- **CXR: loops of air-filled intestine in thorax, mediastinal shift, and cardiac dextroposition**
- Upper GI: intraluminal contrast in the thoracic cavity
- Echo: associated cardiac defects

Treatment
- **All congenital diaphragmatic hernias require surgical repair**
- Preoperative care
  - NGT, mechanical ventilation, spontaneous respiration, and permissive hypercapnia
  - Immediate repair has no immediate beneficial physiologic effect on lung function
  - Alkalosis improves pulmonary HTN (NaHCO$_3$, THAM)
  - Increase arterial pressure with dopamine/milrinone; reduces right to left shunt
  - Consider nitric oxide (pulmonary vasodilator) for worsening pulmonary HTN
- **Extracorporeal membrane oxygenation (ECMO)** if:
  - Requires and fails high-frequency ventilation: pre-ductal PaO$_2$ <50, PIP 25–30
  - Intractable hypotension: MAP <35 while on FiO$_2$ 1.0, PIP 25–30, + pressors
  - Causes progressive anasarca; surgical repair within 24 hours or post-ECMO
- Operative details
  - Median or left subcostal laparotomy/laparoscopy/thoracoscopy
  - Carefully reduce abdominal viscera

- Dissect posterior diaphragmatic rim
- Close primarily if possible with interrupted sutures
- If unable to close defect: Gore-Tex patch or transversus abdominis flap
- If abdomen not amenable to primary closure, then skin flap closure
- Thoracoscopic repair is also increasingly popular in selected patients; notably, those without baselie hypercarbia (which would be worsened by CO_2 insufflation)
- Insufflation of chest, if tolerated, can increase space in abdomen and make reduction of hernia contents easier
- Follow-up: RSV prophylaxis (Synagis), influenza immunization, CT head, EEG, ophthalmology evaluation, and brain stem auditory response
- Prognosis: survival 50–80% in symptomatic patients at tertiary centers with ECMO
  Complications: Gore-Tex patch susceptible to recurrent hernias, persistent hydrothorax

---

23-4: Pediatric Neoplasms

Wilms' Tumor

Epidemiology
- Second most common abdominal tumor in children
- Mean age at diagnosis: 3 years
- Associated anomalies: sporadic aniridia, isolated hemihypertrophy, and genital anomalies
  - Denys–Drash (nephropathy, renal failure, male pseudohermaphroditism, and Wilms)
  - Beckwith–Wiedemann syndrome (visceromegaly, macroglossia, omphalocele, and hyperinsulinemic hypoglycemia of infancy)
  - WAGR (Wilms, Aniridia, Genitourinary malformation, and mental Retardation)
- Histologic subtypes determine overall prognosis, recurrence rate, response to adjuvant therapy, and treatment algorithm (unfavorable histology: anaplastic)
- Wilms tumor suppressor genes: WT1, WT2; metastasizes to lung

Clinical Presentation
- **Large asymptomatic flank mass** in healthy toddler which **does not cross midline**
- Abdominal pain (30%), hematuria (12–25%), and hypertension (25%)
- Seldom invades surrounding organs; compresses adjacent structures
- Intravascular tumor thrombus (renal vein and IVC) (4%)

Staging System (Children's Oncology Group)
- Stage I: limited to kidney and excised without rupture or biopsy; capsule intact
- Stage II: extends through capsule, removed with clear microscopic margins; tumor penetrates renal capsule or invades renal sinus vessels
- Stage III: gross or microscopic residual tumor in setting of incomplete resection, biopsy prior to removal, tumor rupture, incomplete resection, lymph node metastases within abdomen, or incompletely removed tumor thrombus
- Stage IV: hematogenous metastases or extra-abdominal lymph node metastases
- Stage V: bilateral disease note, each side is staged independently

Imaging
- **Abdominal US**: hydronephrosis, multicystic kidney disease, tumor infiltration of renal vein and IVC, and blood flow
- CT abdomen: classically "pushes away" normal parenchyma creating the "claw sign," can also detect bilateral tumor, local invasion, and intravascular spread
- CT chest (lung metastases, present in 13–15% of patients)
- MRI abdomen

Treatment
- **All suspected Wilms tumors should be resected, however:**
  - If tumor massive in size or resection necessitates removal of adjacent organs (liver, spleen, and pancreas), mass should be biopsied and operation aborted; if tumor extends above hepatic veins, is bilateral, or in a solitary kidney, primary repair should not be pursued
  - In these cases, preoperative chemotherapy is preferred, with surgery reserved for good response
  - Stage V (Bilateral) Wilm tumor is treated by 3 drug preoperative chemotherapy with vincristine, dactinomycin, and doxorubicin followed by surgical resection within 12 weeks of diagnosis
- Operative details
- Generous subcostal or thoracoabdominal incision
  - Full intra-abdominal inspection; palpate liver, contralateral kidney, IVC
  - Mobilize colon off anterior kidney and tumor prior to controlling renal hilum
  - As tumor mobilized, transect ureter close to bladder

- If tumor located at upper pole of kidney, resect adrenal gland
- If tumor located at lower pole of kidney, adrenal gland may be spared
- Most tumor rupture occurs during posterior dissection off of the diaphragm
- May resect portion of diaphragm if necessary
- Lymph node sampling
  - Adjuvant treatment: based on post-resection histologic findings and staging
  - Stages I and II: vincristine and dactinomycin, no radiation
  - Stage III: vincristine, dactinomycin, and doxorubicin + radiation (local, tumor bed)
  - Stage IV: vincristine, dactinomycin, and doxorubicin + radiation (local, lung field)
  - Neoadjuvant therapy (requires biopsy): tumor in solitary kidney, bilateral tumors, tumor in horseshoe kidney, intravascular extension above intrahepatic IVC, and respiratory compromise secondary to diffuse metastatic disease

Neuroblastoma
Epidemiology
- **Most common extracranial solid tumor in children**
- Arises from sympathetic neuroblast cells derived from the neural crest
- **Tumor located anywhere sympathetic cells are found: adrenal gland (40–60%) > retroperitoneum (20%) > mediastinum (10%) > pelvis (2–6%) > neck (2%)**
- Local extension with vascular encasement and invasion of surrounding structures
- Metastases: liver and bone
- Spontaneous regression possible
  Staging is by International Neuroblastoma Risk Group (INRG) using Image Derived Risk Factors (IDRF)
- L1: localized tumor within one bod compartment without IDRFL2: local–regional tumor with one or more IDRF, ipsilateral contiguous body compartments
- M: Distant metastases, contralateral body compartments extension by infiltration or by lymph nodes
- MS: L1 or L2 primary with age <18 months and metastases confined to skin, liver, or bone marrow. **Image Derived Risk Factors** include encasement or invasion into vascular structures, airway, adjacent organs or bone.
- **Age** is a significant risk factor with patients <18 months having improved survival
- **Other adverse risk factors** include N-MYC amplification, unfavorable tumor histology, and DNA ploidy

Clinical Presentation
- **62–70% metastatic, 25% localized, and 10% Stage IVS**
- Usually asymptomatic; mass may be present
- Systemic symptoms: malaise, weight loss, fever, sweating, and diarrhea or constipation
  - Metastatic symptoms: bone/joint pain, periorbital ecchymosis, and proptosis
  - Hypertension (catecholamine secretion and renal artery compression)
- **Opsomyoclonus syndrome** (2–3% of neuroblastomas and 50% have neuroblastoma)
  - Opsoclonus: rapid involuntary eye movement
  - Myoclonus: brief involuntary muscle twitching
  - Cerebellar ataxia, dysphasia, mutism, lethargy, drooling, and strabismus
  - Treatment: tumor resection; glucocorticoids, adrenocorticotropic hormone; IVIG
- Urine metabolites (85%): vanillylmandelic and homovanillic acid
- Biochemical markers
  - Neuron-specific enolase: >15 ng/mL abnormal; >100 ng/mL advanced
  - Lactate dehydrogenase: <1,500 U/mL improved survival
  - Ferritin: >142 ng/mL, Stages III–IV

Imaging
- Prenatal US: detects only 3%
- Abdominal US: solid vs. cystic mass; mixed pattern with calcification and necrosis
- CXR: identification of mediastinal mass
- CT abdomen/chest: adrenal tumor, displacement of renal parenchyma, not replacement; determine site, consistency, and relation to adjacent structures
- MRI abd/chest: soft tissue changes, bone/liver involvement, and intraspinal extension
- Bone scan (MIBG/technetium): identify metastatic skeletal disease
- Tissue biopsy

Treatment
- **Tumor burden should be reduced as much as is safely possible**
- Thoracic tumors
  - Standard thoracotomy usually sufficient: apical tumors may require "trap-door"
  - Usually lie in costovertebral angle with encasement of major vessels uncommon

- Upper thoracic ganglia excision may affect stellate ganglion (postoperative Horner's syndrome)
- May be difficult to resect intraspinal portion of dumb-bell thoracic tumors
- Abdominal tumors
  - Upper transverse or thoracoabdominal incision
  - In Stages III and IV disease, tumor often encases great vessels and visceral tissues
  - Subadventitial plane may be used to dissect tumor off the vessels
  - Partial diaphragmatic resection is often necessary
  - Acceptable to incise tumor during resection; piecemeal removal not uncommon
- Adjuvant therapy
  - Neoadjuvant chemotherapy +
  - Radiation for residual disease (Stages III, IV) and hepatomegaly (Stage IVS)
  - Total body irradiation followed by bone marrow transplantation: advanced

Hepatoblastoma
Pathophysiology
Tumor growth and metastasis: local growth via direct extension, intrahepatic lymphatic and vascular channels; can extend into hepatic veins and vena cava. Extrahepatic metastasis to regional lymph nodes in porta hepatis, hematogenous spread to lungs, bone, and bone marrow.
- Classification (of epithelial origin): fetal (well-differentiated), embryonal (immature and poorly differentiated), mixed epithelial, mesenchymal, and anaplastic
- Associated anomalies: Beckwith–Wiedemann syndrome, prematurity, TPN cholestasis, and familial polyposis

Incidence and Clinical Presentation
- Usually <4 years old; more common in right lobe of liver
- Most common primary pediatric hepatic malignancy
- Incidence is increasing (doubled in last 30 years)
- Associated with toxic exposures, maternal tobacco exposure, certain maternal medication use, prematurity
- Right upper quadrant mass that moves on respiration (90%)
- Nausea and vomiting from compression of stomach, weight loss, and anemia
- Precocious virilization (rare, hCG secretion)
- Laboratory values: LFTs may be elevated, AFP, and ferritin elevated (90%)

Diagnostic Studies
- Liver US: anatomic relationships, cystic vs. solid, and extension into vasculature
- CT torso: evaluate mass; metastatic workup, and preoperative staging

Treatment
- Surgery for all tumors
- Primary resection for localized disease (segmentectomy and lobectomy)
- If multicentric or large (>50%): initial biopsy, neoadjuvant chemotherapy, and delayed primary resection (75% become resectable)
  - If tumor not responsive and still unresectable: orthotopic liver transplant
- Intraoperative US
- Consider hepatic artery chemoembolization
- Postoperative care: monitor for hypoglycemia, hypoalbuminemia, and hypoprothrombinemia
- Adjuvant chemotherapy (doxorubicin) after ~3 weeks (after hepatic regeneration)

Postoperative Staging (Children's Cancer Study Group)
- Overall survival 70%
- Stage I: completely resected (80–100% survival)
- Stage II: microscopic residual disease (80–100% survival)
- Stage III: biopsy only or tumor rupture
- Stage IV: metastatic disease

Rhabdomyosarcoma
Incidence
- Most common pediatric soft tissue sarcoma (50%)
- Bimodal distribution with younger patients (ages 2–6) likely to have embryonal histology and older patients (teenage years) likely to have alveolar histology
- Associated genetic syndromes: Beckwith–Wiedemann syndrome, neurofibromatosis, Li–Fraumeni syndrome, and basal cell nevus syndrome

Pathophysiology
- **Highly malignant: involves local structures early**

- Metastasizes by hematogenous and lymphatic routes:
  - Lung (50%) > nodes (33%), bone (35%) > liver (22%) > brain (20%) > breast (5%)
- MDM2 oncogene expression: multidrug resistance

Pretreatment TNM Staging System—Based on Primary Site
- Stage I: orbit, head and neck, and genitourinary
- Stage II/III: bladder/prostate, extremity, head/neck, parameningeal, trunk, and retroperitoneum
- Stage IV: any primary site with metastatic disease

Imaging
- CT of affected area: determine anatomic relationships and primary/metastatic disease
- Lymph node biopsy: staging and tissue diagnosis

Treatment
- **Resect all primary tumors with wide local excision and clear margins**
- Perform re-excision for microscopic residual disease or after radiotherapy in stage III
- Patients are placed into low-risk, intermediate-risk, and high-risk treatment categories according to tumor site, histology, tumor size, pre-treatment TNM stage, clinical group (localized, completeness of resection, lymph nodes, and margins), and age of patient
- Adjuvant treatment
  - Chemotherapy: vincristine, actinomycin D, cyclophosphamide, and irinotecan
  - Radiotherapy for locally advanced tumors: reduce local recurrence
- Overall survival >75%; 5-year survival of metastatic disease <30%

Sacrococcygeal Teratoma
Clinical Presentation
- If prenatally diagnosed, C-section to prevent intravaginal trauma and tumor rupture
- Visible mass at coccyx at birth (unless intrapelvic)
- Female predelection, older patients have worse prognosis
- Currarino Triad: Sacral malformation, presacral mass, and anorectal malformation
- More severe presentation: prematurity, high-output cardiac failure, DIC, tumor rupture and bleeding (high mortality), and intrapelvic causing urinary obstruction

Imaging
- Prenatal US: often makes diagnosis
- Plain film: rule out spinal defects and observe presence of calcifications
- Abdominal US: determine intrapelvic/intra-abdominal component
- AFP: increased malignant rate if elevated

Treatment
- All sacrococcygeal teratomas should be resected
- Aspiration of cystic component in utero to aid in atraumatic delivery
- Adjuvant therapy indicated: adolescents, unresectable tumors, and malignancy

Complications
- Tumor rupture/hemorrhage upon delivery
- Large tumors can cause high output cardiac failure, nonimmune hydrops fetalis
- Fecal/urinary incontinence
- Lower limb weakness
- Recurrence: failure to resect coccyx and larger more solid tumors
  - Often within 3 years: monitor AFP and physical examination every 3 months
  - Treat with platinum-based chemotherapy and local radiation

---

23-5: Congenital Pulmonary and Chest Wall Abnormalities

Bronchogenic Cyst
Pathophysiology
- Arises from the foregut endoderm and lined with respiratory bronchial epithelium
- Mucus-filled wall usually contains cartilage
- Tends to be centrally located, can develop into abscess cavities
Parenchymal cysts: abnormality of pseudoglandular stage of lung development

Clinical Presentation
- Recurrent coughing, wheezing, and pneumonia
- Newborn: acute respiratory distress if large cyst and compressing adjacent structures
- Asymptomatic: usually present in early adulthood

Treatment
- Resect all bronchogenic cysts
- Wedge, lobectomy, or simple cystectomy

Congenital Cystic Adenomatoid Malformation
Pathophysiology
- Abnormality of branching morphogenesis of the lung: excessive proliferation of bronchial structures without cartilage
- **Communicates with tracheobronchial tree, but lack of normal alveoli leads to very poor gas exchange from these lesions**
- **Arterial supply and venous drainage via pulmonary circulation**

Clinical Presentation: Varied
- Majority occur in lower lobes and are unilateral
- In modern era, most lesions are diagnosed in utero
- Fetal hydrops with compromised pulmonary function (40%) → respiratory distress at birth (IVC and cardiac compression)
- Rarely cyst can rupture after birth causing pneumothorax
- One-third present later in life with recurrent pneumonia

Surgical Treatment and Perioperative Care
- Resect all congenital cystic adenomatoid malformations with complete lobectomy
- Resection also important to reduce risk of future malignancy
- In utero resection or aspiration is possible if lesion enlarges, progressive hydrops fetalis, and impending in utero death (specialized centers)

Pulmonary Sequestration
Pathophysiology
- **No communication with tracheobronchial tree**
- **Blood supply derived from systemic circulation**

Clinical Presentation
- Intralobar: recurrent pneumonias in same segment in adolescence; possible high-output cardiac failure from shunting (left-to-right shunt)
- Extralobar: respiratory distress, less commonly recurrent infection

Treatment
- Indications
  - Symptomatic disease (respiratory distress, infections, and CHF): immediate repair
  - Asymptomatic intralobar disease: elective resection to prevent infections
  - Asymptomatic extralobar disease may not require resection
- Intralobar disease: complete lobectomy
- Extralobar disease: simple resection of lesion

Pectus Excavatum
Epidemiology
- **Most common congenital chest wall deformity (88%)**
- Associated disorders: marfanoid features (19%), mild scoliosis (18.4%), severe scoliosis (11.4%), and Ehlers–Danlos syndrome (2.2%)
- Pathophysiology: depression deformity of the chest wall

Clinical Presentation
- History: dyspnea, exercise intolerance, chest pain, and palpitations
- Present at birth but progresses with growth, leading to increased cardiopulmonary symptoms as chest wall becomes more rigid

Indications for Surgery
- **$2 parameters: CT index >3.25, PFTs indicating restrictive/obstructive disease; heart compression/murmurs, MVP, cardiac displacement or conduction abnormality; progression of deformity with physical symptoms; and failed Ravitch or Nuss procedure**

Pectus Carinatum
Epidemiology
- Associated disorders: congenital heart disease
- Pathophysiology: overgrowth of costal cartilages leads to forward buckling and secondarily deforming pressure on body of sternum
- Chondrogladiolar (more common): "Chicken breast"
- Chondromanubrial: "Pouter pigeon breast"

Treatment
- Indication for surgery: improve cosmesis (>90%), usually in preadolescent years
- Non-operative management: exercise, posture program, and orthotic bracing

- Procedure: costochondral resection
  - Transverse osteotomy of anterior sternum
  - Bilateral cartilage resection (to prevent recurrence)
  - Preservation of perichondrium (new cartilage growth)
- Support bar for 4–6 months

23-6: FOREIGN BODY

Clinical Presentation
- **Tracheobronchial foreign bodies:** sudden onset of choking or coughing—most lodge in bronchi, typically on the right, 10% above the carina; wheezing and rhonchi, possible decreased breath sounds; **frequently food (peanuts)**
- **Esophageal foreign bodies:** sudden onset of choking, drooling; can present with respiratory distress since objects tend to lodge **just below the cricopharyngeus muscle** impinging on the airway; **frequently coins**
- **Gastrointestinal foreign bodies:** once in stomach, most ingested foreign bodies pass through GI tract in 5 days
  - Sites of potential obstruction: pylorus, ligament of Treitz, ileocecal valve, undiagnosed Meckel diverticulum, and appendix

Treatment
- **All lodged objects should be removed**
- Laryngeal: Heimlich maneuver; direct laryngoscopy and removal with McGill forceps in OR under close monitoring and sedation if necessary
- Tracheobronchial: rigid bronchoscopic removal with forceps or Fogarty catheter retrograde removal; food particles sometimes require fragmentation
  - If object too distal and not amenable to bronchoscopic retrieval, thoracotomy required, pending identification of type of foreign body
  - Postoperative CXR to exclude pneumothorax
- Esophageal: rigid endoscopy; after removal of object, reassess the esophageal wall.
- Postoperative CXR to exclude pneumomediastinum
- Gastrointestinal: if object still in stomach after 4 weeks, retrieve via gastroscopy
  - If object lodges distally (ligament of Treitz, ileocecal valve) and causes obstruction or significant GI hemorrhage, may require laparotomy and enterotomy

ROBOTIC SURGERY

PARTHA BHURTEL • GEORGIOS ORTHOPOULOS • OMAR YUSEF KUDSI

24-1: HISTORY OF ROBOTIC SURGERY

- Unimation Puma 560 robot 1985: Kwoh et al. used it to obtain CT-guided brain biopsies (Unimation PUMA 560, 1985)
- Automated Endoscopic System for Optimal Positioning (AESOP) 1993: a voice activated robotic arm used to manipulate an endoscopic camera
- ROBODOC 1992: designed to achieve greater precision in total hip replacement surgeries—the first surgical robot approved by the FDA
- ZEUS 1998: a master–slave system that consisted of three robotic arms attached to the operating table operated remotely from a surgeon console with three-dimensional (3D) visualization and computer enhancement. The system-filtered tremors and provided 3D vision
- The first trans-Atlantic robotic-assisted laparoscopic cholecystectomy was performed by Marescaux et al. in 2001 using the ZEUS system.

24-2: ADVANTAGES OF ROBOTIC SURGERY

- High-definition, 3D visualization of surgical anatomy.
- A robotic arm manipulates the camera. This helps provide a steady view which is controlled by the surgeon.
- Wristed surgical instruments (EndoWrist) with 7 degrees of freedom mimicking human wrist and hands akin to open surgery in a minimally invasive setting.
- Intuitive instrument manipulation and increased dexterity: The instrument tip movements are synchronous with the surgeon's hand.
- Elimination of fulcrum effect: The instrument tips move in the same direction as the surgeon's hand unlike with conventional laparoscopy where the surgeon must move the hand in opposite direction of the instrument tip motion secondary to the fulcrum effect.
- Elimination of physiologic tremors and scaling of motion using software and hardware filters makes fine and precise movements possible.
- Improved ergonomics. Surgeon is able to sit comfortably and operate from a remote console. There are four customizable parameters and multiple ergonomic adjustments, which could help reduce surgeon fatigue.
- Provides all the advantages of laparoscopic surgery, viz. smaller incisions, decreased postoperative pain, shortened hospital stay, decreased risk of infection, better cosmesis.

24-3: DISADVANTAGES OF ROBOTIC SURGERY

- High cost: High establishment cost along with required maintenance costs. The robotic surgical instruments expire after a set number of clinical uses thus adding to the cost. However, the reimbursement for robotic procedures is at the same rate as conventional laparoscopic surgery.
- Bulky and difficult to maneuvre especially in today's already crowded operating rooms
- Require docking and undocking if working in multiple areas of the abdomen
- Learning curve associated with use of the robotic platform
- Absence of haptic feedback
- Given the complexity of the robotic system, there is increased opportunities for technological failures.
- Increases communication requirements between members of the operating team
- Could result in reduction of the ability to maintain vision in the operative field with potential blind spots

24-4: THE DA VINCI SYSTEM

- A master–slave system consisting of a surgeon console, vision cart, and a surgical/moveable patient cart
- Surgical console:
  - Located far from the patient table
  - It contains:
    - A stereoscopic viewer that provides high-definition, 3D images of the surgical field with adjustable magnification.

- Master controller: designed so that each hand can control a robotic arm and the instrument placed in it. They have clutch buttons that disengage the robotic arms enabling the surgeon to reposition the controllers without moving the instruments.
    - Foot pedals that consist of the master clutch and pedals that allow the surgeon to control robotic arms, camera, and the energy sources.
    - A touch pad that functions as the control unit of the surgical console
  - Surgeon sits at the console and controls the movements of the robotic arms, 3D camera, and the wristed instruments.
  - Surgeon receives high-definition, real-time 3D image into the stereo viewer.
  - The wristed instruments are aligned with the master controller and thus with the surgeons' hands. Movement of the surgeon's hand and the instruments are synchronous and there is no fulcrum effect.
  - The newer systems have dual console for an assistant surgeon.
- Vision cart
  - Consists of video monitor, processor, light source, insufflator, etc.
  - Holds a dual light source and two separate high-definition cameras in a single casing that generate a 3D image of the surgical field. The camera has digital zoom capabilities allowing for true depth perception and high magnification.
  - Manipulated by a robotic arm controlled by the surgeon. This allows for a steady view of the operative field.
- Patient cart
  - Consists of four arms: one for the camera and three other arms for placing wristed instruments. The arms interface with the patient directly at the operating table. After docking, the arms engage various surgical instruments including graspers, needle drivers, electrosurgical and suction devices.

Basic Surgical Setup

- Initial access and trocar placement
  - Either the Veress needle technique, optical view trocar or an open "cut-down" approach can be used to gain access into the abdominal cavity to establish pneumoperitoneum.
  - Triangulation of the surgical field: It is important to place left and right instruments on either side of the camera to achieve triangulation of the surgical target with respect to the camera and the working arms. With regards to robotic surgery, aligning the central column of the surgical cart, surgical target, and the camera provides maximal visualization.
  - A minimum of 6–8 cm distance must be maintained between the camera port and the trocars. Adequate spacing prevents the robotic arms from interfering with each other.
  - A minimum distance of 8 cm is recommended between the trocars and the surgical field.
  - The trocars should be inserted until the black markings are seen. These markings represent the point that enables maximal movement with minimal tissue truama.
  - Trocar lengths: 11 cm (standard) and 16 cm (bariatric).
  - Trocar diameters: 8.5 and 12 mm. Currently, 0- or 30-degree scopes are available.
- Docking the robot
  - The operating table is placed into the optimal position for the planned procedure. Further changes in the position are not possible after the robot is docked.
  - The motorized surgical cart is driven into the optimal position by an assistant.
  - Robotic arms are then attached/coupled to their cannulas to complete the docking.
- Inserting the instruments
  - The tip is inserted first into the trocar and loaded onto the robotic arm by snapping them into the mechanical rotors.
  - Once the light starts blinking in the robot arm, instruments are manually directed under vision into the surgical field. Once in satisfactory position, the arm is locked. Once properly loaded, subsequent instrument exchanges are facilitated by "guided instrument exchange" as the system recalls the postion and orientation of the instrument prior to the exchange.
- The team must be trained to quickly undock the robot and provide the surgeon with necessary instruments, should a need to convert to conventional laparoscopic or open surgery arise.

24-5: CURRENT APPLICATIONS OF ROBOTICS IN SURGERY

- Current applications: The FDA has currently approved the da Vinci system for use in general, cardiac, colorectal, gynecologic, head and neck, thoracic, and urologic surgical procedures.
- Robotic surgery has enabled increased adoption of minimally invasive surgery techniques, especially, in urology and gynecology.
- Robotic surgery has showen clear benefit in radical prostatetomy over both open and laparoscopic techniques by decreasing complications, length of hospital stay, better urinary continence and erectile function recovery, and increased rate of free surgical margins.
- Robotics in foregut surgery
  - Robotic surgery has been shown to be safe and feasible for Heller myotomy, Nissen fundoplication, and minimally invasive esophagectomy.
  - It has been able to achieve acceptable oncologic dissections for esophageal cancers.
  - Some studies have shown a lower incidence of esophageal perforation with the use of robotic platform compared to the laparoscopic approach for Heller myotomy.
  - It has demonstrated comparable outcomes but longer operating times and higher costs for Nissen fundoplications.
- Robotics in gastric cancer
  - Studies have shown comparable morbidity, mortality, and the number of lymph nodes retrieved per level between robotic and laparoscopic gastrectomies. Robotic surgery is associated with significantly less blood loss and a shorter hospital stay.
- Robotics in bariatric surgery
  - Enhanced suturing with robotic surgery helps perform manual gastrojejunal anastomoses within reasonal operative time frame. This has been shown in a case-controlled study to be cost effective due to avoidance of use of mechanical staplers.
- Robotics in hepatobiliary/pancreatic surgery
  - No obvious benefit has been demonstrated for robotic multiport cholecystectomy. It is useful for developing familiarity with the robotic platforms by surgeons early in their learning curve.
  - Robotic hepatectomy is feasible. Lack of randomized trails prevents significant conclusions to be drawn comparing open versus laparoscopic versus robotic procedures. A comparative study between robotic and laparoscopic hepatetcomy has shown that robotic approach resulted in high percentage of hepatectomies being completed in a minimally invasive fashion.
  - Pancreaticoduodenectomy, distal/central/total pancreatectomy, pancreatic enucleation, Appleby and Frey procedures have been described. As with hepatectomies, lack of randomized controlled trials prevent drawing conclusions about the superiority of robotic approach.
- Robotics in colorectal surgery
  - No obvious benefit has been demonstrated in robotic colorectal surgery in comparision to standard laparoscopic approach.
  - Robotic surgery may be beneficial in cases involving rectal and pelvic dissection and has been described as an enabling technology as the 3D visualiztion and wristed instruments offer advantages in the limited space. Early results have shown trends toward better sexual or bladder function in rectal surgery.
  - Has been shown to be safe and feasible in combination with transanal minimally invasive surgery.
- Robotics in hernia surgery
  - Robotic platform has been shown to be safe and feasible in ventral hernia repair. Studies have demonstarted shorter length of stay with robotic ventral hernia repair compared to open.

24-6: EVOLVING TECHNOLOGIES

- Single-site surgery: Single-site platform was approved in 2011 for cholecystectomy.
  - The single-site port is made of silicone and can be placed through a 2.5-cm incision. Port has five lumens: three straight lumens for the 3D HD camera, insufflation adaptor and 5-mm assistant port, and two curved lumens that cross the midline for the 5-mm curved robotic cannulae that allow passage of semi-rigid instruments.

- The curved cannulae cross at the middle of the port. This establishes the abdominal wall as the fulcrum and allows for triangulation. The design allows for separation of arms outside the abdominal wall thus maximizing motion.
  - The software compensates for the crossed instruments and thus the left robotic arm instrument is controlled by the right hand and vice versa.
  - Single-site surgery has shown to be feasible in multiple surgeries, viz. cholecystectomy, multiple urological and colorectal procedures.
- FireFly Imaging System
  - The system allows opportunities to perform fluorescence-guided surgery.
  - It is made possible by an optical system that is capable of emitting near-infrared (NIR) laser light alongwith an ability to switch between white light and NIR light in real time.
  - Indocyanine Green is used for the purpose.
  - Currently, it is used for fluorescent cholangiography, evaluation of bowel stump perfusion, lymph node mapping, sentinel lymph node biopsy, and urologic procedures.
- Table motion
  - Lack of ability to change table positions has required docking and redocking for multiple-quadrant abdominal robotic surgery
  - Integrated table motion has been developed for the da Vince Xi system which is Intuitive Surgical's latest robotic-assisted surgical system
  - The Trusystem® 7000dV table is synchronized in movement with the da Vinci surgical system.
  - It provides optimal table position so that gravity assists in anatomic exposure
  - Maximizes reach and access to target anatomy
  - Helps reposition the table during the procedure and thereby helps improve anesthesiolgists' ability to care for the patient

---

24-7: FUTURE DIRECTIONS

- Multiple robotic systems are currently under development aimed at conducting complex procedures through single ports or natural orifices, e.g., the Single-Port Orifice Robotic Technology (SPORT™) Surgical System (Titan Medical Inc., Toronto, ON, Canada).
- Systems that provide haptic feedback, e.g., Amadeus Composer™ (Titan Medical Inc., Toronto, ON, Canada).
- Miniature robots that can be placed in vivo and directed to perform tasks.

25-1: UROLOGIC TRAUMA AND INJURIES

Ureteral Injury
- Most commonly from gynecologic surgery—higher risk associated with hysterectomy, C-section, and laparotomy for pelvic inflammatory disease. Occurs during vasculature dissection.
- Treatment:
  - In trauma, ureteral laceration repair during laparotomy in stable patients. Temporary urinary drainage in unstable patients. Ureteral stenting, or resection and primary repair for traumatic ureteral contusions.
    - **Lower third of the ureter:** reimplantation into bladder ± psoas–hitch procedure (optional antireflux ureteral anastomosis to minimize potential damage to upper urinary tract)
    - **Mid-ureteral injuries:** primary end-to-side ureteroureterostomy if no significant loss of viable ureter between proximal and distal ends or transureteroureterostomy
    - **Upper ureteral injuries:**
      - Nephrostomy tube in ipsilateral kidney: primary ureteroureterostomy
      - Auto-transplantation of kidney if there is extensive loss of ureter
      - Ileoureteral replacement if extensive loss of ureter, especially if solitary kidney

Always drain the site of repair, keep a tension-free anastomosis, surround repair with fat or omentum if at a high risk for infection

Urethral Injury
- Epidemiology: occurs in 4–14% of pelvic fractures
- Clinical presentation: blood at urethral meatus, inability to urinate, a high-riding prostate
- Diagnosis: high clinical suspicion; retrograde urethrography
- Classification
  - Posterior urethra (above urogenital diaphragm)
    - Type I: urethral stretch
    - Type II: urethral disruption proximal to the urogenital diaphragm
    - Type III: proximal and distal disruption of urogenital diaphragm
  - Anterior urethra (below urogenital diaphragm)
- Treatment
  - Posterior injuries: early endoscopic realignment with a stented Foley
    - Suprapubic catheterization with delayed antegrade and retrograde endoscopic repairs or open surgical repair if realignment not possible
  - Anterior injuries: primary realignment with Foley catheterization
    - Suprapubic catheterization followed by delayed open surgical repair if severe

Renal Parenchymal Injury
- Diagnosis: CT imaging, intravenous pyelogram
- Injuries
  - Renal vein: repair if stable, otherwise ligate
  - Renal artery: repair in stable patients, otherwise nephrectomy
  - Pedicle avulsion: nephrectomy
  - Extravasation: repair, parietal resection, or nephrectomy
- Perform urinary drainage (stent, percutaneous drain, percutaneous nephrostomy tube) in patients with urinoma, fever, pain, infection, fistula, or ileus.

Perinephric hematoma: explore if there is contrast extravasation or expanding hematoma

Bladder Injury
Diagnosis: retrograde cystography in stable patients who have gross hematuria and a pelvic fracture, a concern for bladder injury, or a pelvic ring fracture with clinical signs of bladder injury
- Extraperitoneal female: Foley catheter
- Extraperitoneal male: suprapubic cystostomy
- Intraperitoneal: primary repair and suprapubic cystostomy

Other Injuries
Penile fracture: clinical presentation of penile bruising, swelling, "cracking" or "snapping" during intercourse, and detumescence. Needs surgical exploration and repair
Genitourinary infection and burns: surgical exploration and debridement

Testicular rupture: scrotal exploration and debridement with tunica closure and/or orchiectomy of nonsalvageable testicle

Penile amputation: Wrap amputated penis in saline soaked gauze, place on ice. Immediate reimplantation

25-2: OBSTRUCTION

Obstructive Uropathy
- Etiology
  - Benign prostatic hypertrophy
  - Urethral stricture
  - Bladder neck contracture
  - Cancer of the prostate or bladder
  - Bladder calculi
  - Neurogenic bladder

Benign Prostatic Hypertrophy (J Urol. 1992;148(5):1549–1557)
- Clinical presentation: urinary frequency, nocturia, hesitancy, urgency, and weak stream
- American Urological Association Symptom Score: score ranges from 0 to 35
  - Based on degree of incomplete emptying, frequency, intermittency, urgency, weak stream, straining, and nocturia
- Physical examination: abdomen, genitalia, and digital rectal examination
- Lab tests: urinalysis, serum prostate-specific antigen, and serum creatinine
- Clinical testing: uroflowmetry, assessment of postvoid residual, and urodynamics
- Medical treatment
  - **Alpha-adrenergic antagonists** (terazosin, doxazosin, tamsulosin) to reduce smooth muscle tension in the prostate
  - **5-Alpha-reductase inhibitors** (finasteride) to reduce prostate size
- Surgical treatment
  - **Transurethral resection of prostate:** laser vs. traditional (if <80–100 g)
  - **Transurethral resection of prostate syndrome:** due to hyponatremic solution used during procedure
    - Hyponatremia causing mental confusion, nausea, vomiting, hypertension, bradycardia, and visual disturbance
    - Treatment: Lasix and normal saline
- Open prostatectomy: preferred when prostate weighs more than 100 g

25-3: NEOPLASMS

Renal Cell Carcinoma
- Epidemiology: 80–85% of all primary renal neoplasms; 2:1 male-to-female ratio
- Risk factors: smoking, von Hippel–Lindau syndrome
- Clinical presentation: asymptomatic until advanced
  - **Classic triad: hematuria, flank pain, and palpable abdominal mass**
- 25% have metastases at diagnosis, many with paraneoplastic syndromes
- Diagnosis: incidental finding on a CT performed for other reasons
  - Enhancement of lesion, thickened irregular walls, septa, and multiloculations
- Treatment
  - Stage I or II (limited to kidney): partial vs. radical nephrectomy
  - Stage III: surgery with removal of any IVC thrombus
    - Invasion into adrenal or perinephric tissues but not beyond Gerota fascia
    - Enlarged abdominal lymph nodes
    - Invasion of the renal vein or inferior vena cava
  - Stage IV: surgery only for palliative care or in clinical trials
    - Distant and/or extensive lymph node metastases, tumor beyond Gerota fascia
  - Generally not responsive to chemotherapy or radiotherapy

Bladder Cancer
- Risk factors
  - Transitional epithelium: smoking, industrial solvents, aniline dyes
  - Squamous cell: chronic Foley use, bladder stones, bilharzias infection
- Pathology: transitional epithelium (90%); squamous cell (7%)
- **Clinical presentation: gross or microscopic hematuria in 70–95%**
- Diagnosis and staging: cystoscopy with transurethral resection
- Staging: depth of invasion
- Treatment: determined by stage, grade, size, and number of tumors detected
  - Low-grade superficial tumors: transurethral resection

- Muscle-invasive tumor (stage T2 or higher): radical cystectomy +/– chemotherapy
  - Intravesical BCG to reduce the rate of recurrence and progression
  - Radical cystectomy requires the creation of a urostomy or neobladder from small or large intestine for the diversion of urine; most commonly an ileal conduit using ileum 15–20 cm proximal to ileocecal valve

Prostate Cancer
- Epidemiology: most common cancer in men, the second most common cause of cancer death in men
- Risk factors: increased age, African-American ethnicity, family history, high dietary fat intake
- Diagnosis: prostate-specific antigen **>4.0 ng/mL**; transrectal ultrasound biopsy; Gleason score
- Metastatic workup: CXR, bone scan, and pelvic CT
- Treatment
  - Small, localized, well-differentiated cancer: active surveillance or external beam radiation or radical prostatectomy or brachytherapy
  - Moderately differentiated cancer: radiation therapy or radical prostatectomy +/– pelvic lymphadenectomy
  - Locally advanced disease (T3): neoadjuvant hormone therapy, then external beam radiation, option of tumor debulking
  - Castrate resistant prostate cancer (when the androgen receptor continues to work despite medical castration)
    - Observation and continued medical therapy if nonmetastatic
    - Abiraterone with prednisone, enzalutamide, docetaxel, or sipuleucel-T if the patient has low to no symptoms and good functional status
    - Vitamin D and calcium for fracture prevention
    - Radium-223 if the patient has symptoms from bony metastasis
    - Abiraterone with prednisone, cabazitaxel, or enzalutamide for patients who are relatively healthy and have received prior docetaxel therapy
    - Palliative care if failed docetaxel therapy and poor functional status

Testicular Cancer
- Epidemiology: most common malignancy in men 15–35 years of age
- Pathology: seminomas or nonseminomatous germ cell tumors (NSGCT)

Testicular Cancer—Diagnosis
- CT and chest radiography to identify distant and nodal metastasis
- Serum markers
- **Alpha-fetoprotein:** elevated 80–85% of NSGCT, not seminomas
- **Beta-human chorionic gonadotropin:** elevated 80–85% of NSGCT, <20% of seminomas
- **Lactate dehydrogenase**

- Clinical presentation: nodule or painless swelling in one testis
- Treatment: radical inguinal orchiectomy with high ligation of spermatic cord
- Seminomas
  - Radiation to para-aortic nodes regardless of CT involvement
  - Add chemotherapy for nodal involvement (cisplatin based)
  - Retroperitoneal lymph node dissection for residual retroperitoneal disease
- Nonseminomas
  - If normal para-aortic nodes on CT: retroperitoneal lymph node dissection followed by chemotherapy (platinum based)
  - If nodes enlarged on CT: chemotherapy first, then nodal dissection
- Surveillance: follow tumor markers to detect patients with persistent occult disease

25-4: Stone Disease
- Risk factors: low urine volume, hypercalciuria, hyperoxaluria (enteric hyperoxaluria and short bowel syndrome), hyperuricosuria, dietary factors (high oxalate, low calcium, and low sodium), history of prior nephrolithiasis, and type I renal tubular acidosis
- Epidemiology
  - Prevalence: 3–12% over lifetime
  - Types of stones: 80% calcium stones, either calcium oxalate or calcium phosphate
    - Other: struvite and cystine stones
- Clinical presentation: pain when stone enters and/or obstructs ureter
  - Waves or paroxysms due to ureteral spasm/distention

- Starts in flank and radiates to the front upper abdomen for kidney-related pain or to the groin for ureter-related pain
- Diagnosis: microscopic hematuria and noncontrast CT
  - Plain abdominal film, ultrasound, and intravenous pyelography; other diagnostic modalities
- Medical treatment: pain medication, hydration, Flomax, steroids, and alpha-blockers
- Surgical treatment
  - Renal and proximal ureteral stones <2 cm: extracorporeal shock wave lithotripsy (contraindications: acute UTI, urosepsis, uncorrected coagulopathy or bleeding disorder, pregnancy)
  - Stones >2 cm: percutaneous lithotripsy
  - Rarely open surgery

25-5: OTHER SURGICAL CONSIDERATIONS

Enterovesical Fistula
- More common in men than women
- Usually from diverticular disease
- Can present with pneumaturia and fecaluria
- Diagnose with CT imaging; need cystoscopy to exclude bladder cancer and colonoscopy to exclude colon cancer
- Surgical treatment consists of removal of fistula tract, bladder wall repair, and colic resection with or without diverting colostomy

Testicular Torsion
- **Surgical emergency**
- Clinical signs include horizontal testicular lie, high-riding testicle, pain, tenderness; swelling
- More common on the left testicle
- Ultrasound to evaluate arterial flow, testicular perfusion
- Immediate surgical exploration
  - Orchiopexy if viable testicle
  - Orchectomy if nonviable
  - Orchiopexy for contralateral side to reduce torsion risk
- 20% testicular viability if detorsion after 12 hours; no testicular viability if detorsion after 24 hours

26-1: BENIGN GYNECOLOGIC CONDITIONS

Pelvic Inflammatory Disease

Definition: spectrum of inflammatory disorders of the upper female genital tract, including any combination of endometritis, salpingitis, tubo-ovarian abscess (TOA), and pelvic peritonitis, due to ascension of micro-organisms from the cervix and vagina

Epidemiology

- **Leading cause of infertility**
- Etiology: sexually transmitted diseases (many from untreated asymptomatic infections)
  - *Neisseria gonorrhea*: 33–50% of pelvic inflammatory disease (PID)
  - *Chlamydia trachomatis*: ~60% of salpingitis (PID precursor)
  - Vaginal flora (anaerobes, *Gardnerella vaginalis*, *Haemophilus influenzae*, enteric gram-negative rods, and *Streptococcus agalactiae*)

Clinical Presentation

- May be asymptomatic
- Fever, cervical motion tenderness, lower abdominal pain, new or different vaginal discharge, painful intercourse, and irregular menstrual bleeding
- Symptoms usually after recent sexual activity
- Complications: TOA, infertility, ectopic pregnancy, chronic pelvic pain

Diagnosis

- **Diagnosis based on clinical findings**
- Bimanual pelvic examination: abnormal cervical or vaginal mucopurulent discharge, cervical motion tenderness and/or adnexal tenderness, and abundant WBC on saline microscopy of vaginal secretions
- Documented cervical infection with *N. gonorrhea* or *C. trachomatis*
- Endometrial biopsy: histopathologic evidence of endometritis
- Transvaginal ultrasound or MRI: thickened, fluid-filled tubes, +/– free fluid in pelvis or tubo-ovarian complex, tubal hyperemia
- Laparoscopy: 65–90% positive predictive value (PPV) for tubal disease or abscess

Differential Diagnosis (DDx) of PID
• Appendicitis
• Enteritis
• Ectopic pregnancy
• Septic abortion
• Hemorrhagic or ruptured ovarian cysts
• Ovarian malignancy
• Ovarian torsion
• Degeneration of myoma

Management

- Antibiotics: empiric, broad coverage to include *N. gonorrhea* and *C. trachomatis*
  - Mild or moderate PID: parenteral and oral therapy have equal clinical efficacy, and thus oral is preferred unless specific indication for parenteral
    - Indications for parenteral therapy: TOA, pregnancy, severe illness, nausea/vomiting, unable to follow or tolerate outpatient oral regimen, no clinical response to oral therapy
- Oral regimens
  - Ceftriaxone 250 mg intramuscularly in a single dose **plus** doxycycline 100 mg orally twice a day for 14 days, with or without metronidazole 500 mg orally twice a day for 14 days **or**
  - Cefoxitin 2 gram intramuscularly in a single dose **plus** probenecid 1 gram orally in a single dose **plus** doxycycline 100 mg orally twice a day for 14 days, with or without metronidazole 500 mg orally twice a day for 14 days **or**
- Parenteral regimens: continue for 24–48 hours until clinical improvement, then transition to oral regimen for 14-day course
  - Cefotetan 2 g IV q12 h or Cefoxitin 2 g IV q6h plus Doxycycline 100 mg q12h
  - Clindamycin 900mg IV q8h plus Gentamicin loading dose 2 mg/kg, followed by maintenance dose 1.5 mg/kg every 8 hours
  - Unasyn 3 g IV q6h + Doxycycline 100 mg q12h

Uterine Fibroids (Leiomyomas)
Epidemiology
- **Most common neoplasm in females:** affects 70–80% of women by age 50
- Typically do not progress to sarcoma, but sarcoma may be found in 0.05–0.28% of surgeries for myometrial mass

Clinical Presentation
- Menorrhagia, bulk symptoms (pelvic pressure, urinary frequency), infertility
- **Fibroids are hormone dependent** (estrogen and progestin receptors)
  - May enlarge rapidly during the first trimester of pregnancy and regress after menopause

Diagnosis
- Physical examination: enlarged uterus with irregular contour
- Imaging: pelvic ultrasound is standard; MRI can be helpful for surgical planning
- DDx of enlarged uterus: adenomyoma or adenomyosis, sarcoma, endometrial carcinoma, pregnancy
- Pathology
  - Arises from overgrowth of smooth muscle and connective tissue of the uterus
  - Round, well circumscribed, but not encapsulated, solid nodules, varied in size and shape

Treatment
- **Asymptomatic: no treatment indicated**
- Menorrhagia: hormonal therapy, NSAIDs, uterine artery embolization, or myomectomy
- Pelvic pressure/bulk symptoms: myomectomy or hysterectomy (definitive)

Ovarian Cysts
Epidemiology
- Adnexal masses are found in females of all ages
- Prevalence of cysts in women age 25–40 is 6.6%
- Simple cysts <10 cm typically resolve spontaneously

Clinical Presentation
- Most are asymptomatic
- Most common: dull aching, or severe, sudden, and sharp pain in lower abdomen, pelvis, vagina, lower back, or thighs; may be constant or intermittent
- Other: fullness, heaviness, pressure, swelling, or bloating in abdomen; pain during or shortly after the beginning or end of menstrual period; irregular periods or abnormal uterine bleeding or spotting; change in frequency or ease of urination; and difficulty with bowel movements

Diagnosis
- Physical examination: low sensitivity for diagnosing adnexal masses
- **Transvaginal ultrasound: imaging modality of choice**
- Definition by ultrasound: any ovarian follicle larger than 2 cm
  - Simple cyst: unilocular, uniform thin wall surrounding a single cavity, no internal echoes
  - Complex cyst: multilocular, thickening of the wall, projections into lumen or on surface, or abnormalities within the cyst contents

Treatment
- **Most simple cysts do not require treatment**
- Indications for surgery: persistent simple ovarian cysts larger than 5–10 cm, complex cysts, severe symptoms from endometriosis, torsion, rupture if evidence of ongoing bleeding
- Goals of surgery: confirm diagnosis, assess for malignancy, peritoneal washings for cytology
  - Remove entire cyst intact, frozen section, interrogate other abdominal organs
  - If premenopausal, goal is to excise cyst alone with preservation of ovary, unless malignancy discovered
  - If postmenopausal, oophorectomy
- Endometrioma (osis)
  - Medical: achieve an anovulatory state
  - Laparoscopy: removal of endometriomas, ablation or excision of endometriotic implants, and lysis of adhesions

Types of Ovarian Cysts			
	Clinical Presentation	Pathology	Treatment and Complications
Functional or simple cysts (Graafian follicle or follicular cyst)	• Asymptomatic • Spontaneously resolves • **Most common ovarian cyst**	Thin-walled, lined by one or more layers of granulosa cell, and filled with clear fluid	**Rupture can create sharp, severe adnexal pain (Mittelschmerz), occurs in middle of menstrual cycle**
Corpus luteum cyst	• Asymptomatic • If large enough: intermittent torsion • Oral contraceptives prevent formation	Fluid-/blood-filled corpus luteum after ovulation	Usually does not require surgical intervention
Hemorrhagic cyst	• Adnexal pain (rapid stretching of ovarian capsule 2/2 bleeding)	Small blood vessel in wall breaks, blood enters the cyst	If ruptures can lead to hemoperitoneum; surgery if evidence of ongoing bleeding or unstable, but typically not needed. Treat with transfusion
Ovarian teratoma (complex cyst)	• 10–20% of all ovarian neoplasms	**Parenchymal cell types representing usually all three germ layers** (hair, endocrine tissue, fat, teeth, skin, and muscle)	• Torsion (3.2–16%) • Malignant (0.1–2%) transformation • Rupture • Infection • Hemolytic anemia.
Endometrioma (complex cyst)	• Ovary most frequent site of endometriosis	Ovary enlarges with cystic, blood-filled spaces	• If very large: increased torsion • Rupture: spills material into pelvis, onto surface uterus, bladder, and bowel

Ovarian (Adnexal) Torsion
Epidemiology
• **Gynecologic surgical emergency**
• **#1 suspect: dermoid tumors;** rarely malignant tumors, secondary to adhesions, pregnancy (ovarian enlargement + laxity of the supporting tissues of the ovary)

Clinical Presentation
• Sudden, severe, unilateral lower abdominal pain, worsens intermittently over hours
• Nausea and vomiting (70%)
• Fever: late symptom when ovary necrotic

Diagnosis
• Tender adnexal mass (50–90%), but absence does not exclude diagnosis
• Pelvic ultrasound with Doppler: ovarian enlargement 2/2 impaired venous/lymphatic drainage
  • **Absence of arterial blood flow diagnostic,** but arterial perfusion may be preserved early on with only obstruction of venous and lymphatic flow
  • Color Doppler sonography helps predict viability of adnexal structures
  • If normal ovarian size, then high negative predictive value

Surgical Treatment
• **Laparoscopy: uncoil torsed ovary, ovarian cystectomy, and possible oophoropexy**
• Salpingo-oophorectomy if severe vascular compromise, peritonitis, or tissue necrosis

Ectopic Pregnancy
Definition: fertilized ovum implants in any tissue other than the uterine wall

Epidemiology
- Prevalence in women who present to ED with the first trimester pain/bleeding: 6–16%
- Location: **fallopian tube most common;** 2% cervix, uterus, or intra-abdominal
- Risk factors
  - Prior tubal damage of any origin (history of PID, history of ectopic pregnancy)
  - Prior tubal ligation
  - Adhesive disease from prior surgery or intra-abdominal inflammatory process (endometriosis)
  - In vitro fertilization

Clinical Presentation
- Mean of 7 weeks after the last normal menstrual period
- Early signs (mild): lower abdominal pain, pain on urinating or defecating, and vaginal bleeding
- Late signs: severe pain as fallopian tube distends, vaginal bleeding from falling progesterone levels, and internal bleeding from hemorrhage of affected tube

Diagnosis
- **Suspect in any female with lower abdominal pain or unusual bleeding who is sexually active and positive pregnancy test**
- Vaginal ultrasound: gestational sac located in the fallopian tube.
- BhCG test: No intrauterine pregnancy with BhCG > 3,000 IU/mL
- Cullen sign: bruising around umbilicus indicates rupture
- Uncertain diagnosis: repeat blood work/ultrasound in a few days; diagnostic laparoscopy

Treatment
- Medical: methotrexate (disrupts growth of developing embryo)
- **Indications for surgery: if evidence of rupture, ongoing bleeding**
  - Salpingostomy: incise affected tube and remove only the pregnancy **or**
  - Salpingectomy: remove the affected tube with the pregnancy
- Complications: hemorrhagic shock; infertility (10–15%)

26-2: UROGYNECOLOGY
Pelvic Organ Prolapse
Definition: descent of one or more pelvic structures (uterus or vaginal apex, anterior vagina, or posterior vagina)

Epidemiology
- Prevalence: symptomatic prolapse in ~6–8% of women
- Risk factors: genetic predisposition, parity, menopause, advancing age, prior pelvic surgery, connective tissue disorders, obesity, chronic constipation

Clinical Presentation
- Symptoms: feeling of a bulge or protrusion through vaginal opening; difficulty voiding or urinary retention

Diagnosis
- Pelvic examination consistent with prolapse
- **Sometimes prolapse only visible with Valsalva or cough**
- Treatment: indicated when symptomatic
- Nonsurgical: pessaries, pelvic floor muscle exercises (Kegels)
- Surgical:
  - Procedure choice depends on location of prolapse (cystocele, rectocele, uterine, vault), surgeon and patient factors
  - Sacrocolpopexy (open, laparoscopic, robotic), transvaginal vault suspension procedures (uterosacral ligament, sacrospinous), anterior and posterior colporrhaphy, colpocleisis (obliteration of vagina)

Stress Urinary Incontinence
Epidemiology
- Risk factors: obesity, multiparity, history of vaginal delivery
- Prevalence: ~15% of women age 25–84

- History: leakage of urine with increases in intra-abdominal pressure (e.g., coughing, sneezing, laughing)

Diagnosis
- Positive cough or Valsalva stress test
- Urodynamic testing helpful if lack of clear diagnosis based on history and physical examination
- DDx: urge incontinence, overflow incontinence, UTI (exclude with urinalysis), neurologic disorder, fistula, vaginitis, drug-induced
- Treatment: depends on patient preference and impact of SUI on quality of life
- Conservative (first line): weight loss, pelvic floor muscle exercises (Kegels)
- Other: Pessary, urethral bulking agents
- Surgery: urethral sling (vaginal), colposuspension (open or laparoscopic)

26-3: MALIGNANT GYNECOLOGIC CONDITIONS

Ovarian Neoplasms
Epidemiology
- Most common cause of cancer death from gynecologic tumors in the United States, average age at diagnosis in United States is 63 years old
- Pathology: 95% epithelial origin
- Prognosis: 46% 5-year survival, closely related to the stage at diagnosis
  - Long-term survival correlates with amount of residual tumor after the first operation
  - Extent of residual disease outweighs stage in its prognostic importance

Clinical Presentation
- Early disease: minimal, nonspecific, or no symptoms
- Late disease: symptoms from metastases to gastrointestinal tract or omentum, ascites
- Symptoms: bloating, abdominal distention, vague crampy abdominal pain, abnormal vaginal bleeding, heavy feeling in pelvis, central weight gain, and/or peripheral weight loss, nausea/vomiting, and bowel obstruction
- Signs: ascites, pleural effusion, and abdominal and/or pelvic mass

Diagnosis
- Laboratory tests: CBC, chemistry panel, LFTs, albumin, and transferrin
  - **CA-125: can be normal with early disease; abnormal result can be from benign and/or nonovarian disease; levels >200–300 usually malignant disease**
- Imaging: pelvic ultrasound or CT vs. MRI if uncertain diagnosis; CXR to evaluate for effusions
- Procedures: **no FNA or percutaneous biopsy of adnexal mass**
  - Diagnostic paracentesis for ascites or diffuse carcinomatosis if no obvious mass
  - Diagnostic and staging laparotomy/laparoscopy
- DDx:
  - Nonovarian intra-abdominal cancer (pancreatic, gastric, and colorectal)
  - Benign adnexal mass: ovarian cysts (see above) and uterine fibroids (see above)
  - Irritable bowel syndrome
  - Gallbladder disease
  - Diverticular disease

Surgical Management
- Gold standard: midline laparotomy for resection and complete surgical staging
- Laparoscopy: thin, young women with small lesions, stage I disease, where ovary can be removed without rupture
- **Intensive staging: peritoneal cytology + multiple peritoneal biopsies + omentectomy + pelvic and para-aortic lymph node sampling**
- Cytoreductive surgery: goal is to reduce tumor burden to no visible disease; however, optimal tumor debulking is defined as reduction of implants to ≤1 cm
- Interval debulking: questionable if improves survival. Do after chemotherapy

Chemotherapy
- Postoperative: cisplatin/carboplatin + paclitaxel
- Intraperitoneal: cisplatin if optimally debulked disease and Stage II/III
- Neoadjuvant: 2–3 cycles and then re-evaluate for surgical cytoreduction

Ovarian, Fallopian Tubal, and Peritoneal Cancer Staging System (FIGO Staging System)

Stage I: Tumor growth limited to the ovaries or fallopian tubes
- IA: limited to one ovary (capsule intact) or fallopian tube with no ascites or tumor on external surface
- IB: limited to both ovaries (capsules intact) or fallopian tubes with no ascites or tumor on external surface
- IC: IA or IB with tumor on surface of one or both ovaries or fallopian tubes, capsule rupture, ascites with malignant cells, and positive washings
  - IC1 surgical spill
  - IC2 capsule ruptured before surgery
  - IC3 malignant cells in ascites or peritoneal washings

Stage II: tumor involves one or both ovaries or fallopian tubes with pelvic extension or peritoneal cancer
- IIA: extension of growth or metastases to uterus and/or tubes and/or ovaries
- IIB: extension to other pelvic tissues

Stage III: tumor involving one or both ovaries with peritoneal implants outside the pelvis and/or positive retroperitoneal nodes, superficial liver metastases
- IIIA: grossly limited to pelvis but histologic proof of microscopic disease on abdominal peritoneal surfaces and/or positive retroperitoneal lymph nodes
- IIIB: confirmed implants outside of pelvis on the abdominal peritoneal surface; no implant exceeds 2 cm in diameter and/or positive retroperitoneal lymph nodes
- IIIC: abdominal implants larger than 2 cm (includes extension of tumor to capsule of liver and spleen) and/or positive retroperitoneal lymph nodes

Stage IV: distant metastases, pleural effusion with positive cytology, and parenchymal liver metastases
- IVA: pleural effusion with positive cytology
- IVB: parenchymal metastases and metastases to extra-abdominal organs (including inguinal lymph nodes)

Uterine Neoplasms

Epidemiology
- Most common cancer of the female reproductive tract in the United States
- Pathology: endometrial cancer (95%) of which 80% are endometrioid adenocarcinoma; nonendometrioid adenocarcinoma (clear cell, serous), squamous, and undifferentiated make up the rest
  - Other: uterine sarcoma (4%) (carcinosarcomas or mixed homologous Müllerian tumors), leiomyosarcomas, and endometrial stromal sarcomas

Clinical Presentation
- **75–90% present with postmenopausal vaginal bleeding**
  - Only 3–20% of women with postmenopausal bleeding have a gynecologic malignancy; most of these have endometrial cancer
- Less than 5% are diagnosed incidentally when the patient is asymptomatic
- Symptoms of advanced disease: purulent genital discharge, lower abdominal pain, pelvic cramping, weight loss, anorexia, anemia, and change in bladder or bowel habits

Risk Factors for Endometrial Cancer

Unopposed and/or Increased Levels of Estrogen
- Obesity
- Exogenous estrogen w/o periodic progestin in postmenopausal women
- Tamoxifen
- Nulliparity
- Infertility
- Early menarche
- Late menopause
- Diabetes
- History of endometrial polyp

Diagnosis
- No recommended screening for asymptomatic women
- Labs: CBC, chemistry panel, LFTs, CA-125, and clotting profile
- Histologic diagnosis: endometrial biopsy, endometrial curettage, or hysterectomy specimen
- **Dilation and curettage (D&C): definitive technique for diagnosis**

- Hysteroscopy: guides directed biopsies of suspicious areas (evaluates endocervical canal)
  - Concern exists regarding transtubal intraperitoneal expulsion of cancer cells
- **Transvaginal ultrasound:** excludes other pelvic pathology that might contribute to postmenopausal bleeding
- Additional imaging is necessary only when surgical staging not planned

---

Staging Uterine Carcinoma (FIGO Staging System)

- Stage I: tumor confined to corpus uteri
  - IA: tumor limited to endometrium or invades less than one-half of myometrium
  - IB: tumor invades one-half or more of the myometrium
- Stage II: tumor invades stromal connective tissue of cervix but not beyond uterus
- Stage III: tumor involves serosa and/or adnexa
  - IIIA: tumor involves serosa and/or adnexa
  - IIIB: vaginal involvement or parametrial involvement
  - IIIC1: lymph node metastasis to pelvic lymph nodes
  - IIIC2: lymph node metastasis to para-aortic lymph nodes
- Stage IV: extending outside true pelvis or involving mucosa of bladder or rectum
  - IVA: invasion into mucosa of bladder or intestine
  - IVB: spread to distant organs (including inguinal lymph nodes)

Surgical Treatment
- **Total hysterectomy with bilateral salpingo-oophorectomy with pelvic and para-aortic lymph node dissection,** usually via minimally invasive approach (e.g., laparoscopic or robotic). Radical hysterectomy only indicated when gross cervical involvement in order to accomplish cytoreduction.
- Debulking: increased median survival, even for advanced stage cancer

Radiation
- Definitive treatment for medically inoperable patients at all stages, improves survival
- Postoperative after staging: intermediate-risk patients
  - Reduces recurrence but does not improve survival
  - High-risk patients unlikely to be cured without radiation

Chemotherapy/Hormonal Therapy
- Chemotherapy: serous histology, advanced stage or recurrent disease; multiple regimens
- Hormonal therapy: may be used in setting of nonoperative candidates or in those in whom radiation is contraindicated
  - Types of hormonal treatment: progestins and tamoxifen

Cervical Neoplasms
Epidemiology
- Second most common malignancy in women worldwide; more common in Hispanic, African-American, and Native American women
- Leading cause of cancer-related death among women in developing countries
- Pathogenesis
  - **Human papilloma virus (HPV) viral DNA detected in more than 99.7% of squamous intraepithelial lesions and invasive cervical cancers**
  - High infection rate, but most clear spontaneously within months to a few years
    - Low risk: HPV 6b, 11 (low-grade dysplasia, never found in invasive cancer)
    - High risk: HPV 16, 18 (50–80% of dysplasia; up to 70% of invasive cancer)
- Risks of carcinogenesis: high-risk HPV infection and persistent infection, age at first intercourse, multiple sexual partners, promiscuous male partners, history of sexually transmitted diseases, immunosuppression, poor nutritional status, and smoking
- Pathology: squamous cell carcinoma (69%), adenocarcinoma (25%)

Clinical Presentation
- Abnormal Papanicolaou smear
- First symptom: abnormal vaginal bleeding, usually postcoital
- Other symptoms: vaginal discomfort, malodorous discharge, and dysuria
- Late symptoms indicate local organ involvement: constipation, hematuria, fistula, and obstruction

Diagnosis
- Physical examination: normal early-stage; later-stage cervix with gross erosion, ulcer, mass

- Bimanual examination: bulky mass, bleeding in advanced disease
- Pap smear cytology, colposcopy with directed biopsies; cystoscopy, proctosigmoidoscopy
- CBC, chemistry panel, LFTs, and CXR for staging
- MRI if stage IA2 or IB1 to determine surgical candidacy; CT abd/pelvis: mets to liver, lymph nodes, other organs, and evaluate for hydronephrosis/hydroureter

Cervical Cancer Staging System (FIGO Staging System)

Stage I: limited to the uterus
- IA: diagnosed only by microscopy; no visible lesions
- IA1: stromal invasion <3 mm in depth and ≤7 mm in horizontal spread
- IA2: stromal invasion between 3 and 5 mm with horizontal spread ≤7 mm
- IB: visible lesion or a microscopic lesion with more than 5 mm of depth or horizontal spread of more than 7 mm
- IB1: visible lesion 4 cm or less in greatest dimension
- IB2: visible lesion more than 4 cm

Stage II: invades beyond uterus but not to pelvic wall or lower third of vagina
- IIA: without parametrial invasion, but involves upper two-thirds of vagina
  - IIA1: visible lesion 4 cm or less, involving upper two-thirds of vagina
  - IIA2: visible lesion more than 4cm, involving upper two-thirds of vagina
- IIB: with parametrial invasion

Stage III: extends to pelvic wall or lower third of vagina
- IIIA: involves lower third of vagina
- IIIB: extends to pelvic wall and/or causes hydronephrosis or nonfunctioning kidney

Stage IV: extends beyond true pelvis or involves bladder or rectal mucosa
- IVA: spreads to adjacent organs
- IVB: distant metastasis (extrapelvic lymph nodes, liver, lung, and bone)

Treatment
- Early stage (Stage IA or IB1): generally surgery
  - Stage 0 (precancer): loop electrosurgical excision procedure, laser, conization, and cryotherapy
  - Stage IA: total hysterectomy, conization (IA1), modified radical hysterectomy with pelvic lymphadenectomy (IA2)
    - Intracavitary radiation for patients who are not surgical candidates (Stage IA)
  - Stage IB1: radical hysterectomy with bilateral pelvic lymphadenectomy
    - Radical hysterectomy: removal of uterus, cervix, upper half of vagina, and parametria
- Locally advanced (Stage IB2–IVA): chemoradiation
  - Stage IB2–IVA: radiation + cisplatin-based chemotherapy
    - Radiation: brachytherapy plus external beam radiation
- Recurrent or metastatic cervical cancer:
  - Stage IVB and recurrent cancer: chemotherapy
  - Total pelvic exenteration: consider if isolated central pelvic recurrence
  - Palliative radiation: control bleeding, pelvic pain, and/or urinary or bowel obstructions

ANESTHESIA

BIJAN J. TEJA • STEPHANIE B. JONES

The anesthesiologist today—perioperative physician
• Roles include preoperative evaluation, intraoperative management, postoperative care, pain management, and critical care

---

27-1: TYPES OF ANESTHESIA

• General anesthesia: deepest level of anesthesia, patient unarousable even with painful stimulus, typically requires endotracheal tube or LMA
• Monitored anesthesia care: ranges from minimal sedation/anxiolysis to deep sedation, but patient should respond purposefully to repeated or painful stimuli. Airway instrumentation usually not required
• Epidural: catheter placed in epidural space; local anesthetic +/- opioid infused to maintain anesthesia
• Spinal: usually single injection of local anesthetic +/- opioid into the dural sac (between L1 and S2) typically providing 1–3 hours of analgesia depending on dose and local anesthetic agent
• Regional: local nerve block for intraoperative anesthesia and/or postoperative analgesia

Preoperative Evaluation
• H&P, allergies, previous anesthetic issues, family history of problems with anesthesia (e.g., malignant hyperthermia)
• Last meal/drink: for elective cases, wait 8 hours after heavy meal, 6 hours after light meal, 4 hours after breast milk, 2 hours after clear liquids. It is acceptable to administer premeds such as acetaminophen or gabapentin with a sip of water before procedure.
• Review labs, ECHO and EKG results, previous type and screen results if available (presence of antibodies may complicate cross-matching)
• See chapter on preoperative evaluation for more on risk stratification and specific comorbidities
• Airway evaluation includes Mallampati classification (Fig. 27-1), dental assessment (prominent, loose or chipped teeth), mouth opening, neck range of motion. Also, mandibular protrusion, thyromental distance, and hyomental distance.
  • Predictors of difficult mask ventilation: presence of a beard, BMI >26 kg/m^2, lack of teeth, age >55, history of snoring
  • Predictors of difficult intubation: high Mallampati score, short neck, receding mandible, prominent maxillary incisors, history of difficult intubation

Figure 27-1 Mallampati Classification (From Diepenbrock, N. *Quick Reference to Critical Care*, 4th ed. Philadelphia, PA: Lippincott Williams & Wilkins, 2012.)

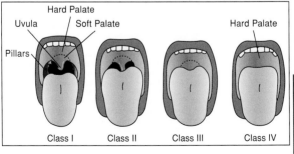

ASA PS Classification	Definition	Examples, including but not limited to:
ASA I	Normal, healthy patient	Healthy, nonsmoking, no or minimal alcohol use
ASA II	Patient with mild systemic disease	Mild diseases without substantive functional limitations: current smoker, social alcohol drinker, BMI 30–40, well-controlled DM or HTN, mild lung disease. Pregnancy is also included in this category
ASA III	Patient with severe systemic disease	Substantive functional limitation, one or more moderate to severe diseases: poorly controlled DM or HTN, COPD, BMI ≥40, alcoholic hepatitis, ESRD on dialysis, MI >3 mo ago, TIA, CAD/stents
ASA IV	Patient with severe systemic disease that is a constant threat to life	MI <3 mo ago, ongoing cardiac ischemia, severe valvular dysfunction, sepsis, DIC, ARDS
ASA V	Moribund patient who is not expected to survive without the operation	Ruptured AAA, massive trauma, intracranial bleed with mass effect, ischemic bowel in the face of significant cardiac disease or multiorgan failure
ASA VI	Patient declared brain-dead, organs are being removed for donor purposes	

Adapted from, American Society of Anesthesiologists (ASA) Physical Status Classification. www.asahq.org, accessed July 5, 2016.

*The addition of "E" denotes emergency surgery, i.e., a delay in treatment would lead to a significant increase in the threat to life or body part.

General Anesthesia

Induction

- Preoxygenation allows longer time to intubate before patient desaturates. Usually give 100% O_2 by facemask until end tidal O_2 >80%
- Induction techniques
  - Standard IV induction: typically begin with IV lidocaine and/or opioid to blunt sympathetic response to laryngoscopy, followed by sedative–hypnotic induction agent (propofol most common). Once consciousness lost, begin mask ventilation and give neuromuscular blocking agent. Mask ventilate until patient adequately paralyzed, then intubate (~45 seconds for succinylcholine or until patient fasciculates; ~1–3 minutes for rocuronium depending on dose).
  - Rapid sequence: similar to IV induction but without mask ventilation. Usually for patients at risk of aspiration (emergency surgery without adequate NPO time, severe reflux, pregnancy, etc.). Succinylcholine or high-dose (1.2 mg/kg) rocuronium is given immediately after induction agents to achieve intubating conditions rapidly before O_2 desaturation.
  - Inhalation: often for pediatric patients without established IV access. Use sevoflurane +/− nitrous oxide by facemask to induce because less pungent.
- Induction agents
  - Propofol: most popular agent; facilitates binding of GABA to its receptor, among other effects; very rapid onset. Single-dose effect terminates within minutes because of rapid redistribution. Disadvantage is hypotension due to drop in SVR, preload, and contractility. Safe in CKD and cirrhosis. Often avoided in patients with severe CAD or cardiac valvular disease due to hypotension.
  - Etomidate: mimics GABA. Advantage over propofol is that CO, contractility, and SVR are well maintained. Disadvantages include high frequency n/v (aka "evomidate"), less rapid recovery/more postoperative malaise than propofol and adrenal suppression (more common when used as an infusion in the ICU).
  - Methohexital: barbiturate. Binds GABA receptor. Unlike other induction agents, it does not have anticonvulsant properties. It is thus used to induce anesthesia for electroconvulsive therapy. Disadvantage is longer recovery time and more postoperative malaise than propofol.
  - Ketamine: NMDA antagonist. Advantage is preserved respiratory drive. Excellent adjunct, but rarely used as sole induction agent. Large boluses avoided in patients

with cardiac disease because of increases in SBP, HR, and CO. Also causes disturbing dreams and delirium; risk of this reduced by coadministration of benzodiazepine.

- Opioids
  - Bind mu (μ), kappa (κ), delta (δ), and sigma (σ) receptors. Primary effect is on CNS, but these receptors are found on somatic and sympathetic nerves as well.
  - Side effects include depression of GI motility, sedation and decreased respiratory drive.
  - With the exception of remifentanil, which is metabolized in the plasma, all opioids depend primarily on the liver/CYP system for biotransformation. Excretion is by kidney and biliary system.

	Time to Peak (IV)	Half-Life of Single Dose	Typical Dose
Morphine	20 min	~2 h	2–5 mg
Hydromorphone	10–20 min	~2 h	0.5–1 mg
Fentanyl	A few minutes	~30 min	1–3 mcg/kg
Remifentanil	A few minutes	3–10 min	1–2 mcg/kg

  - Morphine/hydromorphone: long half-lives facilitate pain control in postoperative period. Good choices for induction if you expect the patient to require postoperative pain control.
  - Fentanyl: much shorter half-life with single dose because of rapid distribution into fat. Infusion or high number of repeated doses cause drug accumulation and prolonged elimination time.
  - Remifentanil: rapidly metabolized by plasma esterases, thus does not accumulate in blood/fat like other narcotics with continuous infusion or repeated doses.
  - Alfentanil/sufentanil: more rapid onset of action and shorter duration of action than fentanyl.
  - Infusions or large doses of fentanyl analogues (remifentanil in particular) can cause opioid-induced hyperalgesia, in which the patient becomes more sensitive to painful stimuli and can require much larger doses of opioids for postoperative pain control.
  - Meperidine: used primarily for the treatment of perioperative shivering. Unique because it has minor local anesthetic properties in addition to narcotic properties. Its metabolite, normeperidine, is excreted by kidneys, can cause seizures in patients with CKD.
- Commonly used neuromuscular blocking agents
  - Succinylcholine: the only depolarizing agent still in use. Consists of two joined acetylcholine (ACh) molecules, which depolarize the muscle by binding the ACh receptor. Rapid onset (30–60 seconds) and rapid metabolism by serum pseudocholinesterase (duration <10 minutes). Raises serum potassium by 0.5 in healthy patients. Contraindicated in patients with hyperkalemia, burn injuries, massive trauma, many neurologic disorders, myopathies, and children/adolescents (risk of undiagnosed myopathy), because of risk of life-threatening potassium elevation in these patients. Also, patients with homozygous atypical pseudocholinesterase (incidence 1/3,200) can be paralyzed for 4–8 hours due to slow metabolism.
  - Rocuronium: nondepolarizing agent; ACh receptor antagonist that prevents muscle depolarization. Rapid-onset (dose-dependent, 1–3 minutes), duration 20–35 minutes, or longer in patients with renal failure.
  - Cisatracurium: also nondepolarizing. Slower onset (3–5 minutes), duration 20–35 minutes. Degraded spontaneously by Hofmann elimination (independent of liver and kidney function), thus often used in patients with severe renal failure rather than rocuronium.
- Adjunct medications
  - Common adjuncts include ketamine (see induction agents), lidocaine (see epidural/spinal), and benzodiazepines (see MAC).

Airway Management

- Intubation techniques: Options for placing an endotracheal tube include standard direct laryngoscopy, as well as video laryngoscopy and fiberoptic intubation for more difficult cases. An overview of direct laryngoscopy technique with a Macintosh (Mac) blade is provided below:
  1. Adjust bed height so patient's face is at the level of your xiphoid cartilage
  2. Extend head (assuming no c-spine pathology) once induced. This often opens the mouth.
  3. If mouth does not open adequately with head extension, manually open it using counter pressure of the right thumb on the mandibular teeth and right index finger on the maxillary teeth.

4. Insert the blade with your left hand just right of midline. You may need to roll the lip away with your left index finger to prevent bruising if it gets caught under the blade with insertion.
5. Deflect the tongue to the left as you advance the blade toward the epiglottis. Your blade should advance to the base of the tongue, just shy of the epiglottis, to allow you to bring the epiglottis up and expose the vocal cords.
6. **Lift** along the axis of the handle to bring the laryngeal structures into view (Fig. 27-2). **Do NOT use the blade as a lever** (pull the handle up with a rigid wrist, rather than rotating the blade with the patient's teeth as a fulcrum—rocking the blade on the patient's teeth can cause injury).
7. Hold the ET tube in your right hand like a pencil. Advance it gently along the right side of the mouth to avoid obscuring your view.
8. Once the proximal end of the balloon cuff is 1–2 cm past the vocal cords, remove the laryngoscope.
9. Inflate the cuff with the minimum volume required to prevent a leak of positive pressure, usually ~25 cm H_2O (overinflation can cause mucosal ischemia of the tracheal wall).

Figure 27-2 Cormack and Lehane classification. (From Wolfson, AB. *Harwood-Nuss' Clinical Practice of Emergency Medicine*, 5th ed. Philadelphia, PA: Lippincott Williams & Wilkins, 2010.)

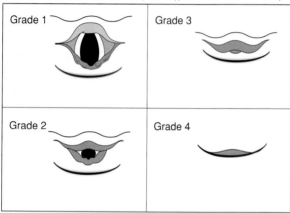

- Laryngeal mask airways (LMAs): These devices sit above the glottis and are generally less invasive and sometimes easier to place than endotracheal tubes. Many sizes and types are available. The disadvantage is that they provide incomplete protection from gastric aspiration, so are relatively contraindicated in patients at risk for aspiration (e.g., pregnancy, hiatal hernia). Other relative contraindications are reduced pulmonary compliance (e.g., restrictive airway disease requiring peak inspiratory pressures greater than 30 cm H_2O, which can leak around the device), and pharyngeal pathology. Spontaneous ventilation may be maintained; pressure support or controlled ventilation may be used as well. Routine use of controlled ventilation with LMAs is controversial.
- LMAs are a life-saving rescue device in patients with difficult airways (situations where patient cannot be ventilated or intubated) and are prominently included in the ASA Difficult Airway algorithm.

Maintenance
- Anesthesia can be maintained either with volatile anesthetics or total intravenous anesthesia (TIVA). TIVA is usually performed with propofol and a narcotic. TIVA is more expensive and depth of anesthesia is more difficult to monitor but TIVA is sometimes needed (e.g., cases requiring jet ventilation or neuromonitoring, patients at risk of malignant hyperthermia, etc.)
- Volatile anesthetic concentrations are standardized to minimum alveolar concentration (MAC), which is the alveolar concentration of an inhaled anesthetic that prevents movement in 50% of patients in response to surgical incision.

- MAC decreases with age, acute alcohol intoxication, and hyper or hypothermia, among others.
- MAC increases with chronic alcohol abuse and acute cocaine use, among others.
- Volatile agents

	Wake-Up Time	BP	CO	1 MAC (%)	Notes
Sevoflurane	Moderate	↓	↓	2.0	Requires 2 L/min gas flow minimum to prevent accumulation of compound A, which may be nephrotoxic (based on rat models)
Isoflurane	Slow	↓↓	N/C	1.2	Slowest wake-up time due to higher solubility, usually used only when patient will stay intubated after surgery
Desflurane	Fast	↓↓	↓ or N/C	6.0	Accelerates HR/RR with rapid increase in concentration. Noxious for awake patients. Most negative environmental impact
Nitrous Oxide	Fast	N/C	N/C	105	Combine with other agent since not potent enough to be used alone. ↑ risk of PONV. Expands air containing spaces so contraindicated in bowel obstruction, pneumothorax, etc.

N/C, no change.

- Modes of ventilation: see Critical Care, ventilator management
- Standard monitors: include pulse oximetry, FiO_2 analyzer, continuous EKG, BP monitoring, end-tidal CO_2 capnography, ventilator disconnect alarm, temperature probe (if change in patient temperature may be reasonably expected)
- Arterial lines: Allow continuous BP monitoring and facilitate drawing of labs/arterial blood gases. Also allows measurement of variations in pulse pressure (difference between systolic and diastolic pressure) that can help guide fluid resuscitation.
- BIS (bispectral index): Two-channel EEG, analyzed to provide an indicator of wakefulness on a proprietary scale of 0–100. Sedation is between about 65 and 85, general anesthesia is between about 40 and 65. Most often used for TIVA cases. Efficacy in preventing awareness under anesthesia is controversial.
- Train-of-four monitoring: Monitors degree of neuromuscular blockade. Not perfect: four twitches without fade can still mean that 50% of ACh receptors are antagonized. Newer quantitative accelomyography monitors are improving detection of residual paralysis. Need 1–2 twitches minimum before reversing blockade with acetylcholinesterase inhibitor to be confident that reversal will be adequate.
- CVP: Approximates right atrial pressure. Very low values (<5 cm H_2O) may indicate volume depletion; elevated values (>10 cm H_2O) may reflect volume overload or poor ventricular compliance.
- PA pressures: see Critical Care
- Pressors/inotropes: see Critical Care
- Common intravenous antihypertensives:

	Mechanism	Onset Time	Half-Life	Notes
Labetalol	Blocks α1, β1, and β2 receptors	2–5 min	4 h	
Metoprolol	Selectively blocks β1 receptors	10 min	3–4 h	Acts more on HR than BP
Esmolol	Selectively blocks β1 receptors	2–10 min dose dep.	2–9 min dose dep.	Acts more on HR than BP
Hydralazine	Releases NO, ↑ cGMP	5–20 min	1–4 h	
Nitroglycerine	Releases NO, ↑ cGMP	<1 min	3–5 min	Primarily venous vasodilator, good for CHF since reduces preload

Nitroprusside	Releases NO, ↑ cGMP	<2 min	2 min	Can cause methemo-globinemia or cyanide toxicity
Nicardipine	Ca channel blocker	2 min	~8 h	Primarily arterial vasodilator
Fenoldopam	D1 dopamine receptor agonist	5–10 min	~30 min	Preserves GFR despite ↓ BP

- Blood products: see Perioperative Management

Emergence
- Reversal agents: two options for reversing neuromuscular blockade from nondepolarizing agents (e.g., rocuronium) are cholinesterase inhibitors (e.g., neostigmine) and the new relaxant-binding medication sugammadex.
- Cholinesterase inhibitors like neostigmine increase ACh, which competes with ACh antagonists. They will not provide adequate reversal unless the patient has at least 1–2 twitches before administration. Neostigmine is given in combination with an anticholinergic (e.g., glycopyrrolate) that serves to counteract undesirable muscarinic effects, particularly bradycardia.
- Criteria for extubation:
  - Neuromuscular blockade has worn off or has been adequately reversed.
  - Patient either deeply anesthetized ("deep extubation") or awake/following commands ('awake extubation'). Avoid extubating under light anesthesia because of increased risk of laryngospasm.
  - Rough indicators of adequate respiratory function include tidal volume >5 cc/kg, vital capacity >10 cc/kg, PaCO$_2$ <50, RR <25.
  - Pressor use/hemodynamic instability is a relative contraindication depending on severity of patient condition.

Monitored Anesthesia Care (MAC)
- Ranges from minimal sedation/anxiolysis to deep sedation, but patient should respond purposefully to repeated or painful stimuli to be considered MAC. No volatile anesthetics (e.g., sevoflurane) are used for MAC cases. Instead, patients are kept sedated with IV medication boluses and/or infusions.
- Common MAC medications:
  - Propofol, ketamine, opioids: see induction agents in General Anesthesia
  - Dexmedetomidine: α-agonist similar to clonidine with greater affinity for α$_2$-receptors, and shorter half-life (2–3 hours vs. 12–16 hours). Advantage over propofol is that respiratory drive and ventilation are preserved. Disadvantage is that bradycardia (and hypotension) can occur, particularly with infusions, and half-life is much longer than propofol.
  - Midazolam: IV benzodiazepine, binds to same GABA receptor as barbiturates but at a different location. Very good amnestic (only impairs memory after it is given—no retrograde effect). Disadvantage is long half-life and respiratory depression.
- See General Anesthesia section for information on monitors and antihypertensives used in anesthesia.

Epidural/Spinal
Anatomy
- Needle path for midline approach: skin, superficial fascia, deep fascia, supraspinous ligament, interspinous ligament, ligamentum flavum (dense ligament before loss of resistance). For spinal, continue through dura.
- Epidural catheters are placed in epidural space (loss of resistance after passing through ligamentum flavum identifies epidural space)
- Spinal injections are administered in dural sac (free-flowing CSF identifies intrathecal space)

Local Anesthetics
- Two types: esters (chloroprocaine, benzocaine, cocaine) undergo rapid ester hydrolysis, thus very short acting. Amides (lidocaine, bupivacaine—all with two 'i's in their names) are metabolized by the liver, and thus last longer.
- Duration of action: chloroprocaine < lidocaine < mepivacaine < ropivacaine < bupivacaine
- Epinephrine 5 mcg/mL prolongs effect and reduces systemic absorption/toxicity, allowing higher doses (less effect on duration with bupivacaine and ropivacaine)
- Bupivacaine has the lowest therapeutic index (i.e., the lowest margin of safety before neurologic/cardiac toxicity). Also, cardiac toxicity occurs soon after neurologic

toxicity, thus there is less "warning" before cardiac arrest. It is a very useful medication, however, due to its long duration of action.

- Maximum doses

	Plain (mg/kg)	With Epi (mg/kg)	Duration (min) for Local Infiltration	Duration (min) for Epidural Anesthesia
Chloroprocaine	11 (max 800 mg)	14 (max 1,000 mg)	15–30 plain 30 w/ epi	45–60 plain 60–90 w/ epi
Lidocaine	3–5 (max 300 mg)	7 (max 500 mg)	30–60 plain 120–360 w/ epi	80–120 plain 120–180 w/ epi
Bupivicaine	2.5 (max 175 mg)	2.5 (max 200 mg)	120–240 plain 180–240 w/ epi	165–225 plain 180–240 w/ epi
Ropivicaine	2–3 (max 200 mg)	2–3 (max 250 mg)	120–240 plain 180–240 w/ epi	140–180 plain 150–200 w/ epi

Contraindications
- Absolute: patient refusal, bleeding diathesis, severe hypovolemia, elevated ICP/intracranial mass, infection at injection site, severe aortic/mitral stenosis (spinal)
- Relative: severe aortic/mitral stenosis (epidural), uncooperative patient, severe spinal deformity

Risks
- Hypotension: due to loss of sympathetic tone. Usually responds to phenylephrine (restores vascular tone) and fluids.
- Postdural puncture headache: incidence ~1% with spinal or routine epidural (~50% if dura punctured unintentionally with large bore epidural introducer needle). Leakage of CSF though dural puncture site believed to stretch cerebral veins causing headache. Key feature is positional nature (headache present when sitting up/standing, significantly improved lying flat). Conservative management (pain control, caffeine) often successful. Refractory or severe cases tx with epidural blood patch (~80% success: first attempt; ~95% success: second attempt).
- High block: rare, but can result in respiratory compromise if severe. Usually from epidural catheter accidentally placed in subdural space, or from local anesthetic overdose.
- Intravascular injection can cause neurologic symptoms (delirium, seizures) and cardiac arrest.
- Failed block: epidural failure often due to malposition of epidural catheter (e.g., in soft tissue from false loss of resistance, or unilateral block from paravertebral misplacement). Spinal failure less frequent because location can be confirmed by visualizing free flowing CSF; however, needle can move prior to medication injection.
- Backache: unclear association since 25–30% general anesthesia patients have postoperative backache. Usually mild/self-limited. Tx with acetaminophen, NSAIDs.
- Epidural abscess/hematoma: rare (<1/1,000), but any worsening back pain or progressive neurologic deficit should be investigated with stat MRI (preferred) or CT.

Regional
Common Nerve Blocks
- Usually performed with ultrasound or nerve stimulation to confirm needle position

Block	Nerves	Most Common Indication	Notes/Risks
Interscalene	C5–C7 nerve trunks (frequently spares ulnar nerve/ C8–T1 roots)	Shoulder/upper arm surgery	100% incidence of ipsilateral phrenic nerve block—avoid in patients with borderline resp. status
Supraclavicular	Brachial plexus divisions (frequently spares axillary and suprascapular nerve)	Procedures at or distal to elbow	Highest risk of pneumothorax. 50% incidence of ipsilateral phrenic nerve block—avoid in patients with borderline resp. status
Infraclavicular	Brachial plexus cords	Procedures distal to elbow	Risk of ptx, but less than supraclavicular

Axillary	Brachial plexus branches	Procedures distal to elbow	Axillary and musculocutaneous nerves branch before block site, thus not anesthetized
Femoral	Femoral nerve (upper thigh/inner leg, saphenous nerve)	Hip, thigh, knee, and ankle procedures	Usually inadequate for surgical anesthesia, but helps with postoperative pain control
Sciatic	Sciatic nerve (posterior thigh, lateral leg/foot, tibial, and common fibular nerves)	Hip, thigh, knee, ankle, and foot procedures	High sciatic block is adequate for some knee surgeries
Obturator	Obturator nerve (medial thigh/knee)	Hip and knee procedures	Usually combined with femoral and sciatic blocks for certain knee procedures
Popliteal fossa	Popliteal nerve	Foot and ankle procedures	Combine with femoral (or saphenous) block to anesthetize ankle joint
Ankle block	Saphenous and sural nerves + lateral plantar, medial plantar and medial calcaneal branches of tibial nerve	Foot procedures	Can anesthetize all five nerves with fewer than five needle punctures. Can block selectively depending on surgical site
Intercostal block	Selected intercostal nerves	Thoracic surgery	Well vascularized. Fastest systemic absorption of local anesthetic and thus highest risk of systemic toxicity
Transversus abdominis plane block	T7–T12 spinal, ilioinguinal and iliohypogastric nerves	Abdominal surgeries (requires bilateral block for midline incisions)	Nerves travel between internal oblique and transversus abdominis muscles. Can be performed by anesthetist or surgeon to help with postoperative pain control

Local Anesthetics
- Rate of systemic absorption inversely related to vascularity: IV > tracheal > intercostal > paracervical > epidural > brachial plexus > sciatic > subcutaneous
- Adding sodium bicarbonate speeds block onset and also decreases pain during subcutaneous infiltration.
- See epidural/spinal section for local anesthetic types

Contraindications
- Absolute: patient refusal, bleeding diathesis, infection at injection site
- Relative: sepsis, uncooperative patient, poor baseline function of target nerve (if present, carefully document baseline deficits prior to block)

Risks
- Toxicity of local anesthetics: from overdose or intravenous/intra-arterial injection (delirium, seizures, cardiac arrest)
- Transient or chronic paresthesia
- Block failure
- Local infection/abscess: <1%
- Peripheral nerve injury: Very rare (~1/10,000)

Postoperative Care
- Information on postoperative nausea/vomiting (PONV) and pain control below. See postoperative care and critical care sections for more on other postoperative issues.

Nausea/Vomiting Prevention and Treatment
- Several studies show that PONV is one of patients' greatest fears
- Four biggest risk factors: female gender, postoperative opioid use, nonsmoking status (smoking is protective), history of PONV or motion sickness

- Sample PONV prevention algorithm:
  - One risk factor: usually give ondansetron at the end of case
  - Two risk factors: give dexamethasone after induction (assuming no contraindication) and ondansetron at the end of case
  - Three or four risk factors: consider TIVA (propofol is antiemetic) rather than inhaled agents, give dexamethasone and ondansetron assuming no contraindications
- Antiemetic agents: ondansetron, haloperidol, dexamethasone, and TIVA with propofol each independently reduce PONV risk by 25%
  - Ondansetron: antagonist at $5\text{-}HT_3$ receptor, found in GI tract and brain, mediates n/v. Give at the end of surgery or as rescue agent. Most common side effect is headache (<3%).
  - Haloperidol: block dopamine receptors that contribute to PONV. Can prolong QT but generally safe at low doses given for PONV in patients without baseline pro-longed QT. Give at the end of surgery or as rescue agent.
  - Dexamethasone: mechanism unknown. Give after induction (more effective if done early in the case). For prevention only, not for treatment. Pushing dose in awake patient may cause severe perineal pruritis, so wait until asleep or inject slowly. Although chronic steroid use increases wound infection risk, almost all studies have shown no increased risk from single dose. Relatively contraindicated in diabetics due to hyperglycemia and in patients with active infections.
  - Phenothiazine/prochlorperazine (Compazine): affect multiple receptors (histaminergic, dopaminergic, muscarinic). Given as rescue agents. May also cause extrapyramidal and anticholinergic side effects.
  - Promethazine (Phenergan): anticholinergic and antihistaminergic. Sedating. Given as rescue agent.
  - Metoclopramide: Primarily promotes gastric motility. Also blocks dopamine receptors in the chemoreceptor trigger zone of CNS. Less effective in treating PONV at usual doses of 10–20 mg (only reduces n/v significantly at 1–2 mg/kg)
  - Scopolamine patch: anticholinergic. Usually used for prevention since 2–4 hour onset time. Potent sedative, which may prolong awakening. Also can cause dry mouth, amnesia and sometimes delirium.

Pain Control
- Multimodal analgesia (i.e., treatment with multiple classes of analgesics) is the gold standard for pain control. Using modalities other than opiates can reduce opioid requirements significantly and reduce opioid side effects such as n/v, constipation, and delirium.
- Acetaminophen: reversible COX inhibitor (predominantly COX-2). Can reduce opioid requirements by as much as 40%. IV form is ~$20 per dose but is often appropriate for patients with severe pain not yet awake enough to swallow.
- Ibuprofen: reversible COX-1 and 2 inhibitor. Contraindicated in patients with active bleeding, peptic ulcers, and those with hyperkalemia or severe renal impairment.
- Ketorolac: reversible COX-1 and 2 inhibitor. Provides higher level of analgesia than acetaminophen and ibuprofen. IV form available (less expensive than IV acetaminophen, ~$2 per dose). Contraindications same as for ibuprofen. Ask surgeon before giving due to concern for increased bleeding risk (although meta-analyses show no increased risk). Do not administer for procedures where bleeding could be rapidly fatal (i.e., neurosurgery).
- Gabapentin/pregabalin: similar structure to GABA, but do not bind GABA receptors; exact mechanism unknown. Helpful as an adjunct to decrease narcotic use. Can cause dizziness and sedation. Pregabalin is more expensive, but has quicker onset (1 hour vs. 3–4 hours), similar half-life, and more reliable absorption/pharmacokinetics.
- Tizanidine/baclofen/cyclobenzaprine: antispasmodics are helpful for pain associated with sprains, muscle spasms or contractures. Tizanidine is a centrally acting α_2-agonist, baclofen is a GABA agonist, and cyclobenzaprine has an unknown mechanism. Do not discontinue baclofen abruptly as doing so can cause delirium and even rhabdomyolysis.
- Opiates: see opioid section under General Anesthesia. A conversion table for IV and oral opioids is provided below. Note that when switching agents, doses are often decreased by at least 25% to adjust for incomplete cross-tolerance.

	IV	IV to PO Conversion	PO
Morphine	10 mg	x2–3	20–30 mg
Hydromorphone	1.5 mg	x5	7.5 mg
Oxycodone	N/A		15–20 mg
Codeine	N/A		200 mg
Hydrocodone	N/A		30 mg

Malignant Hyperthermia

- Prevalence <1/10,000
- Caused by mutation of the ryanodine receptor (receptor responsible for Ca release from sarcoplasmic reticulum)
- Episodes triggered by potent inhaled anesthetics (not nitrous oxide) or succinylcholine
- Clinical manifestations include masseter muscle rigidity, tachycardia, and hypercarbia. Hyperthermia is a late sign. Patients can also have dark colored urine due to myoglobinuria from rhabdomyolysis.
- Mortality 5–30% even with prompt recognition/treatment
- Treatment includes discontinuing triggering agent, administering dantrolene and providing supportive care. Can call MH hotline at 1–800–644–9737 to consult on-call physician.

SAYURI JINADASA • ALOK GUPTA

"What would you like to close with, doctor?"

When asking for sutures, there are three general pieces of information that are important to convey in your request: suture size, suture type, and suture needle.

28-1: SUTURES

There are varying types and sizes of sutures and their use depends on the type of tissue being repaired and the time duration intended for the suture to stay in place.

Suture Size

Sutures are sized in the United States following the United States Pharmacopeia (USP) method, which takes into account knot security, tensile strength, and suture diameter. Gauge varies from #12-0 to #4, going from the thinnest to the thickest diameter. For example, #2, #1, 0, 00, 000, etc. are a list of suture sizes in decreasing diameter. To simplify the vernacular, 00000 is colloquially referred to as "5-0." This is an easy way to remember that 7-0 is smaller than 2-0, for example.

The following table lists common suture sizes used in surgery cases listed in the smallest to largest diameter gauge:

Common Suture Sizes and Uses	
USP Standard	**Common Uses**
6-0	Common for use in vascular graft sewing
5-0 4-0	Used for larger vessel repair or skin closure
3-0 2-0	Skin closure when there is a lot of tension, closure of muscle layers or repair of bowel
0 1	Used for closing of abdominal fascia, various orthopedic procedures

Suture Material

Four main classifications of suture material:
- **Physical:** size (diameter), number of filaments, tensile strength, coefficient of friction
- **Handling:** pliability, packaging memory, knot slippage, tissue drag
- **Biocompatibility:** degree of inflammatory reaction and propensity for wound infection, allergic reactions
- **Biodegradation:** tensile breaking strength and mass loss, biocompatibility of degradation properties

The two most practical properties of suture material are whether or not they are absorbable and whether they are mono- or multifilament.

Absorbable vs. Nonabsorbable

Absorbable suture materials are those that are naturally degraded and absorbed by the body over time by way of hydrolysis (synthetic sutures) and enzymatic degradation (natural sutures).
- Use for suturing internal tissue or in patients who cannot return for suture removal
- Dissolution time depends on suture type, size, and type of tissue
- Examples: surgical gut suture, Vicryl, Monocryl, Polydiaxonone Suture (PDS)

Nonabsorbable sutures are made of materials not readily broken down by the body.
- Used when a suture may be removed after a certain period of time (e.g., nylon sutures to close a superficial laceration) or when they can or need to be left permanently (e.g., vessel repair or bowel anastomosis)
- Fibroblasts encapsulate or wall off nonabsorbable sutures
- Provoke less of an immune response and cause less scarring than absorbable sutures; therefore are used where cosmetic outcome is important
- Examples: silk, nylon, stainless steel, polyester, prolene

Monofilament vs. Multifilament

Monofilament sutures are composed of a single smooth strand.
- Cause less drag through tissue and therefore are less traumatic
- More likely to slip, therefore approximately 5–7 knots are required when tying

- Crush and crimp easily, creating weak spots that lessen tensile strength

Multifilament sutures consist of multiple fibers braided or twisted together.
- Provides increased tensile strength and pliability
- Increased drag and trauma on the tissues
- Less likely to slip, therefore requires only 3–4 knots when tying
- Can be coated with different materials that can decrease drag and make it easier to slide knots into place (this may compromise knot security)

Synthetic vs. Natural
Frequently Used Sutures
Monocryl: absorbable, synthetic, monofilament; ideal for subcuticular closures

Nylon: nonabsorbable, available as mono- or multifilament, synthetic; because of their elasticity, particularly well-suited for retention and skin closure
- Monofilament nylon sutures have memory (a tendency to return to their straight state); therefore, more throws are required for knot security compared to braided nylon sutures

PDS: absorbable, monofilament, synthetic; ideal for secure fascial closures

Prolene: nonabsorbable, monofilament, synthetic; used in general soft tissue approximation and/or ligation
- Causes minimal tissue reaction and does not adhere to tissue

Silk: nonabsorbable, multifilament, natural; used for bowel anastomoses, vessel ligation, suturing drains in place

Stainless steel: nonabsorbable, available as mono- or multifilament, synthetic, nonabsorbable; often used for sternal closure
- Disadvantages associated with handling: possible cutting, pulling, or tearing of patient's tissue or injury to surgeon

Surgical gut (catgut): absorbable, monofilament, natural; indicated in general soft tissue approximation and/or ligation
- **Plain:** consists of purified collagen derived from animal intestines; breaks down enzymatically and tensile strength is maintained for 7–10 days; completely absorbed within 70 days
- **Chromic:** plain gut treated with chromium salts that result in prolonging tensile strength to 10–21 days and absorption time to over 90 days

Vicryl: absorbable, multifilament, synthetic; used in general soft tissue approximation and/or ligation

Dissolution Time
The dissolution time of suture material depends on
- type of material
- blood supply to the tissue
- structure of the tissue
- degree of fluid accumulation on the suture material

Suture Type Dissolution Times	
Suture	**# Days**
Monocryl	90–120
PDS	180–210
Plain gut	70
Chromic gut	90
Vicryl	55–70

Miscellaneous
Pledgeted suture: suture supported by a small, flat, nonabsorbent pad (pledget) so that the suture will not tear through tissue; used routinely in valve replacement operations.

The strength of a **knotted** suture decreases by approximately 50% due to the stresses from bending and twisting that are introduced into the suture when knotting.

Anatomy of a Needle

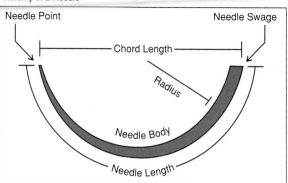

Point: sharpened part of the needle that first penetrates the tissue
- Determines ease of penetration and the initial size and shape of the hole made in tissue
- **Blunt tip:** sharp enough to penetrate fascia and muscle but not skin; also can be used to suture friable tissue such as kidney or liver
  - minimizes risk of needle stick injury

Diameter: gauge or thickness of the needle wire; select based on the tissue to be sutured; finer diameter for softer tissue (e.g., bowel) and wider diameter for tougher tissue

Body: portion which is grasped by the needle holder

Curvature
- The curvature of the needle body comes in a variety of different shapes and sizes, which give the needle different characteristics
- Classified by the fraction of a circle the needle takes up

Basic Needle Shapes

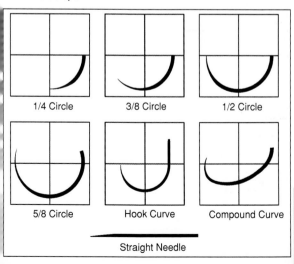

Tapered vs. Cutting

Tapered: body of tapered needles are round in cross section that taper to a point; they separate tissue fibers rather than cut them

- Most atraumatic needle type, therefore used in tissue that can be easily penetrated, e.g., deep fascia closure, bowel, vessels, nerves, tendons
- Not used on skin because of difficulty to penetrate tissue

Cutting: body of cutting needles are triangular in cross section; cut rather than separate tissue and therefore make it much easier to penetrate tough tissue

- Used in areas of tough, fibrous, or dense tissue and for suturing skin
- **Conventional cutting needle:** apex cutting edge is on the inside of the needle curvature
- **Reverse cutting needle:** apex cutting edge is on the outside of the needle curvature
  - Has improved the strength and increased resistance to bending

Needle Point Geometry

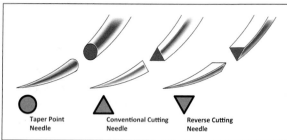

| Taper Point Needle | Conventional Cutting Needle | Reverse Cutting Needle |

Common Needle Codes and Meanings

Code[a]	Meaning	Common Uses
BV	Blood vessel	Blood vessels
CT	Circle taper	Closure of deep tissue layers
SH	Small half (circle)	Bowel closure; closure of tissue layers after breast surgery
UR	Urology	Laparoscopic port site closure

[a]Subtypes of needle shapes are classified by numbers from larger to smaller size.

Which Needle to Use?

- Depends on procedure, tissue type, exposure, and accessibility to tissue being sutured, and surgeon preference
- Goal is to minimize trauma to tissue
  - Should be as slim as possible without compromising strength
  - Stable in grasp of needle holder
  - Able to carry suture material through tissue
  - Sharp enough to penetrate tissue with minimal resistance
  - Rigid enough to resist bending but able to resist breaking
- Care should be taken to match the size of the needle to the size of the tissue bite required

Suture Packaging Guide

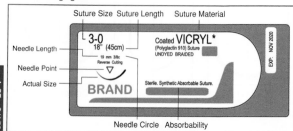

Miscellaneous
Eyed needles: manufactured separately from suture thread
- requires rethreading
- reuse leads to loss of sharpness
- more than a single strand is pulled through tissue, therefore, more trauma and a larger gap is created than is filled by sutures
- Advantage: any needle and suture combination can be achieved

"Pop-offs": Needles designed to come off the suture with a sharp straight tug; commonly used for interrupted sutures, where each suture is only passed once and then tied; risk of needle-stick injury while tying is minimized

---

28-3: SUTURING TECHNIQUE

Needle Holder
- Needle holder should be selected to match the size and strength of the needle being used.
  - If too large, can result in damage to needle and distortion of needle curvature.
- Needles should be grasped at approximately two-thirds of the needle length from the point.
- The needle and holder should be roughly perpendicular.
- The needle tip should enter the target tissue at a 90-degree angle.
- When applying force to achieve passage of the needle through tissue, it should be applied in a direction following the curvature of the needle.
- If placement of the needle in tissue needs to be readjusted, the needle should be removed and re-inserted.

Suture Removal Timing
Different parts of the body heal at different speeds. Common time to remove sutures will vary:
- Face: 3–4 days
- Scalp: 5 days
- Trunk: 7–10 days
- Limbs: 7–10 days
- Foot: 10–14 days

28-4: OTHER WOUND CLOSURE METHODS FOR HEALING BY PRIMARY INTENTION

- Staples
- Steri-Strips
- Adhesives—e.g., Dermabond

DANIEL A. HASHIMOTO • DANIEL B. JONES

29-1: SIMULATION

Types of Procedural Trainers (*Fundamentals of Surgical Simulation*. Springer, 2012)
- Bench-top trainers
  - Animal tissue: can be porcine, chicken, sheep, cow models to practice surgical skills
  - Synthetic models: made of rubber, latex, polyurethane, etc.
- Virtual reality trainers: computer-generated environment for training
  - Part-task trainers: focus on particular tasks such as instrument handling, suturing
  - High-fidelity trainers: allow for simulation of entire procedures such as laparoscopic cholecystectomy, colonoscopy, endovascular procedures, etc.
- Human patient simulators
  - Mannequins: simulate human physiology
- Live animal models
- Cadavers

29-2: FUNDAMENTALS OF LAPAROSCOPIC SURGERY (FLS) **FLS** (http://www.fls-online.org; http://www.flsprogram.org)

The **Fundamentals of Laparoscopic Surgery (FLS)** program is designed to teach principles and techniques in laparoscopic surgery and is a requirement of the American Board of Surgery for board certification. The examination for FLS certification includes a multiple-choice examination and a technical skills examination.

Laparoscopic Technology
Scopes
- Sizes
  - 2–10 mm in diameter
  - 30–45 cm in length
- Angles
  - 0, 30, and 45 degrees

Insufflation
- Gas
  - CO_2 typically used as it is noncombustible, readily absorbed by the body, eliminated with ventilation
    - Diffusion coefficient of CO_2 in blood is 20x that of O_2
    - There is accompanying rise in arterial and end-tidal CO_2 with drop in pH
    - Greatest change is in the first 20 minutes, then reaches steady state
  - Alternate gases include nitric oxide, helium
    - N_2O: decreased acid/base disturbance; less postoperative pain
      - Combustion risk but is not flammable itself
      - Fire hazard is when there is a concomitant bowel injury
    - Inert gases (e.g., helium): eliminate acidosis but are less soluble in blood so increases risk of gas embolus
- Settings
  - Flow: L/min of gas flow into the abdomen
  - Pressure: mm Hg of pressure of the insufflated abdomen (typical range 12–15 mm Hg)
- Troubleshooting the insufflator
  - Low pressure, no flow: standby mode or tank empty
  - High pressure, no flow: kink or block in insufflation tubing
  - Low pressure, high flow: leak in tubing or disconnected tubing

Light Source
- 300 W xenon light source most common
- In translucent cables, points of light show broken fibers

Patient Selection
- ASA 4 and 5 patients may not be appropriate for laparoscopy due to physiologic demands of pneumoperitoneum
- Typical length of trocars for obese patients is >10 cm

Contraindications to Laparoscopy
- Absolute contraindications
  - Inability to tolerate laparotomy
  - Hypovolemic shock
  - Lack of proper surgeon training or institutional support
- Relative contraindications
  - Inability to tolerate GA
  - Longstanding peritonitis
  - Large abdominal or pelvic mass
  - Massive incarcerated ventral or inguinal hernias
  - Severe cardiopulmonary disease
- Not contraindication
  - Diaphragm injury
  - GI Bleed
  - Perforated viscus
  - SBO
  - Trauma
    - Only use laparoscopy if stable
  - Intrauterine/ectopic pregnancy
  - Obesity
  - COPD
  - Renal insufficiency
- Conditions requiring additional preoperative precautions
  - Arterial aneurysms
  - Scars that may suggest increased risk of extensive adhesions or risk of enterotomy
    - Same with the history of peritonitis
  - Umbilical abnormalities
  - History of ventral hernia repair
  - Hepatosplenomegaly
  - Cirrhosis: increased risk of bleeding/ascites leak
  - SBO with bowel dilation

Patient Positioning
Supine: most common position
- Used for cholecystectomy, appendectomy, right colectomy
- Can tuck either or both arms to improve surgeon ergonomics

Trendelenburg and reverse Trendelenburg
- Useful to move bowel out of operative field

Modified decubitus position
- Often used for splenectomy, nephrectomy, adrenalectomy

Lithotomy
- Used for pelvic operations such as hysterectomy, rectal operations

Ergonomic Working Position for Surgeon
- Elbows out <30 degrees
- Elbow bend between 60 and 120 degrees
- Wrist slightly pronated
  - Wrist no more than 2–3 degrees off straight line

Physiologic Changes of Laparoscopy
Pulmonary Physiology
- CO_2 removal mediated by increased minute ventilation
- There is reduced FRC, increased airway pressure, reduced pulmonary compliance from upward pressure on diaphragm

Cardiovascular Changes With Pneumoperitoneum
- Cardiac output (CO) is decreased by reverse Trendelenburg position
  - Decreased by hypovolemia
  - Vagally induced bradycardia can cause low CO
  - If hypotension occurs
    - Desufflate immediately
    - Check insufflator, relaxation, volume status, and other causes of hypotension such as bleeding
- Arrhythmia
  - Most commonly sinus tachycardia
  - PVCs
  - Bradycardia (from vagal response to pressure effects of pneumoperitoneum)

- Increased IVC resistance
  - Venous flow rates drop 26–39%
  - VTE event in lap chole <0.5%
  - Greater risk if duration >1 hour or pelvic procedure
- Oliguria
  - Secondary renin secretion during laparoscopy causing oliguria intraoperatively
  - Urine is an unreliable indicator of fluid status in laparoscopy

Complications
Gas Embolus
- Symptomatic emboli rare (0.015%)
  - Most common presenting symptoms: hypotension, JVD, tachycardia, mill wheel murmur
  - Symptoms can portend sudden cardiovascular collapse
- Management:
  - Place patient left side down in Trendelenburg, this hopefully positions gas embolus in right atrium
  - Give fluid
  - Insert a right IJ line then try to aspirate or break up gas embolus

Hollow Viscous Leak
- Rare occurrence of leak of insufflation gas into hollow viscous such as bowel or bladder
- Keep eye out for bowel distention, bladder distention, air in Foley bag

Bleeding
- Mesenteric or retroperitoneal bleeding can occur on trocar placement
- Aortic or caval injury can occur on trocar placement
- Port site bleeding should be checked at the end of every case on port removal

Intraoperative Events
Establishing Pneumoperitoneum
- Veress needle: blind entry technique using sharp-tip spring loaded needle that acts as conduit for insufflation gas
  - Commonly inserted at LUQ or periumbilical sites
  - Tip should be freely mobile on insertion, saline should flow freely into needle
  - Initial insufflation pressure should be low with low/medium flow of gas
  - Contraindicated if prior abdominal surgery scar or mesh in area of planned entry
- Hasson trocar: open entry technique
- Additional ports should be placed under direct laparoscopic vision

Key Principles of Laparoscopic Surgery
- Visualization is key
  - Ensure scope and port clean at all times
  - Maintain exposure
- Temporary hemostasis can be obtained with direct pressure or grasping a bleeding site
- Surgical energy or laparoscopic suture ligation can be utilized to obtain formal hemostasis
- Convert to open surgery if unsafe to proceed with laparoscopy

| Proficiency Scores to Pass FLS Technical Skills Examination ||
Task	Proficiency Score
Peg transfer	48 sec with no dropped pegs out of view
Pattern cut	98 sec; all cuts within 2 mm of the line
Endoloop	53 sec; no knot slippage, knot within 1 mm of line
Extracorporeal suturing	136 sec; no knot slippage, knot within 1 mm of dots on penrose drain
Intracorporeal suturing	112 sec; no knot slippage, knot within 1 mm of dots on penrose drain

Surg Endosc. 2008;22(8):1887–1893.

The **Fundamentals of Endoscopic Surgery Examination** is an American Board of Surgery requirement for board certification that tests familiarity and facility with endoscopic principles and techniques. It is an examination in two parts: (1) cognitive multiple-choice examination and (2) technical skills examination on a virtual reality simulator.

Endoscopic Technology
* Scope types
  * Video endoscopy
    * Charge-coupled device (CCD) on the end of camera
    * Higher quality image than fiberoptic scope
  * Fiberoptic endoscopy
    * Small fiberoptic glass fibers carry light to transmit images
    * Very easy to break fibers
* Endoscopic channels
  * Working port allows suction, auxillary irrigation, insertion of instruments such as biopsy forceps, snares, brushes
  * Air port allows for insufflation
  * Water port allows for cleaning of lens
* Programmable buttons, suction button, air/water button, up/down controls, left/right controls, umbilical cable

Endoscopy Indications
Upper GI
* Indications for initial endoscopy
  * Failure of PPI therapy
  * Failure of treatment of *Helicobacter pylori* titer
  * Anemia
  * GI bleeding (including hematemesis, hematochezia, melena)
  * Weight loss >10 pounds in 3 months
  * Dysphagia or odynophagia
  * Upper GI obstruction
  * Suspected neoplasm
  * Mucosal irregularities on radiologic imaging
* Indications for surveillance
  * Familial polyposis: q1–2y
  * Esophageal varices after sclero/band: q6–8wk
  * Gastric and esophageal ulcer: q6wk until healed
  * Barrett esophagus
    * Low risk (<3 cm, no dysplasia): every 2 years
    * Moderate (>3 cm, circumferential): yearly
    * High risk (low-grade dysplasia): every 6 months
* Contraindications to upper GI endoscopy
  * Inability to tolerate sedation
  * Hemodynamic instability

Lower GI
* Indications for colonoscopy
  * Colon cancer screening
    * Average colorectal cancer risk
      * Age >50 with repeat at 10-year intervals
    * First-degree relative with colorectal cancer or adenoma and age of onset >60
      * Age 40 with repeat at 10-year intervals
    * First-degree relative with colorectal cancer or adenoma and age of onset <60
      * Age 40 or 10 years before age of onset in relative, whichever is younger
      * Repeat at 5-year intervals
  * Familial adenomatous polyposis (FAP): autosomal dominant inactivation mutation of APC gene that is expressed as adenomatous polyposis of the colon with progression to colorectal cancer
    * Screen with upper and lower endoscopy in teenage years
    * Will ultimately require prophylactic colectomy

- Hereditary nonpolyposis colorectal cancer (HNPCC): autosomal dominant mutation in DNA mismatch repair that conveys increased risk of cancer
  - Begin at age 20 or 10 years before age of onset of colorectal cancer in the youngest relative
  - Repeat at 1–2-year intervals
- GI bleeding
- Unexplained alterations in bowel habits, including prolonged constipation or diarrhea
- Abnormal imaging findings in the colon or rectum
- Assessment of prior colonic anastomoses
- Lower GI indications for surveillance
  - Ademonas and colorectal cancer: interval depends on type and number
  - Inflammatory bowel disease
- Contraindications to lower GI endoscopy
  - Peritonitis

Preprocedure Screening

Pre-endoscopy screening generally follows preoperative screening guidelines.
- Coagulation studies for patients with risk factors for abnormal bleeding
- Hemoglobin if history of anemia
- CXR if history of respiratory problems
- EKG if history of heart disease, arrhythmia
- Pregnancy test if patient is a woman requiring general anesthesia

Complications
Common Complications in Endoscopy
- Upper GI endoscopy
  - Sedation/analgesia-related cardiopulmonary complications
  - Oxygen desaturation
  - Perforation (0.03%)
    - High-risk areas for perforation
      - Cricopharyngeus
      - Pharynx (especially Zenker's diverticulum)
      - Proximal duodenum
    - Signs of perforation
      - Cervical crepitus
      - Abdominal pain
      - Substernal pain
  - Aspiration
    - Risk factors for aspiration
      - Gastric distension
      - Excessive sedation
      - Improper head elevation
      - Incomplete decompression of stomach prior to scope removal
  - Pancreatitis (if ERCP): 3–5% occurrence rate
    - Risk factors for pancreatitis
      - Difficult cannulation
      - Prior hx
      - Precut sphincterotomy
      - Pancreatic duct opacification
      - Normal bili
      - Small bile duct
      - Female gender
      - Younger age
      - Sphincter of Oddi dysfunction
      - Sphincterotomy
  - Death (0.001%)
- Colonoscopy
  - During
    - Arrhythmia
    - Bradycardia
    - Hypotension
    - Hypoxia
    - Missed lesion
  - Postprocedure
    - Bleeding (0.07%)
      - 1% risk of bleeding if polypectomy performed

- Severe abdominal pain without perforation
- Bronchospasm
- Perforation (0.07%)
  - 50% of perforations require surgery
- Death (0.007%)

Patient Preparation
- Upper GI endoscopy does not require a patient to drink a bowel preparation, but NPO status is encouraged for 6–8 hours pre-endoscopy
- Successful colonoscopy is contingent on an adequate bowel preparation to maximize visualization of mucosa
- Iso-osmotic prep: nonabsorbable electrolyte solution that is osmotically balanced to prevent fluid and electrolyte shifts
  - Safe in patients with hepatic, renal, or congestive heart failure
- Hyperosmotic prep: draw water into bowel lumen; smaller volume of fluid to ingest but higher risk of dehydration
  - Magnesium citrate: promotes cholecystokinin release that stimulates fluid excretion and intestinal motility
  - Sodium phosphate: alters fluid and electrolyte balance and risks nephrocalcinosis, hyperphosphatemia, and hypokalemia
    - Contraindicated in CHF, renal failure, acute coronary syndrome, ileus, amongst other conditions

Anticoagulation Management for Endoscopy
- Procedures can be safely performed with an INR between 1.5 and 2.5
- If anticoagulation is short term, elective procedures should be delayed until the completion of anticoagulation term
- Do not use vitamin K to reverse anticoagulation as it can delay return to therapeutic levels

Procedures With Highest Risk of Bleeding
- Sphincterotomy
- Polypectomy
- Dilation
- Percutaneous endoscopic gastrostomy tube placement
- Fine needle aspiration
- Laser ablation and coagulation
- Variceal treatment

Sedation and Analgesia
Anxiolysis
- Anxiolytic only provided to patient

Conscious Sedation (i.e., moderate sedation with analgesia)
- Patient maintains own airway, and hemodynamics remain in equilibrium
- Responds to commands but otherwise depressed level of consciousness
- Can be delivered by the endoscopist
  - Most commonly fentanyl for analgesia/sedation and midazolam for amnesia

Deep Sedation
- Patient does not reliably maintain own airway, and hemodynamic instability can occur
- Painful stimuli needed to provoke response
- Requires anesthesiologist

General Anesthesia
- Patient requires oral airway such as LMA or endotracheal intubation
- Requires anesthesiologist

Monitoring
- Oxygenation: pulse oximetry
- Ventilation: capnography
- Hemodynamics: ECG tracing; periodic, automatic noninvasive blood pressure monitoring

Medications
Be aware that benzodiazepines and opioids have synergistic effects and need to be dose-reduced
- Midazolam: short-acting benzodiazepine
  - Onset of action between 3–5 minutes
  - Titrate in 0.5 mg boluses; usual total dose 2.5–5 mg
  - Risk of hypoventilation, hypotension, paradoxical agitation
  - Flumazenil is antagonist in case of benzodiazepine-induced respiratory depression

- Fentanyl: short-acting opioid
  - Immediate onset of action with 2–4 hour half-life
  - Give in 1–2 ug/kg dosing (dose down if giving with benzodiazepine)
- Remifentanil: ultra-short-acting opioid
  - Naloxone is antagonist in case of opioid-induced respiratory depression
- Propofol: ultra-short-acting sedative, hypnotic, amnestic; has no analgesic properties
  - Causes decreased inotropy, cardiac output, systemic vascular resistance. Increases respiratory depression
  - Cannot be used with patients with egg or soybean allergies
  - No reversal agent

Patient Positioning
Upper GI Endoscopy
- Patient should be positioned in left lateral decubitus position
- In case of GI bleeding, patient can be rotated to right lateral decubitus position to empty fundus of blood

Colonoscopy
- Patient may be left lateral decubitus or prone frog position to start
- Patient may need to be rolled to different positions to optimize passage of the scope to the cecum

Pathology
Polyps
- Hyperplastic or adenomatous
- Sessile, semi-sessile, or pedunculated

Lipomas
- Yellow bulges covered with normal mucosa
- Soft, spongy, and indent (pillow sign)

Colitis
- Often difficult to distinguish type of colitis on visual inspection alone
- Inflammation of mucosa

Diverticulosis
- Outpouching of mucosa from intestinal lumen

Angiodysplasia
- Vascular malformations more commonly seen in right colon

Ischemia
- Can appear similar to resolving inflammation if mild
- Can appear white, blue, black or green if severe
- Most common in watershed area like splenic flexure

Techniques to Control Bleeding
- Nonthermal techniques
  - Submucosal injection
  - Band ligation
  - Endoscopic clips
  - Balloon tamponade
- Thermal techniques
  - Monopolar or bipolar cautery
    - Monopolar has higher risk of full-thickness injury
  - Argon plasma coagulation (APC)

Enteral Access via Endoscopy
Percutaneous Endoscopic Gastrostomy (PEG) Tube
- Indications
  - Inability to take enteral nutrition but with functioning GI tract
  - Gastric decompression for gastric outlet obstruction
  - Reduction of gastric volvulus
- Contraindications
  - Diffuse gastric cancer
  - Ascites

Percutaneous Endoscopic Jejunostomy (PEJ) Tube
- Indications
  - Gastroparesis
  - Gastric atony
  - Reflux and aspiration with gastric feeding
  - Functional gastric outlet obstruction

- Contraindications
  - Ascites

29-4: FUNDAMENTAL USE OF SURGICAL ENERGY (FUSE) (http://www.fuseprogram.org/)

The **Fundamental Use of Surgical Energy (FUSE)** curriculum and examination were designed to inform clinicians, nurses, technicians, etc. on the best practices in the use of electrosurgical, ultrasonic, and other energy devices in the operating room for safe use in patients.

Basic Electricity Terms
- Current (I): flow of electrons
  - Amperes
- Voltage (V): force needed to push charge along a circuit
  - Volts
- Impedance/resistance (R): degree to which the circuit resists electron flow
  - Ohms
- Energy: ability of force to do work
  - Joules
- Power (P): amount of energy per unit of time
  - Watts
- Current density = (Current in amps/area in cm^2)
  - Directly proportional to applied power
  - Inversely proportional to resistance
- Tissue heating = (current density)^2
- Direct current: polarity and flow of electrons remains constant
- Alternating current: electrons oscillate and result in no net flow of electrons
- Duty cycle: proportion of time that a waveform is generated in a given amount of time
  - Cut output has 100% duty cycle
  - Coag output has on average 6% duty cycle

Types of Electrosurgery
- Cautery: destruction of tissue by passive transfer of heat from a heated instrument
- Radiofrequency electrosurgery: conversion of electromagnetic energy into kinetic then thermal energy
- Ultrasonic: Piezo electric transducer vibrates between 23–55 Hz to generate heat

Cellular Effects of Electrosurgery
- Vaporization: intracellular temperature rapidly elevated to 100°C, generating steam that causes cellular rupture through cell expansion
  - "Cut" setting on monopolar cautery
- Desiccation: dehydration through thermally damaged cell wall (45°–100°C)
- Coagulation: "white coagulation" from protein denaturation (50°–100°C)
  - Occurs in conjunction with desiccation
- Fulguration: "black coagulation" that occurs through superficial protein coagulation via carbonization and organic molecular breakdown (>200°C)
  - Requires modulated high voltage waveforms typically produced by the "coagulation" output of the electrosurgical generator and a "no touch" technique
  - Most effective for superficial coagulation of superficial, capillary and small arteriolar bleeding ("ooze")
- Carbonization: breakdown of molecules to sugars and creation of eschar

Electrosurgery Waveforms
- Cut mode: heat quickly to cause cell water to steam and cause cell to explode
  - Unmodulated, continuous waveform with relative low voltage
  - To maximize effect, electrode should not touch tissue directly
- Coag mode: interrupted, high voltage waveform
  - Waveform 94% off, 6% on
- Blend mode: different ratios of cut and coag
  Slower electrode speed often leads to more energy delivery; but if too fast and makes contact with tissue, creates lower current density and zone of desiccation/coagulation
  Low-voltage continuous-wave form application provides most predictable, homogenous seal of vessels compared to coagulation setting which may increase superficial impedance and create heterogeneous coagulation

Mechanisms of Injury

- Dispersive electrode: closes circuit and disperses current from active electrode over a large surface area
  - Partial detachment can cause burns at electrode site
  - Split electrode monitors impedance to both pads and stops working if becomes partially detached
- Current diversion
  - Insulation failure
    - Smaller break = higher current density and current transmission
  - Direct coupling: active electrode comes into contact with another conductor/instrument allow to flow of current down the second conductor
  - Capacitive coupling
    - Risk factors
      - High voltage (coag > blend > cut)
      - High power
      - Open system (electrode not in contact with system)
      - Activation over previously desiccated tissue that now has high impedance
  - Alternate site injuries
    - Antenna coupling: wire to active electrode emits energy to nonactive wires without direct contact
- Active electrode injury
  - Inadvertent activation
  - Direct extension
    - E.g., duodenum, CBD, R hepatic artery
  - Residual heat
  - Collateral injury dependent on voltage, speed, waveform
    - Minimal: low voltage, 100% duty cycle, fast (keep in steam envelope)
    - Modest: moderate voltage 100% duty cycle with moderate speed or high voltage, low duty cycle with slow electrode speed
      High voltages can break the insulating capacity of glove
      Decreased glove resistance with time and exposure to saline (sweat)

Monopolar vs. Bipolar
Monopolar Electrosurgery

- Electrodes: one active and one dispersive electrode
  - Same amount of current at each electrode
  - Dispersive electrode spreads over larger area to reduce risk of thermal injury
- Thermal effect is indirectly proportional to area of current contact
  - Thermal effect proportional to $[\text{Current (I)/Area}]^2 \times \text{Resistance (R)} \times \text{Time (T)}$
- Argon beam fulguration: argon is an easily ionized inert gas that carries current
  - Effective for control of superficial oozing
  - Risk of gas embolus from spraying gas into a blood vessel

Bipolar Electrosurgery

- Resistance is lower in bipolar electrosurgery
- Less lateral tissue damage
  - Risk of outside loop phenomenon where current travels outside of the two blades of bipolar instrument once current no longer passes between them
- Potential hazards of bipolar
  - Inadvertent thermal injury
  - Inadvertent cutting of patent vessels before adequate sealing
  - Improper device function if metal contained within the jaws

Radiofrequency Ablation (RFA)

RFA: subtype of radiofrequency electrosurgery in which alternating current at 375–500 kHz travels through an active electrode, causing ionic agitation from AC heating tissue and causing coagulation

- Continuous low-voltage outputs are used to slowly elevate temperatures to avoid desiccation and increased impedance
- Place dispersive electrodes at 90-degree angle to current
- Vessels in close proximity can cause heat sink effect through uneven delivery of energy
- Can be used in the liver, pancreas, esophagus
  - Cannot be used in perihilar tumors as can lead to biliary ductal strictures
- Requires large or multiple dispersive electrodes due to high-power output that can be generated

Indications for RFA
- Palliation
- Unresectability
- Comorbidities precluding surgery
- Bridge to transplantation

Ultrasonic Devices
Electrical energy converted to mechanical energy to generate heat
Factors affecting ultrasonic energy delivery:
- Tissue tension: increasing tension increases cutting
- Blade excursion (how far the blade travels): increasing excursion increases cutting
- Blade pressure: increasing pressure increases cutting
- Percentage of water in tissue
  Risk of residual heat of the blade causing inadvertent damage
  Thermal spread can be 1–3 mm

Smoke
Residual from electrosurgical devices
- Plume can have benzene, hydrogen cyanide, formaldehyde
- Traditional surgical masks only filter 5-micron particles
  - 77% of surgical smoke content are 1.1 microns or smaller

OR Fires
- Spark, fuel source (e.g., prep, drapes), oxidizer are needed
- Most common sites of fire are the head, neck, face, upper chest
- RACE: Rescue, Alert, Confine, Evacuate
- Steps during fire
  - Stop flow of oxygen to patient before removing breathing circuit
  - Remove burning/burned materials
  - Extinguish fire on burning materials
  - Pull fire alarm
  - Notify administrator
  - Sequester materials involved in fire
  - Restore patient breathing with RA

Surgical Energy in Endoscopy
- Multipolar electrocoaglation (MPEC) probe is commonly used
  - Bipolar device with wound gold electrode
- Blend mode has higher risk of immediate postpolypectomy bleeding while coag has higher delayed bleeding risk
- Postpolypectomy syndrome: full-thickness thermal injury causes localized inflammation and peritonitis without perforation
  - Treat conservatively
- Heater probe: true cautery delivered via heating of a catheter-tip probe

Microwave Ablation (MWA)
Microwave ablation (MWA) does not need dispersive electrode; uses dielectric energy (rapidly reversing polarity)
- Heat transfer occurs by radiation in a sphere as a wave from antenna into surrounding tissue
- Not affected by impedance
- Wavelength is shorter than RFA system
- No air gap between ablation zone and organ
- Types of microwave field zones
  - Surgical: larger diameter without internal cooling device (spherical shape of sphere)
  - Transcutaneous: longer shafts and built in cooling systems to prevent abdominal burns (light bulb–like shape of field)
- Complications
  - Skin burns, hepatic abscess, hepatic infarcts in segment 2–3, hepatic vascular fistula, bile duct injury, hemolysis

Surgical Energy in Pediatric Surgery
- Greater TBSA:volume ratio but less overall TBSA
  - Higher likelihood of injury from overlap
- Greater body water content: greater tissue conductance due to lower impedance
  - Adults: 60% water
  - Term neonates: 75% water
  - Preterm: >75% water

- Increased current density from smaller structures
  - Do not use monopolar cautery in infants <1 pound
- Recommended settings
  - Max power in adolescents: 12–15 Watts
  - Max power in newborns: 8–10 Watts

Dispersive electrodes by weight available in kids:
- Lower limit of weight is 400 g or 1 pound
  - Ok to use adult pads if >30 pounds
- Neonate: place pad on back between scapulae and sacrum
- Infant: back, torso, thigh in large infant

Electromagnetic Interference (EMI)
- Electromagnetic devices such as AEDs, pacemakers are at risk for interference from electrosurgical devices
  - Ultrasonic shears and MWA do not interfere with electromagnetic devices
- Use bipolar when possible over monopolar
  - If using monopolar, consider the following
    - Use "cut" instead of "coag"
    - Avoid crossing leads/dispersive electrode with AED; avoid proximity to AED
      - Be as close as possible to surgical field
    - Use short intermittent bursts vs. long activations
    - Avoid high-voltage arcing/fulguration techniques
- Continuous EKG not sufficient to monitor patient; need pulse oximetry waveform or arterial waveform for perfusion
- Interference risks:
  - Triggering
  - Asynchronous pacing
  - Reprogramming
    - Avoid asynchronous unless patient is pacemaker dependent
      - Pacer-dependent is at greatest risk of EMI
    - Magnet often does not alter pacing function or rate
      - Magnet often disables tachyarrhythmia therapy
      - Never results in asynchronous pacing
    - Turn off rate-adaptive functions
  - Damage to electrical components
  - EMI conduction
    - Have 15 cm between active electrode and generator/leads (procedures above umbilicus)
      - <15 cm or above umbilicus is danger zone
  - Thermal injury at lead–tissue interface
  - If using magnet, must interrogate CIED before discharge

ACS–ASE SKILLS BASED SIMULATION CURRICULUM

ROBERT D. ACTON

30-1: INTRODUCTION

The American College of Surgeons (ACS)/Association for Surgical Education (ASE) Medical Student Simulation Based Surgical Skills Curriculum is a stepwise modular curriculum designed to accelerate the acquisition of universal physician skills needed to be learned by all medical students. As patient safety and quality have been stressed in the United States, students have often been pushed to the side, but yet they are still expected to know how to perform basic physician tasks, but often do not always have a direct means to learn them within early patient events. It is expected that students begin at a higher level of skill and knowledge before first performing a task on a patient. Simulation can help span this divide of expectation and experience by teaching a skill in a stepwise fashion in a safe environment.

To assist students in achieving the goal of learning universal physician skills, the ACS and ASE partnered in developing and publishing an innovative 25-module simulation curriculum for students. The modules are designed to be done by an individual, small or large group. They can be done in a simulation center, class room, or clinic space. The module topics have been confirmed through a formal needs assessment via survey of medical students from five different medical schools as well as surgery clerkship directors.

Further, the modules nicely align with the Entrustable Professional Activities for graduating medical students released by the Association of American Medical Colleges in 2014 (http://members.aamc.org/eweb/upload/Core%20EPA%20Curriculum%20Dev%20Guide.pdf).

30-2: MODULES

The 25 modules are spread across the first 3 years of medical school. They are organized as a typical education may progress, but the modules may be done in any order. Each module is also paired with an assessment tool to help assist the student evaluate their knowledge and acquisition of the skill.

Year 1 modules:
1. Abdominal Exam
2. Basic Vascular Exam
3. Breast Exam
4. Digital Rectal Exam
5. Female Pelvic Exam
6. Male Groin and Genital Exam
7. Universal Precautions
8. Venipuncture and Peripheral IV

Year 2 modules:
1. Basic Airway Management
2. Communication—History and Physical and Case Presentation
3. Foley Bladder Catheterization
4. Intermediate Vascular Exam
5. Nasogastric Tubes
6. Sterile Technique—Gloving and Gowning
7. Surgical Drains—Care and Removal

Year 3 modules:
1. Arterial Puncture and Blood Gas
2. Basic Knot tying
3. Basic Suturing
4. Central Venous Line Insertion
5. Communication—During Codes and Safe and Effective Handoffs
6. Intermediate Airway
7. Intraosseous IV
8. Local Anesthetics
9. Paracentesis
10. Thoracentesis

Module Description

Each module itself is divided into several different sections to facilitate the understanding of the task at hand and practice. Most contain photos of the various steps of each skill to help give a visual understanding and may be paired with a video.

The module components are:

1. Brief overview—describing the module, alternatives, and logistics of the module
2. Objectives—2–4 clear and focused objectives which are linked to the content of the module and the assessment portion of the module
3. Assumptions—basic assumptions of the authors, what prerequisites of prior education or experience do the students require. If the knowledge is extensive, a brief tutorial within the module of the background knowledge
4. Suggested readings—listing of 2–4 suggested readings with specific pages and references
5. Description of the laboratory module—clear and concise description of what will be accomplished within the module. Alternatives on how to do the module and any hint on how to teach the module well or specific training the leader will require
6. Description of techniques and procedure—technical listing in a stepwise manner of the tasks to be performed, including photos.
7. Common errors—description of common errors (why they are errors and how to avoid them) and treatment strategies for complications or problems. Grouped in errors of the skill and errors of the simulation
8. Expert performance video—brief video clip of a person performing the task
9. Supplies and station setup—listing of materials needed for the module including personnel, facility, and models, anticipated budget
10. Suggested module length—time estimate that will take to set up, teach, and perform the module
11. Assessment—evaluation methods that are specifically applicable to the module including checklists or global ratings, as well as adaptation
12. Faculty development—a brief description on how best to teach the module. Suggest the year the module should be taught and how it may be taught differently for different level of learners.

Module Access

The modules may be accessed via the American College of Surgeons, Division of Education webpage. It is specifically located under the section for Medical Student resources and listed as the ACS/ASE Medical Student Simulation-Based Surgical Skills Curriculum, or by going to the following https://www.facs.org/education/program/simulation-based.

Students may apply for and receive an ACS Student username and password that will provide them access to the curriculum. Faculty educators may also obtain access by contacting the ACS if they do not already have an ACS username and password.

ACS/APDS AMERICAN COLLEGE OF SURGEONS/ASSOCIATION OF PROGRAM DIRECTORS IN SURGERY SURGERY RESIDENT SKILLS CURRICULUM

ALI LINSK • TARA S. KENT

31-1: HISTORY AND DEVELOPMENT

(American College of Surgeons Division of Education. ACS/APDS surgical skills curriculum for residents. Available at: http://www.facs.org/education/surgicalskills.html. Accessed February 20, 2017)

- The skills curriculum was developed by the American College of Surgeons (ACS) and the Association of Program Directors in Surgery (APDS) and released in 2007 (https://www.facs.org/education/program/resident-skills)
- Curricular didactic and video content is provided at no cost
- Objective assessments included
- Detailed instructions for setting up simulations

31-2: CURRICULUM OVERVIEW

(American College of Surgeons Division of Education. ACS/APDS surgical skills curriculum for residents. Available at: http://www.facs.org/education/surgicalskills.html. Accessed February 20, 2017)

- Phase 1: Core Skills
  - 16 modules
  - Basic surgical skills
  - Geared towards junior residents
  - Self-guided modules with the help of expert performance videos
  - Breaks down core surgical skills into their individual steps to aid in learning
  - Curriculum includes guidelines for setting up simulations using animal models and other wet lab materials to allow trainees to practice the skills learned during the teaching modules
  - Instructions for setting up Objective Structured Assessment of Technical Skill (OSATS) examinations to assess the residents' progress
- Phase 2: Advanced Procedures
  - 15 modules
  - Advanced surgical skills
  - Geared toward senior residents
  - Step-by-step overview of setting up and performing common surgical procedures
  - Suggested reading for each module to be completed prior to the simulation
  - Video resources from expert surgeons for many of the procedures
  - Instructions for setting up high-level simulations of common surgical procedures using animal models or box trainers/simulators
  - Discussion forums for each module to allow participating institutions to share their experiences with the simulations
- Phase 3: Team-Based Skills
  - 10 modules
  - Resident team building through simulated scenarios
  - Multidisciplinary simulations
  - Curriculum provides patient cases, guidelines for background reading and preparation needed prior to participating, guidelines for simulation centers in terms of equipment and setup, and guidelines for debriefing after participation

31-3: CURRICULUM SPECIFICS

(American College of Surgeons Division of Education. ACS/APDS surgical skills curriculum for residents. Available at: http://www.facs.org/education/surgicalskills.html. Accessed February 20, 2017)

- Phase 1
  - Module 1: Asepsis and Instrument Identification
    - The details of prepping and draping, gowning and gloving, and surgical instrument identification are reviewed

- Module 2: Knot Tying
  - Instrument tie, two-handed knot tying, one-handed knot tying are reviewed with expert videos to provide guidance
- Module 3: Suturing
  - Simple interrupted, simple running, subcuticular interrupted, subcuticular running, and horizontal and vertical mattress suturing techniques are reviewed with expert videos to provide guidance
- Module 4: Skin Flaps
  - Removing dog ears and performing V-Y advancement flap and Z-plasty techniques
- Module 5: Skin Grafts
  - Review of techniques involved in performing split thickness and full-thickness skin grafts
- Module 6: Urethral Catheterization
  - The basics of male and female urethral catheterization are reviewed and common challenges and pitfalls are highlighted
- Module 7: Airway Management
  - Cricothyroidotomy and percutaneous tracheostomy are reviewed with the assistance of expert performance videos
- Module 8: Chest Tube Insertion
  - Procedure indications, steps, common errors, and complications are reviewed
- Module 9: Central Line Insertion
  - Subclavian and internal jugular central line placement and the role of ultrasound guidance are reviewed
- Module 10: Surgical Biopsy
  - Fine needle aspiration biopsy, core needle biopsy, needle-directed breast biopsy, and skin punch biopsy techniques are reviewed
- Module 11: Laparotomy Opening and Closure
  - Detailed, stepwise techniques of opening and closing the abdomen are reviewed, including detailed review of abdominal wall anatomy and common errors made
- Module 12: Basic Laparoscopy Skills
  - Fundamentals of Laparoscopic Surgery (FLS) skills such as peg transfer, pattern cutting, and endoloop are reviewed in addition to other hand–eye coordination box trainer exercises
- Module 13: Advanced Laparoscopy Skills
  - Interrupted and continuous intracorporeal suturing techniques are reviewed with the help of expert performance videos
- Module 14: Hand-Sewn Bowel Anastomosis
  - Double-layer end-to-end hand-sewn anastomosis technique reviewed in stepwise fashion
- Module 15: Stapled Bowel Anastomosis
  - Liner stapler functional end-to-end anastomosis technique reviewed in a stepwise fashion
- Module 16: Arterial Anastomosis
  - Sewing an arterial anastomosis using an artery and a graft is reviewed in a stepwise fashion
- Phase 2
- Module 1: Laparoscopic Ventral Hernia Repair
- Module 2: Open Colon Resection, Lap Right Colon Resection
- Module 3: Laparoscopic Sigmoid Resection
- Module 4: Open Right Colon Resection
- Module 5: Laparoscopic/Open Bile Duct Exploration
- Module 6: Laparoscopic Ventral/Incisional Hernia Repair (Porcine Model)
- Module 7: Laparoscopic Appendectomy
- Module 8: Laparoscopic Nissen Fundoplication
- Module 9: Sentinel Node Biopsy and Axillary Lymph Node Dissection
- Module 10: Open Inguinal/Femoral Hernia Repair
- Module 11: Laparoscopic Inguinal Hernia Repair
- Module 12: Laparoscopic/Open Splenectomy
- Module 13: Laparoscopic/Open Cholecystectomy
- Module 14: Gastric Resection and Peptic Ulcer Disease
- Module 15: Parathyroidectomy/Thyroidectomy
- Phase 3
- Module 1: Teamwork in the Trauma Bay
- Module 2: Postoperative Hypotension
- Module 3: Laparoscopic Crisis

31-4: LITERATURE REVIEW

- Duke University Medical Center (Henry B, Clark P, Sudan R. Cost and logistics of implementing a tissue-based American college of surgeons/association of program directors in surgery surgical skills curriculum for general surgery residents of all clinical years. *The American Journal of Surgery.* 2014;207:201–208) implemented all phases of the program in their general surgery training program, transitioning from inanimate models and simulators to the dry lab and tissue-based cadaveric models described in the ACS/APDS curriculum
  - 100% participation was expected from faculty and residents with once weekly 3-hour sessions of protected time
  - Prospective data gathered on cost and logistics, Likert-type survey data was collected from the residents who participated in this curriculum and compared to survey data collected prior to implementation
  - $110,300 annual operational cost ($3,150/resident), dry lab ($220/module/resident) and animal ($240/module/resident) costs were equivalent with cadaveric modules being the most expensive ($940/module/resident)
  - Resident satisfaction increased from 2.45 to 4.78 on a five-point Likert-type scale
- Six surgical education experts (Korndorffer JR Jr, Arora S, Sevdalis N, Paige J, McClusky DA 3rd, Stefanidis D; PEGASUS Research Group. The American college of surgeons/association of program directors in surgery national skills curriculum: Adoption rate, challenges and strategies for effective implementation into surgical residency programs. *Surgery.* 2013;154:13–20) wrote and circulated a web-based survey to all general surgery program directors in early 2011 with the goals of calculating the implementation rate of each phase of the ACS/APDS curriculum and of understanding any challenges to implementation
  - 117/238 (49%) program directors responded
  - 21% of program directors did not know about the curriculum
  - Approximately 90% of the program directors who were aware of the curriculum felt that it was easy to understand, comprehensive, and likely to improve technical skills
  - Overall rates of implementation were 36% for phase I, 19% for phase II, and 16% for phase III
  - The most common modules to be implemented were suturing, knot tying, chest tube placement, laparoscopic Nissen fundoplication, laparoscopic cholecystectomy, and trauma team training
  - Barriers included lack of protected time for both faculty and residents, lack of personnel, lack of faculty incentives, lack of resident motivation, work-hour restrictions, lack of cadaveric facilities, and the significant cost burden
  - Factors that supported successful implementation included having dedicated simulation center staff, protected faculty and resident time for participation, and the support of the departmental leadership
- The financial, personnel, and time burdens were highlighted in a study that calculated the cost, staff, and hours required to complete all three phases of the ACS/APDS curriculum (Pentiak PA, Schuch-Miller D, Streetman RT, Marik K, Callahan RE, Long G, Robbins J. Barriers to adoption of the surgical resident skills curriculum of the American college of surgeons/association of program directors in surgery. *Surgery.* 2013;154:23–28). These calculations were made based on the description of the curriculum modules on the ACS website
  - The cost for disposable supplies needed for completing the entire curriculum was calculated at almost $33,000/resident and the time for completion of the modules was calculated at 90 hours/resident
  - There are significant additional costs associated with building and staffing a simulation center with the appropriate nondisposable equipment necessary to complete these modules
  - The authors called for modifications to the curriculum that would allow for resource sharing and the use of lower-cost equipment and supplies

APPENDIX I: ENDOSCOPY

MARK A. GROMSKI • KRISTIN RAVEN • MICHAEL CAHALANE

A1: Esophagogastroduodenoscopy (EGD)

Diagnosis
- Upper GI bleed: 95% diagnostic accuracy in the first 24 hours
- Reflux disease
- Stage I: erythema and edema
- Stage II: mucosal erosions and some ulcerations
- Stage III: extensive ulcerations or cobblestone
- Stage IV: fibrosis and stricture, shortening, columnar lined esophagus
- Achalasia
- Dysphagia
- Chronic abdominal pain
- Ulcer disease: gold standard
- Anemia
- Gastric or esophageal malignancies: endoscopy with biopsy or brushing confirmatory in 90–95% of cases. <3% of gastric ulcers evaluated are malignant
- Gastric or esophageal varices

Screening in Patients With Barrett's Esophagus
- Four quadrant biopsies every 2 cm of the Barrett mucosa with at least 10 separate biopsies
- No dysplasia
  - Definition: two esophagogastroduodenoscopies (EGDs) within 1 year with all biopsies showing no dysplasia
  - Follow-up: EGD every 3 years
- Low-grade dysplasia
  - Definition: highest grade of all biopsies on two EGDs within 6 months
  - Follow-up: 1-year interval until no dysplasia x two
- High-grade dysplasia
  - If mucosal irregularity: proceed with endoscopic or surgical resection
  - If flat mucosa: must have repeat EGD with biopsies to rule out esophageal adenocarcinoma within 3 months
  - Follow-up: continued 3-month surveillance

Therapeutic Options
- Dilatation of esophageal strictures
- Esophageal stenting for advanced malignancy
- Sclerotherapy, clipping, and injection for bleeding
- Stapling of esophageal diverticula
- Banding for varices
- Percutaneous gastrostomy tube: low incidence of initial complications. 30–60 day mortality is 20–30%, though death is most often not PEG related

A2: Colonoscopy

Indications
- Screening
- Evaluation of GI bleed: diverticular disease, angiodysplasia, and carcinoma
- Evaluation of colon ischemia following aortic surgery
- Inflammatory bowel disease: evaluation/diagnosis/screening. After 8–10 years of colitis, annual or biannual surveillance colonoscopy with multiple biopsies at regular intervals
- Follow treatment and resolution of diverticulitis

Colonoscopy: Colon Cancer Screening
- Average adults at age 50, then every 10 y if negative
- History of polyps
  - High risk
    - Three or more synchronous adenomas
    - Any advanced adenomas: adenomas ≥1 cm in diameter/villous histology/high-grade dysplasia
    - Rescreen in 3 y

- Low risk
  - 1–2 small (<1 cm) adenomatous polyps with low grade dysplasia
  - Repeat examination in 5–10 y
- Piecemeal removal
  - Sessile adenomas that are removed in pieces
  - Repeat colposcopy in 2–6 mo after adenoma removal
- Family history: 40 y old or first screening 10 y prior to age at diagnosis of family disease (whichever is earlier)
- Previous resection of colonic malignancy
  - Rectal or sigmoid carcinoma: sigmoidoscopy every 6 mo for the first 2 y (anastomotic recurrences)
  - All cancers: colonoscopy every 5 y after surgery (metachronous lesions)

Therapeutic
- Removal of polyps
- Hemostasis of lower GI bleed (sclerotherapy, clipping, injection of bleeding vessels/lesions)
- Endoscopic dilation of anastomotic strictures
- Rectal stents in advanced malignancies
- Decompression on volvulus, ileus

Complications
- Serious: 0.5% (almost always associated with biopsy or polypectomy)
- Perforations: 0.09 per 1,000
- "Postpolypectomy syndrome" in stable patients often being treated with antibiotics and observation
- Bleeding: postbiopsy or postpolypectomy (4.8 per 1,000)

A3: ENDOSCOPIC RETROGRADE CHOLANGIOPANCREATOGRAPHY (ERCP)

Endoscopic retrograde cholangiopancreatography (ERCP): examination of the biliary and/or pancreatic ducts using contrast injected endoscopically through the major or minor duodenal papilla. Two-dimensional black-and-white fluoroscopic images of the biliary tree are produced using this technique, along with the possibility of a variety of interventional techniques.

Extrahepatic Biliary Obstruction
- Visualization of the upper GI tract, ampullary region, biliary and pancreatic ducts
- Cytology brushings and biopsy specimens
- Malignant obstruction of the intrapancreatic portion of the common bile duct: (i) abrupt cutoff; (ii) irregular stenosis; (iii) double-duct sign: proximal obstruction of the common bile and pancreatic ducts
- Placement of endoscopic stents for pancreatic and periampullary tumors
- Complications (6–10%): hemorrhage, pancreatitis, perforation, and cholangitis

Jaundice With Gallstones (When to Do ERCP)
- Preoperatively, followed by cholecystectomy
- Urgent biliary decompression in patients with gallstones, jaundice, and sepsis, often followed by cholecystectomy or cholecystostomy
- Postoperatively, for the management of retained stones
- Endoscopic sphincterotomy (recommended for elderly patients at high risk for complications with CBD exploration)

Jaundiced Patient Without Gallstones (When to Do ERCP)
- Not preferred for biliary drainage in patients with only intrahepatic ductal dilatation, as these patients likely have obstruction in the liver or high in the porta hepatis
- Patients with intrahepatic and extrahepatic ductal dilation and
  - choledocholithiasis: preoperatively, followed by cholecystectomy or
  - no stones and no masses: further evaluation and biopsy of CBD strictures

A4: BRONCHOSCOPY

Diagnosis of Lung Cancer
- Central, endobronchial lesions: sensitivity = 88%
- Peripheral lesions: smaller than 2 cm, 34% sensitivity; larger than 2 cm, 63% sensitivity
- Endobronchial ultrasound has shown potential in increasing the diagnostic yield for peripheral lesions without adding to the risk of the procedure

Removal of Foreign Bodies
- Most foreign bodies are able to be removed with bronchoscope alone or broncho-scopic tools

Infectious Diagnoses
- Ventilator-associated pneumonias (obtain samples) → results of BAL may be too late to influence survival

Longstanding Atypical Infections
- Can take sputum samples and biopsy specimens

A5: MEDIASTINOSCOPY

Invasive Lung Cancer Staging—Diagnose N2 or N3 Nodal Involvement
- N2 disease (Stage IIIA): nodal spread to the ipsilateral mediastinal stations or subcarinal area. Surgery is offered only after preoperative therapy, usually involving a platinum-based regimen of chemotherapy with or without radiation therapy
- N3 disease (Stage IIIB): nodal spread to the contralateral mediastinal lymph nodes or to the supraclavicular nodes on either side. Curative resection is not possible, and surgery is offered only in a multimodality protocol setting
- Mediastinoscopy: >90% accurate in staging the mediastinum in NSCLC, whereas CT scanning misses 15–20% of mediastinal nodal metastasis
- Cautery is generally avoided on the left side of the trachea to avoid injury to the recurrent laryngeal nerve

A6: TRAINING

Fundamental of endoscopic surgery (FES): simulator-based examination developed by the Society of Gastrointestinal and Endoscopic Surgeons (SAGES)
New surgical residency requirements for minimum number of upper and lower endo-scopic evaluations

A7: ADVANCED ENDOSCOPIC TECHNIQUES

**Double-Balloon Enteroscopy: Evaluation of Small Bowel
(Hard to Reach With Standard EGD or Colonoscopy)**
- Allows for biopsy and therapeutic manipulation of small bowel pathology or ability to reach the biliary limb of patients with roux-en-Y postsurgical anatomy
- The technique may be used in either an antegrade approach (initiating the sequence in the duodenum) or a retrograde approach (initiating the sequence in the terminal ileum)
- Due to the length of small bowel that must frequently be examined in double-balloon enteroscopes, the procedure times are often prolonged

Direct Pancreaticobiliary Visualization
- Cholangioscope is inserted into the biliary tree after sphincterotomy and cannulation of the bile duct in a conventional ERCP procedure
- Pancreaticobiliary visualization allows for real-time imaging of the biliary tract while also providing the capability for directed diagnostic and therapeutic maneuvers
- Indications include investigation and biopsy of suspected biliary malignancies and treatment of bile duct stones with lithotripsy
- Complications are primarily related to the initial ERCP

Endoscopic Mucosal Resection (EMR)/Endoscopic Submucosal Dissection (ESD)
- In addition to the removal of early gastric/esophageal cancer and treatment of Barrett's esophagus, endoscopic mucosal resection has also been utilized for removal of large colonic polyps, including flat and sessile polyps
- Mucosa in the area of question is resected and removed, predominantly with either a diathermic snare, band ligator, or needle knife, separating at the submucosal layer
- Usually, a fluid such as methylcellulose or hyaluronic acid is injected to serve as a "cushion" in the submucosal layer to facilitate resection and to decrease the chance of perforation

Endoscopic Ultrasound (EUS)
- Diagnostic and prognostic: staging of esophageal, gastric, rectal, and pancreatic cancers
- Therapeutic: EUS-guided pseudocyst drainage, celiac plexus neurolysis and block, and EUS-guided FNI for directed anticancer treatment have emerged

Natural Orifice Transluminal Endoscopic Surgery (NOTES)
- Scarless, experimental approach to abdominopelvic pathology that combines expertise of endoscopy and minimally invasive surgery.

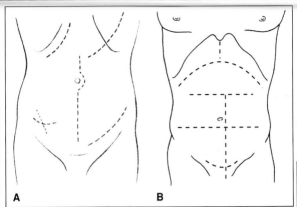

Common types of incisions. **A:** Clockwise from the upper right quadrant are subcostal (Kocher), thoracoabdominal, left lower quadrant (extraperitoneal), vertical midline, and Rockey–Davis (transverse)/McBurney (oblique). **B:** From superior to inferior are bilateral subcostal with vertical T-extension, supraumbilical transverse, infraumbilical transverse, left paramedian, and Pfannenstiel incision.

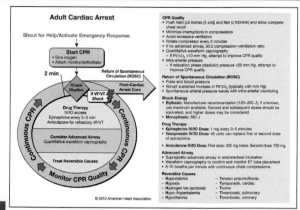

Reprinted with permission from 2010 American Heart Association Guidelines for Cardiopulmonary Resuscitation and Emergency Cardiovascular Care, Part 8: Adult Advanced Cardiovascular Life Support. *Circulation.* 2010;122(Suppl 3):S729–S767. © 2010 American Heart Association, Inc.

Treatable Causes of Pulseless Arrest

The Hs and Ts	
Hs	**Ts**
Hypoxia	Toxins
Hypovolemia	Thrombosis
Hydrogen ions (acidosis)	Pulmonary (PE)
Hypothermia	Cardiac (MI)
Hypokalemia/hyperkalemia	Tension PTX
Hypoglycemia	Tamponade, cardiac

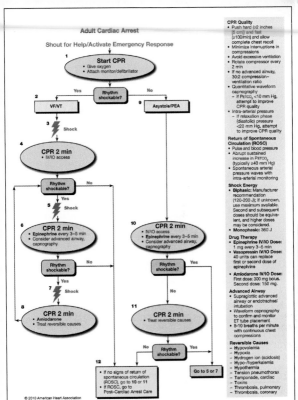

Reprinted with permission from 2010 American Heart Association Guidelines for Cardiopulmonary Resuscitation and Emergency Cardiovascular Care, Part 8: Adult Advanced Cardiovascular Life Support. *Circulation.* 2010;122(Suppl 3):S729–S767. © 2010 American Heart Association, Inc.

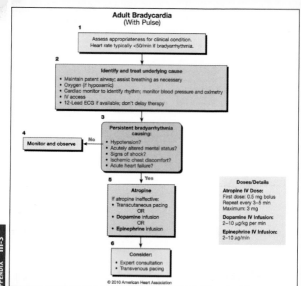

Reprinted with permission from 2010 American Heart Association Guidelines for Cardiopulmonary Resuscitation and Emergency Cardiovascular Care, Part 8: Adult Advanced Cardiovascular Life Support. *Circulation*. 2010;122(Suppl 3):S729–S767. © 2010 American Heart Association, Inc.

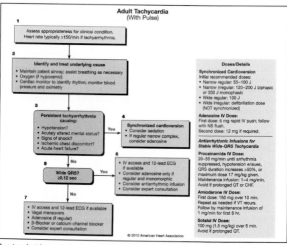

Reprinted with permission from 2010 American Heart Association Guidelines for Cardiopulmonary Resuscitation and Emergency Cardiovascular Care, Part 8: Adult Advanced Cardiovascular Life Support. *Circulation*. 2010;122(Suppl 3):S729–S767. © 2010 American Heart Association, Inc.

Adapted from ATLS 8th Edition, American College of Surgeons

A1: ADVANCED TRAUMA LIFE SUPPORT

Primary Survey	
A	**Airway**—If patient talking, airway OK. Suction, bag mask w/aid of chin lift. May employ airway adjunct (oral or nasal airway), endotracheal intubation, LMA, and surgical airway
B	**Breathing**—Inspect, percuss, auscultate, and palpate chest. ID tracheal deviation or subcutaneous crepitus. Note and treat airway obstruction, hemothorax, tension pneumothorax, cardiac tamponade, and flail chest
C	**Circulation**—Pulses. Hypovolemic shock must be addressed. Initiate two large bore IVs w/LR or NS. Give O-blood, if necessary. Identify sources of hemorrhage. Direct pressure on external hemorrhages. ID hemorrhages from chest, abdomen, pelvis, and long bones
D	**Disability**—Basic neuro-examination with Glasgow Coma Scale calculated. Need to assess level of consciousness, pupils, lateralizing signs, and evidence of cerebrospinal injury
E	**Exposure**—Patient needs to be completely undressed. Use warmed fluids and warm blankets. Note core temperature of patient

Secondary Survey—Do not initiate until primary survey is completed, with all primary issues (ABCDE) addressed
• Secondary survey is a head to toe examination of all organ systems and body parts.

Glasgow Coma Scale						
	1	2	3	4	5	6
Eyes	Does not open eyes	Opens eyes in response to painful stimuli	Opens eyes in response to voice	Opens eyes spontaneously	N/A	N/A
Verbal	Makes no sounds	Incomprehensible sounds	Utters inappropriate words	Confused, disoriented	Oriented, converses normally	N/A
Motor	Makes no movements	Extension to painful stimuli	Abnormal flexion to painful stimuli	Flexion/ withdrawal to painful stimuli	Localizes painful stimuli	Obeys commands

GCS ≤8, severe.
GCS 9–12, moderate.
GCS ≥13, mild.

Drug	Class	Dose	
		Per kg	**Average**
Pressors, Inotropes, and Chronotropes			
Phenylephrine	α_1	10–300 µg/min	
Norepinephrine	$\alpha_1 > \beta_1$	1–40 µg/min	
Vasopressin	V_1	0.01–0.1 U/min (usually <0.04)	
Epinephrine	$\alpha_1, \alpha_2, \beta_1, \beta_2$	2–20 µg/min	
Isoproterenol	β_1, β_2	0.1–10 µg/min	
Dopamine	D β, D α, β, D	0.5–2 µg/kg/min 2–10 µg/kg/min >10 µg/kg/min	50–200 µg/min 200–500 µg/min 500–1000 µg/min
Dobutamine	$\beta_1 > \beta_2$	2–20 µg/kg/min	50–1000 µg/min
Milrinone	PDE	50 µg/kg over 10 min, then 0.375–0.75 µg/kg/min	3–4 mg over 10 min then 20–50 µg/min
Inamrinone	PDE	0.75 mg/kg over 3 min then 5–15 µg/kg/min	40–50 mg over 3 min then 250–900 µg/min
Vasodilators			
Nitroglycerin	NO	10–1,000 µg/min	
Nitroprusside	NO	0.1–10 µg/kg/min	5–800 µg/min
Nesiritide	BNP	2 µg/kg IVB then 0.01 µg/kg/min	
Labetalol	$\alpha_1, \beta_1,$ and β_2 blocker	20 mg over 2 min then 20–80 mg q10min or 10–120 mg/h	
Fenoldopam	D	0.1–1.6 µg/kg/min	10–120 µg/min
Epoprostenol	Vasodilator	2–20 ng/kg/min	
Enalaprilat	ACE	0.625–2.5 mg over 5 min then 0.625–5 mg q6h	
Hydralazine	Vasodilator	5–20 mg q20–30min	
Antiarrhythmics			
Amiodarone	K et al. (Class III)	150 mg over 10 min, then 1 mg/min × 6 h, then 0.5 mg/min × 18 h	
Lidocaine	Na channel (Class IB)	1–1.5 mg/kg then 1–4 mg/min	100 mg then 1–4 mg/min
Procainamide	Na channel (Class IA)	17 mg/kg over 60 min then 1–4 mg/min	1 g over 60 min then 1–4 mg/min
Ibutilide	K channel (Class III)	1 mg over 10 min, may repeat × 1	
Propranolol	β blocker	0.5–1 mg q5min then 1–10 mg/h	
Esmolol	$\beta_1 > \beta_2$ blocker	500 µg/kg then 25–300 µg/kg/min	20–40 mg over 1 min then 2–20 mg/min
Verapamil	CCB	2.5–5 mg over 1–2 min repeat 5–10 mg in 15–30 min prn 5–20 mg/h	
Diltiazem	CCB	0.25 mg/kg over 2 min reload 0.35 mg/kg × 1 prn then 5–15 mg/h	20 mg over 2 min reload 25 mg × 1 prn then 5–15 mg/h
Adenosine	Purinergic	6 mg rapid push if no response: 12 mg → 12–18 mg	

Drug	Class	Dose Per kg	Dose Average
		Dose	
		Per kg	Average
Sedation			
Morphine	Opioid	1-unlimited mg/h	
Fentanyl	Opioid	50–100 µg, then 50-unlimited µg/h	
Thiopental	Barbiturate	3–5 mg/kg over 2 min	200–400 mg over 2 min
Etomidate	Anesthetic	0.2–0.5 mg/kg	100–300 mg
Propofol	Anesthetic	1–3 mg/kg then 0.3–5 mg/kg/h	50–200 mg, then 20–400 mg/h
Diazepam	BDZ	1–5 mg q1–2h then q6h prn	
Midazolam	BDZ	0.5–2 mg q5min prn or 0.5–4 mg then 1–10 mg/h	
Ketamine	Anesthetic	1–2 mg/kg	60–150 mg
Haloperidol	Antipsychotic	2–5 mg q20–30min	
Naloxone	Opioid antag.	0.4–2 mg q2–3min to total of 10 mg	
Flumazenil	BDZ antag.	0.2 mg over 30 sec then 0.3 mg over 30 sec if still lethargic may repeat 0.5 mg over 30 sec to total of 3 mg	
Paralysis			
Succinylcholine	Depolar. paralytic	0.6–1.1 mg/kg	70–100 mg
Tubocurare	nACh	10 mg then 6–20 mg/h	
Pancuronium	nACh	0.08 mg/kg	2–4 mg q30–90'
Vecuronium	nACh	0.08 mg/kg, then 0.05–0.1 mg/kg/h	5–10 mg over 1–3 min, then 2–8 mg/h
Cisatracurium	nACh	5–10 µg/kg/min	
Miscellaneous			
Aminophylline	PDE	5.5 mg/kg over 20 min, then 0.5–1 mg/kg/h	250–500 mg, then 10–80 mg/h
Insulin		10 U, then 0.1 U/kg/h	
Glucagon		5–10 mg, then 1–5 mg/h	
Octreotide	Somatostatin analog	50 µg then 50 µg/h	
Phenytoin	Antiepileptic	20 mg/kg at 50 mg/min	1–1.5 g over 20–30 min
Fosphenytoin	Antiepileptic	20 mg/kg at 150 mg/min	1–1.5 g over 10 min
Phenobarbital	Barbiturate	20 mg/kg at 50–75 mg/min	1–1.5 g over 20 min
Mannitol	Osmole	1.5–2 g/kg over 30–60 min repeat q6–12h to keep osm 310–320	

APPENDIX VI: ANTIBIOTICS

The following tables of spectra of activity for different antibiotics are generalizations. Sensitivity data at your own institution should be used to guide therapy.

Penicillins

Generation	Properties	Spectrum
Natural (e.g., penicillin)	Some GPC, GPR, GNC, most anaerobes (except *Bacteroides*)	Group A streptococci, *Enterococci, Listeria, Pasteurella, Actinomyces,* Syphilis
Anti-Staph (e.g., nafcillin)	Active vs. PCNase-producing Staph Little activity vs. Gram |	Staphylococci (except MRSA), Streptococci
Amino (e.g., ampicillin)	Penetrate porin channel of Gram | Not stable against PCNases	*E. coli, Proteus, H. influenzae, Salmonella, Shigella,* Enterococci, *Listeria*
Extended (e.g., piperacillin)	Penetrate porin channel of Gram | More resistant to PCNases	Most GNR incl. *Enterobacter, Pseudomonas, Serratia*
Carbapenem (e.g., imipenem)	Resistant to most b-lactamases	Most Gram ⊕ and | bacteria including anaerobes, but *not* MRSA or VRE
Monobactams (aztreonam)	Active vs. Gram | but not Gram ⊕	Gram | bacterial infxn in patient w/ PCN or Ceph allergy
b-lact. Inhib. (e.g., sulbactam)	Inhibit plasma-mediated b-lactamases	Adds Staph, *B. fragilis,* and some GNR (*H. influenzae, M. catarrhalis,* some *Klebsiella*); intrinsic activity against *Acinetobacter* (sulbactam only)

Cephalosporins

Resistant to most b-lactamases. No activity vs. MRSA or enterococci.

Gen.	Spectrum	Indications
First (e.g., cefazolin)	Most GPC (incl. Staph & Strep, not MRSA). Some GNR (incl. *E. coli, Proteus, Klebsiella*)	Used for surgical ppx and skin infxns
Second (e.g., cefuroxime, cefotetan)	↓ activity vs. GPC, ↑ vs. GNR. 2 subgroups: Respiratory: *H. influenzae* and *M. catarrhalis* GI/GU: ↑ activity vs. *B. fragilis*	PNA/COPD flare abdominal infxns
Third (e.g., ceftriaxone)	Broad activity vs. GNR and some anaerobes Ceftazidime active vs. *Pseudomonas*	PNA, sepsis, meningitis
Fourth (e.g., cefepime)	↑ resistance to b-lactamases (incl. of Staph and Enterobacter)	Similar to third generation. MonoRx for nonlocalizing febrile neutropenia

Other Antibiotics

Antibiotic	Spectrum
Vancomycin	Gram ⊕ bacteria incl. MRSA, PCNase-producing pneumococci and enterococci (except VRE)
Linezolid	
Daptomycin	GPC incl. MRSA and VRE (check susceptibility for VRE)
Quinopristin/ Dalfopristin	
Quinolones	Enteric GNR and atypicals. Third and fourth generations. ↑ activity vs. Gram ⊕.
Aminoglycosides	GNR. Synergy w/cell-wall active abx (b-lactam, vanco) vs. GPC. ↓ activity in low pH (e.g., abscess). No activity vs. anaerobes.
Macrolides	GPC, some respiratory Gram ⊖, atypicals
TMP/SMX	Some enteric GNR, PCP, *Nocardia, Toxoplasma,* most community-acquired MRSA
Clindamycin	Most Gram ⊕ (except enterococci) and anaerobes (incl. *B. fragilis*)
Metronidazole	Almost all anaerobic Gram ⊖, most anaerobic Gram ⊕
Doxycycline	*Rickettsia, Ehrlichia, Chlamydia, Mycoplasma, Nocardia,* Lyme
Tigecycline	Many GPC incl. MRSA and VRE; some GNR incl. ESBL but not *Pseudomonas* or *Proteus.* Approved for abdominal or skin/soft tissue infections. Check susceptibility if organism isolated.

INDEX

Note: Page number followed by f and t indicates figure and table respectively. Alpha A before page number indicates terms from appendix.